NEUROMUSCULAR TAPING
from Theory to Practice

David Blow

NEUROMUSCULAR TAPING
from Theory to Practice

edi·ermes

NEUROMUSCULAR TAPING from Theory to Practice
by David Blow

Notices

Knowledge and best practice in this field are constantly changing. As new research and experience broaden our understanding, changes in research methods, professional practices, or medical treatment may become necessary.

Practitioners and researchers must always rely on their own experience and knowledge in evaluating and using any information, methods, compounds, or experiments described herein. In using such information or methods they should be mindful of their own safety and the safety of others, including parties for whom they have a professional responsibility.

With respect to any drug or pharmaceutical products identified, readers are advised to check the most current information provided (i) on procedures featured or (ii) by the manufacturer of each product to be administered, to verify the recommended dose or formula, the method and duration of administration, and contraindications.

It lies within the responsibility of practitioners, relying on their own experience and knowledge of their patients, to make diagnoses, to determine dosages and the best treatment for each individual patient and to take all appropriate safety precautions. To the fullest extent of the law, neither the Publisher nor the authors, contributors, or editors, assume any liability for any injury and/or damage to persons or property as a matter of products liability, or arising from negligence or otherwise, or from any use or operation of any methods, products, instructions, or ideas contained in the material herein.

Drawings, Andrea Rossi Raccagni / Edi.Ermes Archive; photos Edi.Ermes Archive

Printed in July 2012 by Arti Grafiche Colombo - Gessate, Milan, Italy
for Edi.Ermes - viale Enrico Forlanini, 65 - 20134 Milan, Italy
http://www.ediermes.it - Tel. +39 02 7021121 - Fax +39 02 70211283

Preface

The history of therapeutic bandaging dates back to Greek and Roman times with that famous episode in the *Iliad* where Achilles bandages Patroclus' arm and dresses his wounds. Bandaging or dressing is, by definition, the application of bandages or dressings over an injured area to limit the damage and encourage healing.

Over the past thirty years, different non-elastic and elastic bandaging techniques have been developed in different parts of the world yet all of these methods are rooted in the same concept: the application of compression to different parts of the body. It wasn't until the 1970s that newer techniques appeared, used mainly in sports, which involved application of an elastic adhesive tape at various tension levels. Here again, the stimulus imparted is compression. In 2003, the Australian acupuncturist David Blow developed NeuroMuscular decompressive and compressive taping technique – concepts that set this technique apart from other types of taping and bandaging. Indeed, this is an innovative rehabilitation technique, based on a different line of clinical reasoning and a new method of application.

NeuroMuscular Taping (NMTConcept) is a biomechanical treatment methodology that exploits compressive and decompressive stimuli to obtain beneficial effects on human musculoskeletal, vascular, lymphatic and neurological systems: each application has clear clinical and rehabilitation objectives. Tape application causes folds in the skin to form during body movement. These folds facilitate lymphatic drainage, encourage blood flow, reduce pain and improve posture by increasing muscle and joint range of motion.

By focusing on specific clinical pictures as they progress through the acute and post-acute to functional stages during rehabilitation, David Blow has created a simple and highly functional method for optimizing treatment outcomes. This technique works toward the achievement of the following objectives: normalization of range of motion, reduction of pain, increase in patient autonomy and biomechanical treatment for reducing inflammation. NMTConcept offers medical and rehabilitation professionals an added resource for optimizing patient response, reducing rehabilitation times and improving the quality of life of the recovering individuals.

NeuroMuscular Taping is a non-invasive and non-pharmacological method that, through the application of adhesive elastic tape with specific mechanical and elastic properties, provides mechanical stimulation capable of creating space within tissue. This space promotes cell metabolism, activates the body's natural healing mechanisms and normalizes neuromuscular proprioception. For these reasons, NeuroMuscular Taping has in recent years achieved significant results in post-surgical orthopedic rehabilitation, neurological rehabilitation of stroke patients, the treatment of spinal trauma and neurodegenerative diseases. The high level of positive results achieved places NeuroMuscular Taping at the cutting edge of new therapeutic techniques.

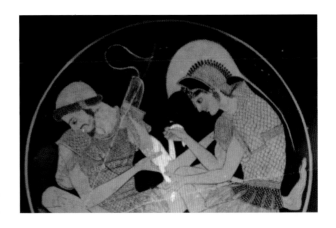

Author

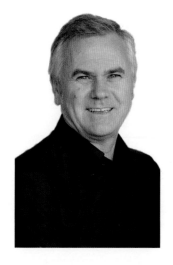

David Blow is the founder and president of the NeuroMuscular Taping Institute, which has been based in Rome since 2003. He is an international instructor of NeuroMuscular Taping in Europe and the United States. He has twenty-four years of therapeutic experience in rehabilitation, including training in Australia, China, Japan, and Italy. In 2003 he developed the innovative NeuroMuscular Taping Concept (NMTConcept) taping technique, which has become popular and is creating significant changes in the field of rehabilitation. The NeuroMuscular Taping Institute is a result of his passion for providing medical professionals working in rehabilitation with protocols that improve patients' overall treatment results and quality of life.

David graduated from the Australian Acupuncture College in 1989 after an internship in Japan rehabilitating patients through acupuncture. He then held an internship at Guang Dong Hospital of Traditional Chinese Medicine for four months, during which he treated many conditions, specializing in treatment for strokes using acupuncture. He brought his experience to Italy and founded the Italian AcuDetox Association and developed programs that treat alcoholism and substance abuse through acupuncture.

In 1999 David came in contact with various taping techniques. He spent the next few years studying these techniques and observed certain limitations from the point of view of rehabilitation. He decided to explore the idea of decompression taping on the skin surface as a form of therapy, based on clinical observations of the dynamics of muscle contraction and extension. Since that time, David has developed the NMTConcept and applied it to treatment to create a clinically validated concept. The NMTConcept is currently used in neurological and orthopedic rehabilitation in both public and private health services in Italy and is becoming a mainstream treatment protocol there.

David has published various case studies and articles and is currently involved in many research projects, including projects involving treatment of multiple sclerosis, Parkinson's disease, pediatric conditions, and neurological conditions as well as oncological rehabilitation and post-surgical rehabilitation. David is the author of the upcoming title *NeuroMuscular Taping – From Concepts to Practice* in English, Italian, Spanish, German, and Korean. However, his principal objective is professional education in medical and physical rehabilitation. He has developed a series of course programs and currently teaches over 1,400 physical therapists, occupational therapists, doctors and nurses each year through continuing education programs and certificate programs in Italy and other European countries.

Since 2008 David has taught 235 continuing-education medical courses with accreditation from the Italian Health Ministry. He recently completed a large-scale government-sponsored project in Italy, in which he taught a course to one hundred physiotherapists in order to integrate the treatment protocol into post-surgical care. David is a scientific referee, consulting professor and authority in continuing education and hospital projects in Italy. He is a visiting professor in the post-master's programs in Sports Traumatology at the University of Pisa and the Agostino Gemelli University Polyclinic and Teaching Hospital of the Catholic University of the Sacred Heart in Rome.

In other European countries David is involved in accredited continuing education programs at University Medical Center Ljubljana, University Medical Center Maribor, and General Hospital Izola in Slovenia, Paprikovac Hospital in Banja Luka, Bosnia, and Bel Medic General Hospital in Belgrade, Serbia. David currently resides in Rome with his wife and two children. He speaks Italian and English. During his spare time, he enjoys sailing, traveling, and Mediterranean cuisine.

to Daniela,
Samila and Valerio

Acknowledgments

Thanks are due to Professor Paolo Castano, University of Milan, Dr. Andrea Foglia and Dr. Cosimo Costantino, University of Parma, for their active collaboration in realizing this book.

A special thank-you goes to Tania Pascucci, Maurizio Mazzarini and Lara Acucella for their contribution to the preparation of the text.

NEUROMUSCULAR TAPING from Theory to Practice

Contents

In the text, before each tape application, the extension of the part to be treated is indicated with the symbol 🎞 and the position of the patient with the symbol ⊤

1

Introduction

ANATOMICAL DIRECTIONS

Correct application of the NeuroMuscular Taping (NMT) technique demands accurate and in-depth knowledge of systemic and functional anatomy. In other words, for this purpose, it is essential to know the position of a muscle, from its origin to its insertion, to be familiar with the skin, the vascular and lymphatic systems and the nervous system, with topographical anatomy and with the subdivision of the body into planes and regions.

The anatomical position of the body (the reference position for anatomical nomenclature) is the erect standing position with the arms at the sides and the palms facing forwards.

The terminology used in this book to describe movements refers to movements of the body from the anatomical position of reference.

BODY PLANES

The position of any part of the human body can be described by reference to three mutually perpendicular planes:
- the sagittal, or median, plane, or plane of symmetry, which divides the body vertically in the anteroposterior direction into two almost symmetrical halves, right and left;
- the frontal, or coronal, plane, which divides the body vertically into two portions, anterior or ventral and posterior or dorsal;
- the transverse plane, which divides the body horizontally into two sections, upper and lower.

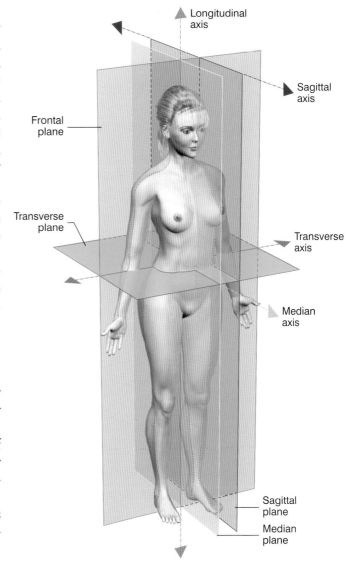

Figure 1.1 Body planes: sagittal plane, frontal plane and transverse plane.

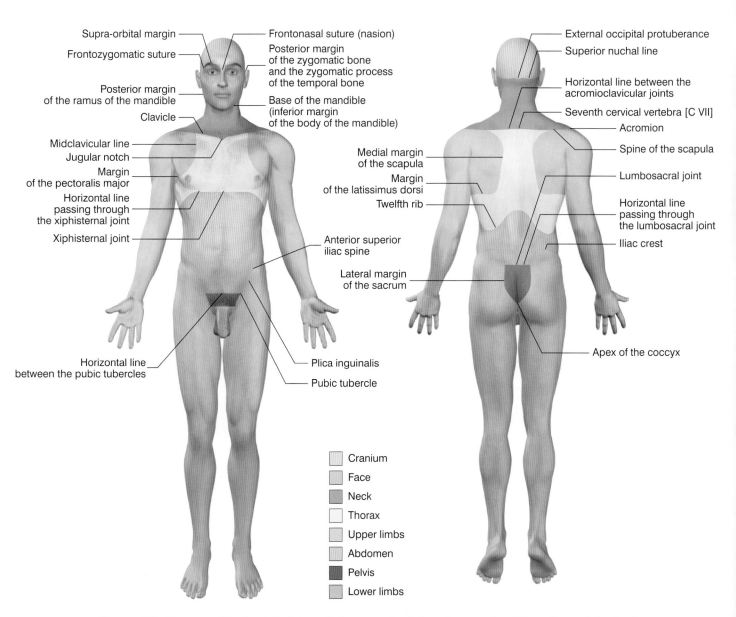

Supra-orbital margin
Frontozygomatic suture
Posterior margin
of the ramus of the mandible
Clavicle
Midclavicular line
Jugular notch
Margin
of the pectoralis major
Horizontal line
passing through
the xiphisternal joint
Xiphisternal joint
Horizontal line
between the pubic tubercles

Frontonasal suture (nasion)
Posterior margin
of the zygomatic bone
and the zygomatic process
of the temporal bone
Base of the mandible
(inferior margin
of the body of the mandible)
Anterior superior
iliac spine
Lateral margin
of the sacrum
Plica inguinalis
Pubic tubercle

External occipital protuberance
Superior nuchal line
Horizontal line between the
acromioclavicular joints
Seventh cervical vertebra [C VII]
Acromion
Spine of the scapula
Lumbosacral joint
Horizontal line
passing through
the lumbosacral joint
Iliac crest
Apex of the coccyx

Medial margin
of the scapula
Margin
of the latissimus dorsi
Twelfth rib

Cranium
Face
Neck
Thorax
Upper limbs
Abdomen
Pelvis
Lower limbs

Figure 1.2 Topographical subdivision of the anterior (**a**) and posterior (**b**) surface of the body.

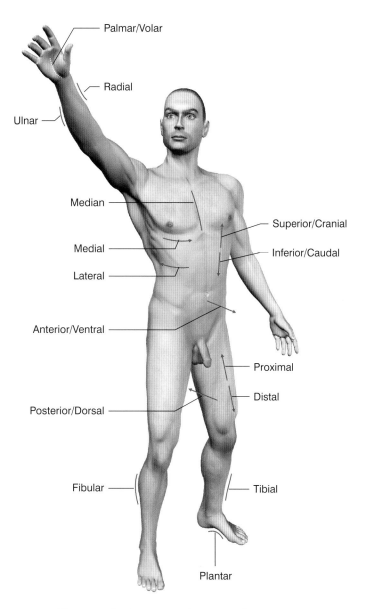

Figure 1.3 Anatomical terms of position.

Terms of Position and Movement

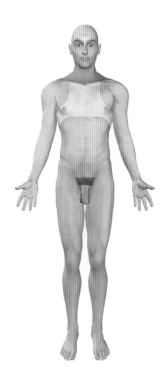

Figure 1.4 Anterior: towards the front or the front of the body.

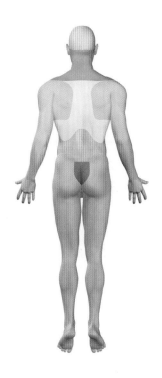

Figure 1.5 Posterior: towards the back or the back of the body.

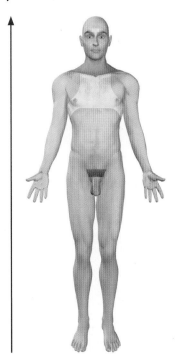

Figure 1.6 Superior: towards the upper part or upwards.

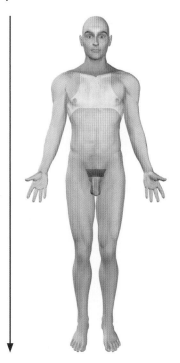

Figure 1.7 Inferior: towards the lower part or downwards.

NEUROMUSCULAR TAPING from Theory to Practice

Terms of Position and Movement

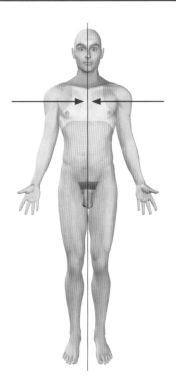

Figure 1.8 Medial: towards the midline of the body or in a medial direction.

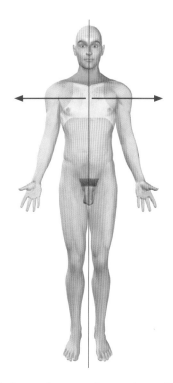

Figure 1.9 Lateral: away from the midline of the body or in the lateral direction.

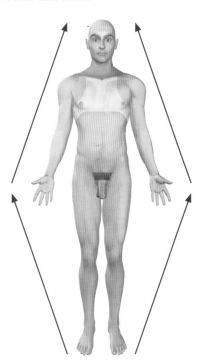

Figure 1.10 Proximal: towards the point of attachment of the limb to the trunk.

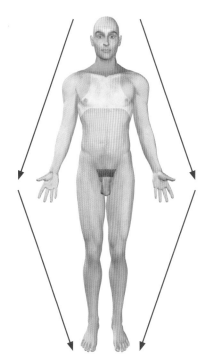

Figure 1.11 Distal: away from the point of attachment of the limb to the trunk.

Terms of Position and Movement

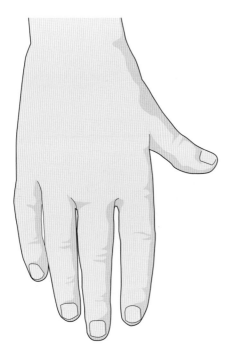

Figure 1.12 Dorsal: in the hand, this term refers to the back part.

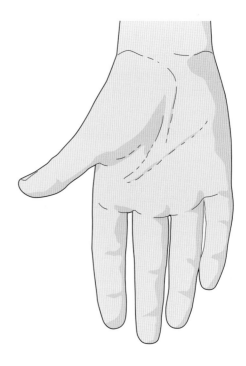

Figure 1.13 Palmar: this term refers to the front part of the hand, or palm.

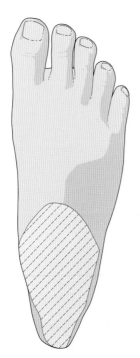

Figure 1.14 Dorsal: in the foot, the term refers to the upper part.

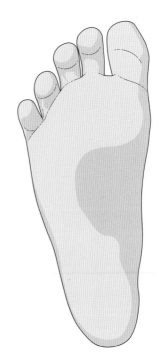

Figure 1.15 Plantar: the term refers to the bottom of the foot, or sole.

Terms of Position and Movement

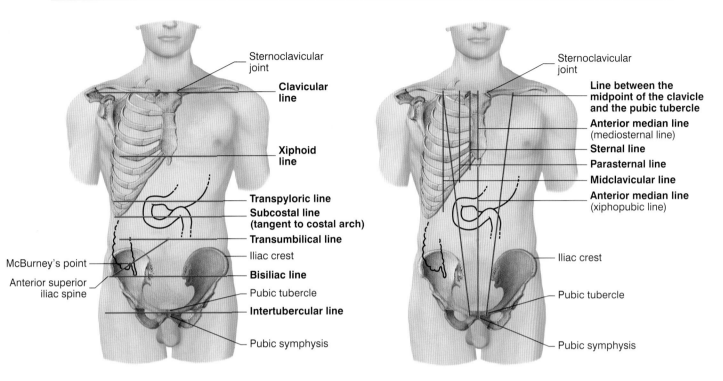

Figure 1.16 Reference lines on the ventral surface of the trunk in relation to the skeleton.

Left figure labels:
- Sternoclavicular joint
- **Clavicular line**
- **Xiphoid line**
- **Transpyloric line**
- **Subcostal line (tangent to costal arch)**
- **Transumbilical line**
- Iliac crest
- McBurney's point
- Anterior superior iliac spine
- **Bisiliac line**
- Pubic tubercle
- **Intertubercular line**
- Pubic symphysis

Right figure labels:
- Sternoclavicular joint
- **Line between the midpoint of the clavicle and the pubic tubercle**
- **Anterior median line** (mediosternal line)
- **Sternal line**
- **Parasternal line**
- **Midclavicular line**
- **Anterior median line** (xiphopubic line)
- Iliac crest
- Pubic tubercle
- Pubic symphysis

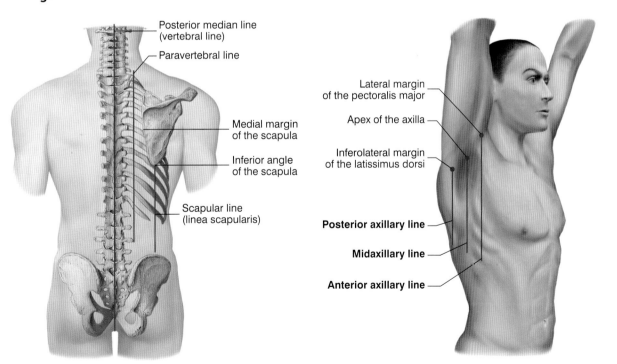

Figure 1.17 Reference lines on the dorsal surface of the trunk in relation to the skeleton.

Labels:
- Posterior median line (vertebral line)
- Paravertebral line
- Medial margin of the scapula
- Inferior angle of the scapula
- Scapular line (linea scapularis)

Figure 1.18 Reference lines on the lateral surface of the trunk: the three axillary lines are shown.

Labels:
- Lateral margin of the pectoralis major
- Apex of the axilla
- Inferolateral margin of the latissimus dorsi
- **Posterior axillary line**
- **Midaxillary line**
- **Anterior axillary line**

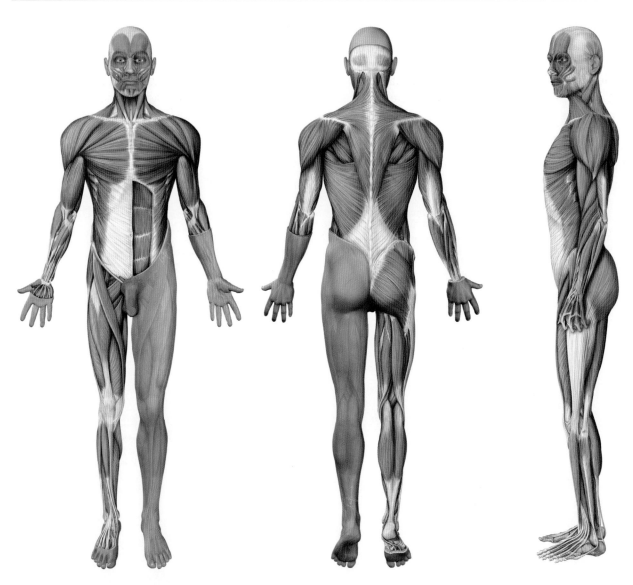

Figure 1.19 Superficial muscles of the human body: **a)** ventral, **b)** dorsal and **c)** lateral views.

The direction of body movements is indicated by the axis around which they occur. The axes of movement are identified by the intersection of the previously described planes.

The transverse axis is located at the intersection of the frontal and transverse planes. The sagittal, or anteroposterior, axis is defined by the intersection the sagittal and transverse planes. The vertical axis is formed by the intersection of the frontal and sagittal planes.

Movements around the transverse axis are called flexion and extension movements; those that occur around the sagittal axis are called lateral inclination movements when referring to the spine, and abduction-adduction movements when referring to the limbs. Movements around the vertical axis are defined torsional when referring to the spine and rotational when they involve the limbs. Rotational movement of the forearm and the hand is called pronation-supination.

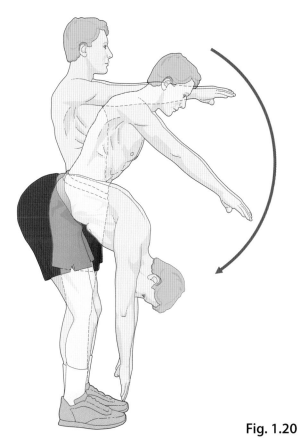

Fig. 1.20

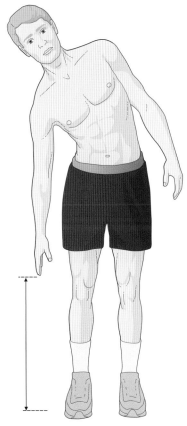

Fig. 1.21

Figure 1.20 Flexion: this term describes the position of a limb, or of the trunk, when it is directed towards the fetal position. Trunk flexion is a forward movement. Elbow flexion refers to movement of the hand towards the shoulder. Knee flexion refers to movement of the foot towards the gluteal muscle. Extension: this refers to the position of a limb, or of the trunk, when it is directed away from the fetal position, i.e., to straighten or bend the trunk backwards or extend the limbs. Hyperextension: this is extension of the limb, or trunk, beyond the normal range of the joint.

Figure 1.21 Lateral flexion or inclination: movement of the head or trunk in a lateral direction.

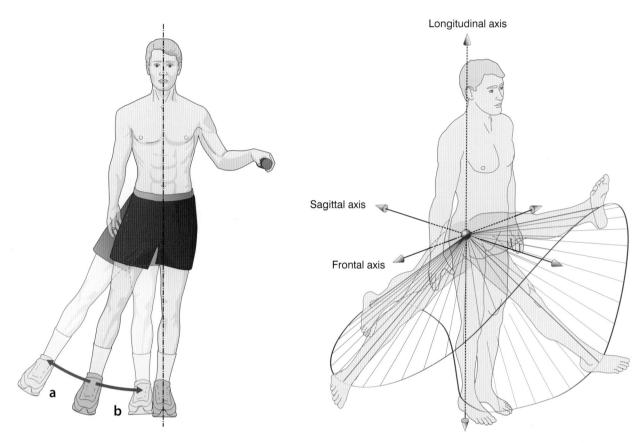

Figure 1.22 **a**) Abduction: movement away from the midline of the body, also of a limb and **b**) adduction: movement towards the midline of the body, also of a limb.

Figure 1.23 Circumduction: circular movement of the distal end of a limb. This is a complex movement of adduction, abduction, flexion and extension.

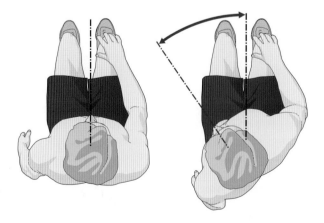

Figure 1.24 Rotation: movement of the limb or trunk about its own longitudinal axis. **a**) Lateral rotation: outward movement away from the midline and **b**) medial rotation: inward movement towards the midline.

Movements of the Body

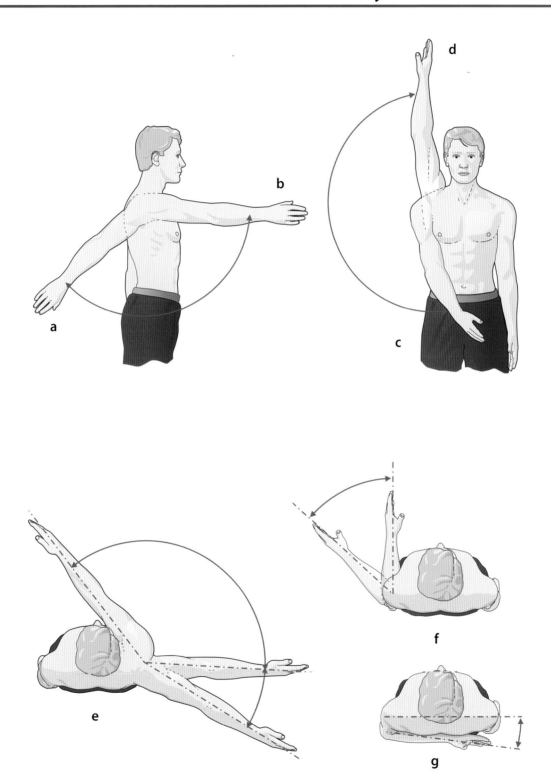

Figure 1.25 Movements of the scapulohumeral joint: **a**) extension, **b**) flexion with anterosuperior elevation, **c**) absolute adduction, **d**) abduction with lateromedial elevation, **e**) rotation in the horizontal plane, **f**) external rotation around the humeral axis and **g**) internal rotation around the humeral axis.

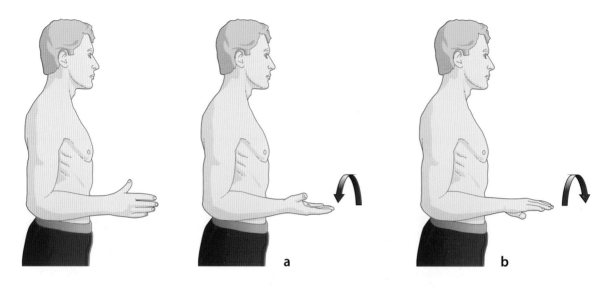

Figure 1.26 **a**) Supination: upward rotation of the palm of the hand and **b**) pronation: downward rotation of the palm of the hand.

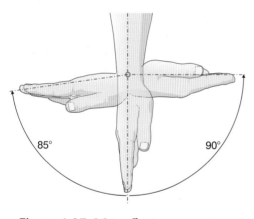

Figure 1.27 Wrist flexion-extension.

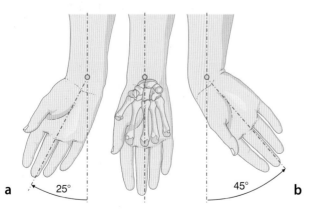

Figure 1.28 Wrist abduction (**a**) and adduction (**b**).

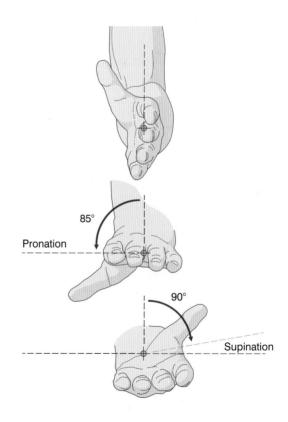

Figure 1.29 Pronation-supination of the wrist.

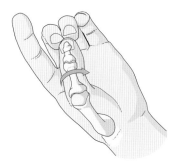

Figure 1.30 Opposition: specific movement of the thumb, which touches the tips of the fingers.

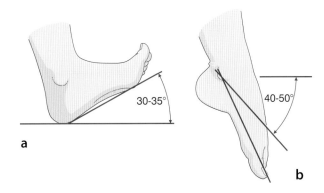

Figure 1.31 a) Dorsiflexion: upward movement of the foot and toes and **b)** plantarflexion: downward movement of the foot and toes toward the floor.

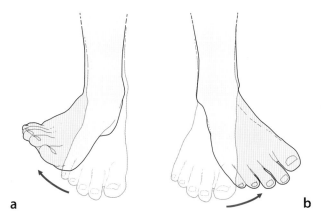

Figure 1.32 a) Eversion: rotation of the sole of the foot towards the outside and **b)** inversion: rotation of the sole of the foot towards the inside.

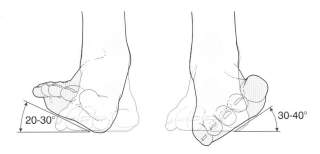

Figure 1.33 Pronation-supination of the foot.

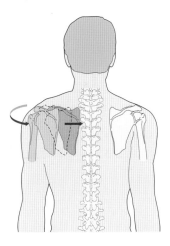

Figure 1.34 Retraction: backward movement in the transverse plane, for example, retraction of the shoulders leading to approximation of the medial edges of the shoulder blades.

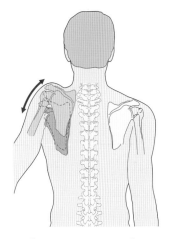

Figure 1.35 Elevation: upward movement of a part of the body along the frontal plane. Lowering: downward movement of a part of the body along the frontal plane.

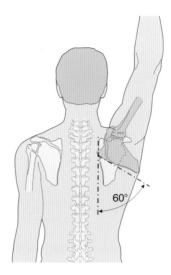

Figure 1.36 Elevation in abduction: raising of the arm in the frontal plane above the head with rotation of the glenohumeral or shoulder joint.

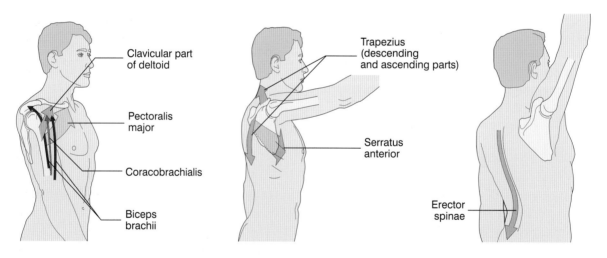

Clavicular part of deltoid

Pectoralis major

Coracobrachialis

Biceps brachii

Trapezius (descending and ascending parts)

Serratus anterior

Erector spinae

Figure 1.37 Elevation in flexion: raising of the arm along the sagittal plane above the head.

2

How NeuroMuscular Taping Works

NeuroMuscular Taping (NMT) is a technique involving the application of elastic adhesive tape to the skin, providing therapeutic effects that are local and direct as well as remote, through reflex pathways. When applied properly, it can reduce pain and facilitate lymphatic drainage through the formation of skin folds.

The NMT technique, unlike traditional non-elastic and elastic taping, is based on the concept of facilitating skin and muscle motion in order to achieve biomechanical therapeutic effects in treated areas. Muscles are among the most important targets for the action of NMT, which also indirectly affects venous and lymphatic circulation and body temperature.

The basic features of NMT differentiating it from other types of taping and bandaging may be summed up as follows:
- The tape used has special characteristics
- Application methods are specific
- Taping techniques can be either **decompressive** or **compressive**.

The tape is comprised of a thin layer of cotton with a wave-like, latex-free, acrylic adhesive coating. A removable paper liner protects the adhesive. Its elasticity is comparable to that of the skin, stretching only lengthwise (approximately 40%), and it is water-resistant. The application method, combined with body motion, induces micro-movements in the tape that stimulate receptors in the skin and underlying layers. These receptors transmit exteroceptive and proprioceptive stimuli to the central nervous system (CNS), triggering reflex muscle responses. Through exteroceptive stimulation, the taping reduces blood and lymph stasis, improves local microcirculation and favors the absorption of edema. Indeed, by lifting the skin, it enlarges interstitial spaces in the tissues, improving circulation and fluid absorption while reducing subcutaneous pressure.

For this to happen it is important, before application, to seek out the muscle and joint motion so as to apply taping that will induce local micro-movements. These will promote decompressive action through the formation of folds during normal body activity. Actually, NMT's distinguishing feature, setting it apart from other types of taping and bandaging, is its unique application method, which may be either decompressive or compressive (Fig. 2.1).

Therefore, the tape may be applied with different degrees of tension, or none at all, depending on the therapeutic effect desired, while its special aerated wavelike structure ensures local breathability.

Use of elastic tape, which is capable of providing external support to muscles, improves muscle function while stimulating nervous system responses to the different structural, biochemical, emotional, and energy stimuli involved in healing. The NeuroMuscular Taping method fulfills the standards for measurability and comparability of therapeutic results as long as the procedures set forth in the training courses are followed.

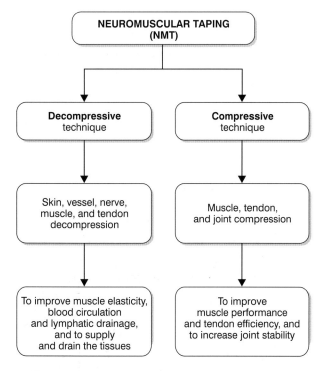

Figure 2.1 Features of NeuroMuscular Taping.

BASIC FUNCTIONS OF NEUROMUSCULAR TAPING

Acting on the skin, muscles, venous and lymphatic systems and on the joints, NMT achieves six major objectives:
• Alleviates pain
• Normalizes muscle tension
• Eliminates lymphatic and venous congestion
• Improves blood vascularization
• Corrects joint alignment
• Improves posture

Therefore, NMT acts on different levels:
• **Sensory**
  – Stimulates cutaneous, muscle, and joint receptors
  – Controls pain

• **Muscular**
  – Restores correct muscle tone
  – Decreases muscle fatigue
  – Increases muscle contraction
  – Decreases excessive muscle relaxation
  – Decreases excessive muscle contraction
• **Lymphatic and hematic**
  – Reduces local inflammation
  – Increases blood circulation
  – Improves lymphatic drainage
• **Articular**
  – Stabilizes at the level of the fasciae
  – Increases range of motion (ROM)
  – Reduces pain

NMT may be used as an adjunctive therapy to both manual and instrumental physical therapy programs, or it can be used as the sole treatment method. Since it provides continuous lymphatic and vascular benefits, its application can facilitate recovery in post-operative and post-trauma situations. The tape used for treatment may be left in place for several days, contains no active substances, and is suitable for use on children, adults, the elderly, and pregnant women. NMT applications can reduce recovery time and improve physical condition.

NMT is used to treat orthopedic and sports related conditions:
• **Muscular**: Elongation injuries, strains, fasciitis (plantar and anterior tibial), functional overloads (of the following muscle groups: quadriceps femoris, ischiocrural - hamstring muscles - semimembranosus, semitendinosus, biceps femoris, thigh adductors, gemelli, anterior and posterior tibialis, quadratus lumborum), and antalgic muscle contracture in low back pain and neck pain
• **Tendinous**: Insertional tendinitis, peritendinitis, tendinosis
• **Articular**: Sprains, contusions, bursitis

As NMT has spread, a variety of uses of the technique in combination with other medical and non-medical disciplines have been noted, improving rehabilitation results when applied to different areas, such as:

- Oncology
- Neurology
- Geriatrics
- Pediatrics
- Posturology

The purpose of this book is to illustrate NMT compression and decompression stimulation techniques, different taping configurations that can be applied to the skin overlying muscle paths, and, finally, to evaluate the possibilities of applying proprioceptive NMT to improve symptoms and mobility in subjects with different conditions. To address these issues, however, it is necessary to be familiar with the neural structures stimulated by NMT applications and their function. Skin folds form on the surface of the body where the tape is applied. These folds, in addition to increasing the interstitial space, stimulate skin receptors and, through these, the muscle fasciae and the nerve receptors in the muscle. The information from these latter receptors is sent to the CNS, which decodes, modulates, and adds to it, finally generating muscle responses. The quality of this information is closely correlated to the type and quantity of receptors present in each square centimeter of skin.

ANATOMY AND PHYSIOLOGY OF EXTEROCEPTIVE SKIN SENSITIVITY

The skin contains many nerve endings, originating from the posterior roots of the spinal nerves, which differ in their structure and in the specific sensory stimuli they detect. These nerve endings are responsible for gathering mechanical (tactile), pain, and thermal sensations. An area of skin innervated by single spinal nerves is called a dermatome (Fig. 2.2).

Although single receptors play an important role in defining stimuli, they do not characterize types of sensitivity by themselves. This is a process that depends on additional inputs and processing at a central level.

Any stimulus reaching the skin activates, in different ways, a series of receptors belonging to different functional categories. Each stimulated receptor sends the CNS an electrical nerve impulse, which ultimately constitutes the spatiotemporal code relating to its stimulation (or perception of the tactile, thermal, or painful event) in that particular moment.

These different codes are decoded (recognized) and processed (integrated) in the CNS, so as to obtain "operational" sensory information, i.e., information useful for planning a motor reaction (response). Therefore, receptors do show functional specialization, but this, as mentioned above, is not linked to specific pathways for the given sensation or to awareness of that sensation.

According to Sherrington, the surface of the skin is a sort of mosaic of sensory areas. Each piece in the mosaic coincides with the site of a receptor or group of receptors. Indeed, it is common knowledge that skin sensitivity is not homogeneous over the entire body, either for quality (type of sensation) or for discrimination of quantity. It is thus possible to draw maps of skin sensitivity to touch, heat, cold, and pain, and to identify specific points for each sensation. However, as stimulus intensity increases, differentiation between the different types of sensitivity diminishes and sensory maps become meaningless. An intense stimulus can induce, contemporaneously, feelings of heat and also of pain, or sensations (usually unpleasant) that are no longer easily classifiable.

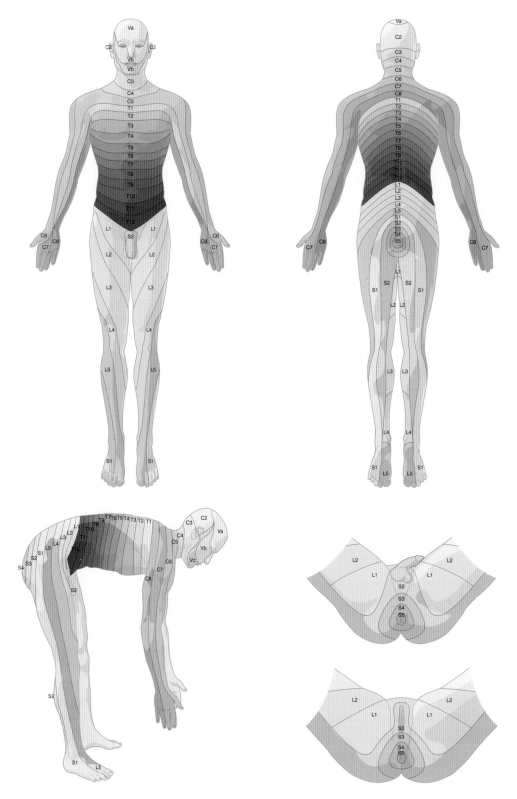

Figure 2.2 Map of the dermatomes of the trunk and limbs.

NEUROMUSCULAR TAPING from Theory to Practice

Table 2.1 Classification of peripheral nerve fibers

Type		Diameter (μm)	Conduction velocity (m/sec)	Fibers	Fibers and sensitive receptor
Ia		12-20	70-120	Myelinated	Neuromuscular spindles
Ib		12-20	70-120	Myelinated	Golgi tendon organs
	A	12-20	70-120	Myelinated	Extrafusal efferent fibers
II	Aα	12-17	70-120	Myelinated	Articular afferent fibers
II	Aβ	6-12	30-70	Myelinated	Other corpuscles including Pacini or Ruffini corpuscles
	γ	2-10	10-50	Myelinated	Intrafusal efferent fibers
III	Aδ	1-6	5-30	Myelinated	Nociceptors, Krause or Pacini corpuscles, perifollicular networks
	B	<3	3-15	Myelinated	Preganglionic efferent fibers
IV	C	1.5	0.5-2	Unmyelinated	Free nerve endings, postganglionic efferent fibers

Classification of nerve receptors

The best-known classification of nerve receptors is probably Sherrington's (developed from Ruffini 1905), based, generally, on the sensory role and topographic distribution of nerve receptors in the body. It identifies:
- **Exteroceptors**, for stimuli from the outside world
- **Interoceptors**, for stimuli from inside the body
- **Proprioceptors**, for stimuli from bones, muscles, tendons, ligaments and joint capsules
- **Teloreceptors**, for stimuli from outside the body that do not physically touch the body (light, sounds)

Equally well known (and equally arbitrary) is the classification based on the forms of energy to which receptors are sensitive:
- **Mechanoreceptors**: Mechanical
- **Chemoreceptors**: Chemical
- **Photoreceptors**: Light
- **Thermoreceptors**: Hot and cold
- **Osmoreceptors**: Changes in osmotic pressure
- **Nociceptors**: Pain (although pain is not actu-ally a form of energy, but the result of CNS information processing)

If a stimulus persists over time, all receptors adapt, some very slowly, others very rapidly. The slower ones include tendon receptors, like the tendon organs (or Golgi tendon organs), which, as long as the stimulus (tendon traction) persists, continue to send signals to the CNS. The receptors of the organs of balance are also slow to adapt and in fact continue firing as long as there is stimulation of the saccule and utricular maculae. It is clear that the need for constant information determines the persistence of the stimulation, precisely because this makes it possible to maintain position, posture, balance and coordination of movements.

Fast-adapting receptors are mainly those in the skin, such as the Pacini corpuscles and the perifollicular networks, which, after the initial burst of action potentials, fall silent, even if the stimulus persists (Fig. 2.3).

Certainly, it would be terrible if, after putting on our clothes first thing in the morning,

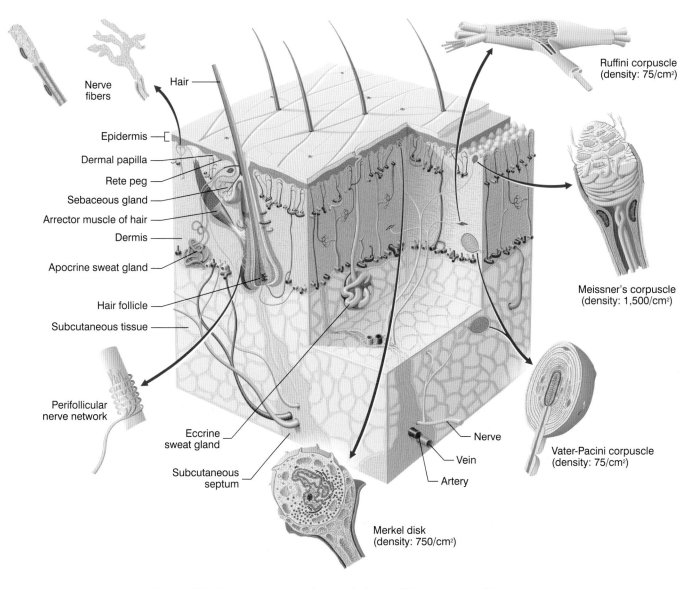

Figure 2.3 Arrangement and morphology of the various skin receptors.

our CNS were to go on being bombarded by the tactile stimuli that garments apply to the skin.

On this basis, then, nerve receptors can be divided into two categories:

- Fast-adapting (FA) receptors
- Slow-adapting (SA) receptors

Almost all receptors bear the names of the authors who first described them during the last century.

Exteroceptive sensitivity

Exteroception is due to stimuli originating outside the body (external stimuli). It corresponds to the tactile, thermal, and pain sensory modes and includes both protopathic and epicritic stimuli.

Exteroceptors (tactile, thermal, and pain) are sensory nerve endings of cranial or spinal nerves, wrapped in connective tissue coverings, which vary in form and consistency depending on the type of stimulus to which they are sensitive. Touch receptors are present practically everywhere, but they are particularly numerous in the glabrous areas of the body (e.g. the skin of the hands, feet, and tongue).

Exteroceptors are present mainly in the skin, and comprise:
- Free nerve endings
- Thermoreceptors and nociceptors
- Perifollicular networks
- Meissner's corpuscles
- Vater-Pacini corpuscles
- Merkel disks
- Ruffini corpuscles
- Krause's corpuscles

Free nerve endings

Free nerve endings are slow conducting, small-caliber with a diameter of less than 1.5 nm, unmyelinated fibers, (C fibers) located in the skin, including the epidermis, although they are quite widespread across all body areas. These C fibers are also to be found, for example, in joint capsules and ligaments, where they are involved in the general reflexogenic activity of joint proprioceptors. They are thought to transmit information related to pain (mechanical insults) and inflammation (chemical insults). Free nerve endings are non-adapting nociceptors (pain receptors), although the pain sensation they transmit can be attenuated by protein neurotransmitters such as endorphins, produced by CNS neurons.

Thermoreceptors

Thermoreceptors are free nerve endings that are almost insensitive to mechanical deformation of the skin. They respond dynamically to small variations in the temperature of an object or of the air in relation to skin temperature, emitting an unvarying static discharge at constant temperatures. Thermoceptor receptive fields are punctiform (1 to 2 mm^2) with sensitivity perception varying by tenths of a degree Celsius. They are divided into thermoreceptors that sense heat and those that sense cold.

The firing rate of *heat thermoreceptors* remains constant at temperatures between 34°C and 36°C. If the temperature rises, discharge frequency increases, peaking at between 41°C and 46°C. When the temperature reaches around 50°C, heat thermoreceptors stop firing and the sensation becomes one of pain. They also stop discharging if the temperature drops below 34°C, when those for cold take over. Conversely, the firing rate of *cold thermoreceptors* increases as the temperature drops below 34°C, stabilizing at 10°C to 15°C. Below this level they fall silent as they stop discharging.

Sudden exposure to high temperatures (above 50°C) or to very low ones can momentarily activate thermoreceptors, even though for a short time identification of the thermal sensation as hot or cold is prevented. At normal temperature conditions (24°C), the CNS is capable of distinguishing changes in skin temperature of just 0.05°C across a skin surface area of one square centimeter. Given that individual thermoreceptors are not endowed with such a fine degree of sensitivity, it is inferred that this fine perception is the result of computations performed by the CNS, integrating and processing the information it receives from the sixteen to twenty-five surface receptors present in that area of the skin.

Nociceptors

Nociceptors are high-threshold receptors that respond only to stimulation at a level of intensity sufficiently high to cause damage to the skin. In general, these are free nerve endings, located in the skin and in the viscera, and they fall into three categories: mechanical, thermal, and polymodal.

Mechanical nociceptors generally respond to mechanical stimuli of an intensity that causes skin damage, such as cuts, piercing, crushing, squeezing, and excessive pressure. Because these nociceptors generally include free nerve endings made up of unmyelinated C-fibers and

Aδ fibers as well, a double pain sensation theory has been proposed, according to which there is dual innervation and thus differing conduction velocities.

Thermal nociceptors are again divided, analogously into normal thermoreceptors, nociceptors for heat, which respond to temperatures above 50°C, and those for cold, which respond to temperatures below 10°C. However, heat receptors also respond to cold, and vice versa, albeit less efficiently.

Polymodal nociceptors, respond to both mechanical and thermal injury, and to chemical substances as well, including those normally produced by damaged tissue. Depending on concentrations, they also respond to substances that can cause pain upon contact or when injected. An important characteristic of polymodal nociceptors is their capacity for sensitization, i.e., to change in response to situations of chronic pain. Indeed, this response gradually weakens over time until it almost disappears. However, the pain may return suddenly when the nociceptors undergo acute stimulation once again. Therefore, polymodal nociceptors' response to chronic pain is a threshold reduction, with typically irregular discharges triggered even by non-painful stimuli.

Perifollicular networks

Perifollicular networks, fairly regular meshes of unmyelinated fibers wrapped around each hair follicle, from bulb to epidermis, react to any stimulation of the hair shaft. Like Meissner's corpuscles and Merkel disks, these are fast-adapting tactile receptors, responsible for superficial tactile sensitivity. Following an initial burst of action potentials, they fall silent, even if the stimulation persists.

Meissner's corpuscles

Along with free nerve endings and Merkel disks, Meissner's tactile corpuscles are the most external and superficial touch receptors in the body and are located in the papillae of the glabrous skin of the fingertips, lips and genital or-

gans. Each corpuscle has an elongated, more or less ovoid shape, with its major axis perpendicular to the surface of the skin. They are made up of a varying number of flattened laminar cells irregularly stacked on one another, between which there is connective tissue and mostly type Ia nerve fiber endings that innervate the corpuscle. Meissner's corpuscles are closely embedded in the connective tissue of their host papilla: hence they are stimulated by the slightest mechanical stimuli on the surface of the fingertips. These corpuscles are high-precision receptors able to distinguish skin vibrations as rapid as 100 Hz and as fine as 10 μm. They are extremely quick to adapt, and stop firing within a few tenths of a second if there are no changes in the force applied to the skin.

Vater-Pacini corpuscles

Vater-Pacini corpuscles, mechanoreceptors widely distributed throughout the body from the deep dermis to the abdominal viscera, are also ovoid in shape, with a thick central (type II) nerve fiber, surrounded by concentric layers of connective tissue. These form a characteristically shaped capsule composed of concentric lamellae, rather like the layers of an onion. They are the largest of the mechanoreceptors, sometimes exceeding 4 to 5 mm in diameter, with a fairly large receptive field of around 25 μm^2. These corpuscles are sensitive to movements as fine as 10 μm, and as rapid as 400 Hz. Hence, they are extremely sensitive to rapid changes in mechanical stimulation, such as quick and intense pressure and vibrations, but not to constant pressure. These rapidly adapting receptors provide deep tactile perception. Some authors have suggested that they act as "movement-limit" sensors in the joints, while others suggest they act as acceleration sensors and fine movement controllers.

Merkel disks

Merkel disks (also known as corpuscles), on the boundary between the dermis and the epidermis, are very superficial and more concentrated in the fingertips, where they have very small receptive fields (around 13 μm^2). With their main function being to perceive sudden skin movement, they are innervated by fast sensory fibers (Ia) and are slow-adapting. They may comprise a single cell (Merkel cell) located in the basal layer of the epidermis covering the dermal papillae, or multiple cells grouped together to form a sort of disk that covers the apex of a papilla. Each individual Merkel cell is innervated by a fast-conducting type Ia sensory fiber with an ending that opens into a cup shape, forming a synaptic contact with the cell in an area rich in vesicles containing chemical mediators such as met-enkephalin and VIP (vasoactive intestinal peptide). A Merkel disk, on the other hand, comprises a group of six or seven Merkel cells, into which the cuplike terminals of branched nerve fibers project.

These corpuscles only respond as perpendicular pressure increases. Highly sensitive, they are activated by movements of just 50 μm, with a dual component response. The first reaction, lasting about 0.5 seconds, is *dynamic* and is characterized by high-frequency discharges, while the second is *static* and is constant, continuing even after the stimulus ends. The latter has a lower discharge frequency and much longer durations of up to eight to ten minutes.

Ruffini corpuscles

Ruffini corpuscles, found in the dermis and also in the locomotor system, are formed by a bundle of collagen and elastic fibers surrounded by a thin capsule, which is "penetrated" by a type IIAb sensory fiber with extensive branching. These corpuscles or bulbs vary greatly in morphology and size. It is believed they are triggered by compression or stretching of the nerve endings due to deformations of the connective tissue within the corpuscle and stretching of the capsule. These slow-adapting mechanoreceptors with large receptive fields of around 25 μm^2 are sensitive to stretching of the skin in a plane tangential to its surface, which triggers a slow, sus-

tained response, consistent over time. If the deformation is perpendicular to the skin's surface, they respond only when directly below the point of stimulation.

They have a fairly high activation threshold, and in fact are not activated unless skin deformation reaches at least 250 μm. Although these bulbs have traditionally been considered (albeit in the absence of any valid proof) to be thermoreceptors (for heat), it is now believed that Ruffini corpuscles perceive skin deformations resulting from joint movements and muscle contractions and that they are actually prevalently proprioceptors. It is not by chance that they are also in the locomotor system.

Krause's corpuscles

There is some debate about these receptors, given that quite different structures are included under this heading. Some are similar to Pacinian corpuscles (Krause's end bulbs) while others are like Meissner's corpuscles (Krause's skeins). The latter are found in different locations, including the dermis (where they are interpreted as being thermoreceptors for cold), in genital mucosa, in ligaments, and in joint capsules. They comprise one or more myelinated fibers penetrating a connective tissue capsule where they lose their myelin sheath and branch out to form a spherical skein. Their function may be to monitor changes in the shape of the structure in which they are located caused by traction, pressure, or other factors. Some authors believe that Krause's corpuscles are neither receptors nor specialized nerve endings, but rather the result of the degeneration of sensory fibers whose peripheral growth has somehow been impeded, followed by their regeneration. Just as Ruffini corpuscles were considered, without proof, to be heat receptors, Krause's end bulbs have been considered cold sensors. It may be surmised that this interpretation arose from the fact that the Italian, Ruffini, lived in a warm country, while Krause, a German, lived in a colder one.

Proprioception

Proprioceptive sensations are due to stimuli coming from muscles, tendons, aponeuroses, joint capsules, and ligaments. Muscles and tendons contain receptors whose task is to inform nerve centers, especially the spinal cord, of the state of contraction or tension to which they are being subjected. These receptors are therefore mechanoreceptors (proprioceptors), which function as transducers of the stretching or contraction of locomotor system organs, transforming the length changes they undergo into nerve impulses that are sent to the spinal cord or brainstem.

Proprioceptors include:
- Free nerve endings
- Ruffini corpuscles
- Muscle spindles
- Golgi tendon organs
- Vater-Pacini corpuscles
- Krause's corpuscles

The paragraphs below do not concern structures already discussed in the cutaneous mechanoreceptors section.

Muscle spindles

Muscle spindles are elongated, tapered structures lying parallel to the muscle fibers in which they are embedded. They comprise around a dozen small muscle fibers (*intrafusal fibers*) within a thin sheath of connective tissue, innervated by both gamma motor and sensory nerve fibers (Fig. 2.4). *Intrafusal fibers*, given this name to distinguish them from muscle fibers proper or *extrafusal fibers*, are smaller than the latter and make no contribution to muscle movement. Each spindle contains three types of intrafusal fiber. Nuclear chains characterize one type, while nuclear bags characterize the other two. *Nuclear chain* fibers are short and fine, with their nuclei arranged, as their name indicates, in a single row or chain. *Nuclear bag* fibers have a larger diameter and are broader at the equatorial region, where their nuclei are located. Based on their functional properties, nuclear bag fibers are defined as either static or dynamic. The latter enable sensory fibers connecting to them to discharge in response to changes in their length, while the former are activated when the muscle has reached and maintains its new length.

A classic neuromuscular spindle contains two nuclear bag fibers, one static and the other dynamic, and a variable number of nuclear chain fibers, usually five. The sensory nerve fibers pass through the capsule into the spindle and terminate in the *equatorial region*, where they wrap around the intrafusal fibers in a spiral. The gamma motor fibers, on the other hand, terminate at the ends of the intrafusal fibers in small "en plaque" motor endings.

When intrafusal fibers are stretched as a result of muscle elongation, the sensory nerve endings located in the equatorial region are activated and increase their firing rate. Gamma motor axons control contraction of the intrafusal fibers, leading to stretching of the equatorial regions. In other words, contraction of the polar regions causes lengthening (active stretching) of the spindle. The resulting deformation of the equatorial region stimulates the sensory endings there, which send signals to the spinal cord or the brainstem. The activity of the gamma motor fibers is always closely related to that of the alpha motor fibers, which innervate the extrafusal fibers. Therefore, through this

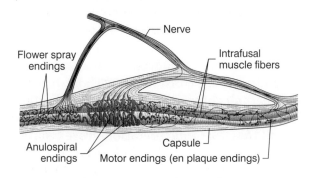

Figure 2.4 Muscle spindle.

mechanism, the gamma fibers regulate spindle sensitivity, since their activation, in keeping the intrafusal fibers stretched, predisposes the spindle to perceive the slightest change in length of the extrafusal fibers, as determined by the alpha fibers. The muscle reaction triggered by the neuromuscular spindles is called the *myotatic reflex* and it opposes excessive stretching of the muscle. The main function of the neuromuscular spindles, therefore, is to monitor the length and speed of stretching of muscle fibers. They are stretch receptors that tell the CNS how far a muscle is being stretched compared to its previous position.

Golgi tendon organs

Golgi tendon organs, located at the junction of the muscle and the tendon (Fig. 2.5), are elongated formations a few millimeters in length that are arranged with one end in the tendon and the other in the muscle. Similar to Ruffini corpuscles, but larger, they are made up of bundles of interwoven collagen and elastic fibers, enveloped by a thin capsule, which is "penetrated" by a large Ib myelinated fiber (sometimes more than one), which loses its myelin sheath and branches around the connective tissue fibers.

Each tendon organ is connected to ten to twenty muscle fibers belonging to different motor units. They are sensitive to the slightest muscle contractions affecting the tendons, monitoring them for relaxation through special interactions between nerve fibers and collagen fibers. They are activated during isometric contraction, when muscle spindles are inactive.

Golgi tendon organs monitor tension that develops in a muscle, inhibiting the action of the alpha motor neurons on the agonist muscles and facilitating the inhibitory action of the motor neurons on the antagonist muscles. Signals generated by the tendon organs arrive at the spinal cord or brainstem where they stimulate neurons that inhibit alpha motor neurons that innervate the muscle from which the impulse

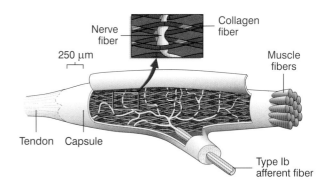

Figure 2.5 Golgi tendon organ.

originated. As a result of this, muscle contraction slows or ceases.

Basically, in the presence of an excessive "amount of force", expressed either through contraction or stretching of muscle fibers, these receptors intervene to inhibit the action. Together with the muscle spindles, these Golgi tendon organs therefore act as servo feedback mechanisms, protecting muscle fibers that are being subjected to excessive loads.

The muscle reaction triggered by Golgi tendon organs is called the *inverse myotatic* reflex or *clasp knife* response. This serves a dual function. On one hand, it is useful for avoiding tendon lesions due to excessively violent contractions, while on the other, it protects muscles from damage due to sudden decreases in applied load. The inverse myotatic reflex therefore opposes excessive shortening of the muscles, in contrast to the normal myotatic reflex triggered by muscle spindles, which opposes excessive stretching of the muscles. Moreover, these proprioceptors, being sensitive to even the slightest tension, are responsible for keeping the CNS (cerebellum) informed of the status of active muscle contraction.

If one group of fibers contracts with greater intensity than the others, Golgi tendon organs intervene, causing the fibers in question to relax and decrease their inhibitory effect on those that are contracting less strongly. The result is smoother and more harmonious motion even at low levels of muscle tension.

Central sensory pathways and their role in perception

Peripheral sensory information enters the CNS through the dorsal roots of the spinal cord and the sensory roots of the cranial nerves, conveyed by the axons of pseudounipolar neurons located in the cerebrospinal ganglia.

In the nerve fibers reaching the spinal cord, a first group of axons, carrying epicritic information, does not enter the gray matter of the posterior horns of the spinal cord, but travels medially and dorsally to them, bending upwards at right angles to form part of the white matter funiculus located in the spinal cord between the two posterior horns. They then terminate in two brainstem nuclei where the first synapses are made.

A second group of axons, which carry the protopathic component of exteroceptive and proprioceptive sensory information, enter the gray matter of the posterior horns of the spinal cord where they synapse with neurons of the sensory pathways, as will be described below.

The epicritic pathway

As noted above, axons that do not enter the gray matter of the posterior horns of the spinal cord travel medially and dorsally to them before taking an upward right-angle turn to join the white matter funiculus situated in the spinal cord between the two posterior horns. These nerve fibers are organized into two separate paired bundles, two on the right and two on the left, called the *gracile* fasciculus and the *cuneate* fasciculus. These bundles project, without synaptic interruption in the spinal cord, up to the brainstem where they terminate in two equal groups of neurons (*nuclei*) located in the medulla oblongata, called the *gracile* nucleus and *cuneate* nucleus. These fibers carry epicritic sensory impulses,

both exteroceptive and proprioceptive, which are sent on to the thalamus, the very high brain relay station, which transmits them to the somatosensory cerebral cortex (postcentral gyrus). Furthermore, axons carrying exteroceptive and proprioceptive epicritic sensory impulses from the head and neck, forming part of the trigeminal and facial cranial nerves, also enter the brainstem and travel to the gracile and cuneate nuclei where, like those mentioned above, they synapse with the neurons there.

The axons of the neurons in the gracile and cuneate nuclei of the medulla oblongata form a paired bundle called the *medial lemniscus*, which leads to the postero-lateral part of the thalamus where the axons find the target neurons to which they transmit the epicritic impulses they are conveying. Finally, the axons of these neurons project to the postcentral gyrus of the cerebral cortex, where the information is finally decoded and processed, and where, if necessary, a response is generated.

It is important to remember that nerve impulses conveyed along nerve pathways are modified to a greater or lesser degree at each synaptic interruption due to the interplay of reciprocal influences (modulations) between synapses and axons of different origins, including systems descending from other centers or from the cerebellar and cerebral cortexes. As a result of this, incoming information is inhibited, reduced, or amplified on each passage. This also applies to the gracile and cuneate nuclei. Any exteroceptive or proprioceptive epicritic information reaching it is amplified or reduced, added or subtracted (i.e. integrated) in accordance with information coming from other sensory afferents, both near and remote, as well as from descending fiber systems.

Finally, afferent inhibition is an additional distinct mechanism designed to enhance the selective-discriminatory capacity of the peripheral sensory system. The physiology of this mechanism is still not completely understood and its presence has to date been confirmed in mammals, but not specifically in humans. Upon application of a mechanical stimulus to a given area, this inhibitory mechanism generates an excitatory response in the same area but an inhibitory response in neighboring areas. Clearly, if a mechanical disturbance eliciting a response from an immediately underlying receptor were also to activate surrounding receptors, the result would be generation of a completely chaotic message

Topographic conservation of stimulus properties

Studies of the projection pathways of peripheral receptors indicate that each columnar group of neurons running through the posterior horns of the spinal cord is responsible for conveying one specific type of sensitivity. The same organizational principle applies to cranial nerve nuclei in the brainstem. It should be recalled that the sensory neurons of the cerebrospinal ganglia are T-shaped, with the peripheral branch of the axon reaching the sensory receptor, where it is stimulated, and the central branch carrying the information to the neurons of the columns in the posterior spinal cord horns. Each column thus receives one type of sensory signal: touch or pressure, tremor or vibration, proprioception or synesthesia. This anatomical and functional specificity also applies to those neurons that do not send their central axon to the posterior horns, but directly to the gracile and cuneate nuclei of the brainstem, where exactly the same specificity is maintained.

In these nuclei, proceeding in the caudal-rostral direction, there are neurons that respond only to touch-pressure, neurons activated by mechanical stimulation of the periosteum (i.e., by deep touch-pressure), and finally, in the most rostral part, neurons stimulated only by joint mechanoreceptors. This arrangement is the same in the posterior horns, with proprioceptive sensitivity at a superficial level and tactile sensitivity at a deep level.

This rigid and precise pattern of the axons conveying information about the location, form, quality, and temporal sequence of the stimuli affecting the body from its various parts is therefore one of the most significant aspects of the epicritic sensory route, the *spino-bulbo-thalamo-cortical pathway*. It gives, at the cortical level, a precise reproduction of the attributes of the original stimuli, converted into patterns of nerve activity distributed over time and in space. In particular, the peripheral pattern or representation is maintained with strict *somatotopy* up to the cortical level. Because the nerve fibers carrying sensory information from various parts of the body (skin and locomotor system) project to regions of the post-central gyrus, which conserve the original somatotopy, it is possible to recognize, in the cerebral cortex of this gyrus, the areas for the head, neck, upper limbs, trunk, lower limbs, and so on.

This does not mean that each peripheral point is represented by a specific point of the cortex, but rather that the cortical representation area is proportional to the density of the peripheral receptors therein. Therefore, the representation of the body projected on the cortical postcentral gyrus does not reflect the relative dimensions of different body parts. Actually, the hands, tongue and lips, which are rich in sensory receptors but physically small-sized parts of the body as a whole, occupy a larger area of the brain than the trunk and lower limbs, which have fewer receptors. If one draws a faithful representation of the extent of the different cortical projection areas for the different parts of the body, the resulting figure has very large hands, a huge mouth with enormous lips, a small trunk and so on. This grotesque little monster is known as the *sensory homunculus* (Fig. 2.6).

Mechanoreceptive differentiation is thus conserved along the entire epicritic pathway (medial lemniscus, thalamus, and cerebral cortex). The information coming from an individual part of the body is differentiated into "cog-

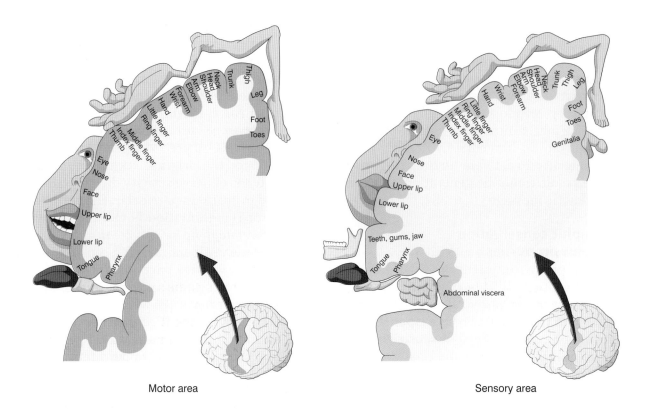

Motor area   Sensory area

Figure 2.6 The motor and sensory areas of the cerebral cortex, located respectively in the precentral gyrus and the postcentral gyrus, are specialized, and each part can be associated with a specific part of the body. Drawing the parts of the body in proportion to the extent of their representation in the cerebral cortex results in a sort of distorted caricature of a human figure, a motor or sensory homunculus. This is because the area of the cerebral cortex reserved for each part of the body is proportional to the precision with which that part is monitored and controlled, i.e., to its degree of innervation, not to its size.

nizant" information about external reality – used to examine the external environment and obtain as faithful a map of it as possible – and "cognizant" information about one's own body, used to generate an accurate map of the body and, specifically, of the part from which a particular piece of information is coming.

The cortical projection area for skin sensitivity lies in the intermediate portion of the postcentral gyrus, while proprioceptive sensation, also in the postcentral gyrus, is located in the lower end of its central sulcus (*sulcus of Rolando*) and in the part closest to the parietal association cortex.

The protopathic pathway

As mentioned above, a second group of axons, which transmit the protopathic component of exteroceptive and proprioceptive sensation, enters the gray matter of the posterior horns of the spinal cord to form synapses with the neurons there.

The spinal cord gray matter is organized into *laminae*, according to the types and quantities of neurons that each part contains, and the types, quantities and arrangement of the nerve fibers and systems of synapses. Nine laminae have been identified: ten if the gray matter around the central canal is included. The laminae are numbered according to their position using Roman numerals starting from the tip of the posterior horns. The first six laminae are the posterior horns containing second-order neurons, i.e., those with which the central branches of the T-shaped ganglionic neurons form synapses.

Lamina I (marginal nucleus or *Lissauer's zone*) is thin, with few small neurons but rich in variously crossing fibers. Lamina II (*substantia gelatinosa of Rolando*) contains small neurons and receives only unmyelinated fibers. Lamina III, more developed and richer in neurons than the previous laminae, also receives unmyelinated C fibers, small-caliber myelinated Aδ fibers, and large-caliber myelinated Aβ fibers and functionally is a single unit with the substantia gelatinosa of Rolando. Lamina IV is highly developed and has widespread neurons, which also receive myelinated fibers. Their axons go on to form the large *spinothalamic tract*, which conveys a large proportion of protopathic exteroceptive information. Lamina V is well developed, with small neurons and few nerve fibers in its medial part, but large neurons with many nerve fibers in its lateral part. This lamina receives collateral branches of ganglionic neurons that convey cutaneous and proprioceptive information. Lamina VI, at the base of the posterior horn, is activated specifically by cutaneous and joint stimuli. Lamina VII, which is part of the intermediate column or zone of the spinal cord gray matter, is very voluminous and protrudes into the anterior horn. It contains two important groups of neurons. The first, located medially, forms the posterior or dorsal thoracic nucleus (*Clarke's column*), which receives proprioceptive information and gives rise to the dorsal spinocerebellar tract (*Flechsig's tract*). The second contains pregangleonic sympathetic nuclei in the toracolumbar region and forms the intermediate lateral horn or column.

Axons forming the system that conveys protopathic information have their first synaptic relay at the level of the second-order neurons of the posterior horn laminae. The medial portion of these axons is made up of myelinated fibers, practically all of which terminate in lamina IV. The intermediate portion also terminates directly at the neurons of lamina IV while the lateral portion of small myelinated Aδ fibers and unmyelinated C fibers goes as far as lamina I. Having entered lamina I, these latter fibers bend upwards or downwards and travel through it for a short distance before entering, in a progressive manner, lamina II (substantia gelatinosa of Rolando), to terminate on the neurons found there. From the substantia gelatinosa, information is diffused to various levels of the spinal cord, both in the same neuromere and to different neuromeres.

By integrating the differentiated information reaching them, the neurons of the substantia gelatinosa of Rolando modulate both pain and non-pain sensory afferents. They do this by means of the inhibitory action exerted by small-caliber fibers and the excitatory action exerted by large-caliber fibers, that, from the T-shaped ganglionic neurons, travel directly to lamina IV neurons, which give rise to the spinothalamic pathways. If one also considers that the substantia gelatinosa of Rolando receives afferents not only from the ganglionic neurons, but also from the brainstem (the regions around the aqueduct of the midbrain, or aqueduct of *Sylvius*, and the third ventricle, exerting an inhibitory action through the reticulospinal fibers), it is easy to appreciate the important role played by this spinal structure in the monitoring and control of protopathic afferents, particularly thermal-pain afferents.

Gate control theory

The excitatory-inhibitory organization so far described provides the anatomical basis underlying the theory of pain sensitivity modulation or gate control theory (GCT), proposed by

Melzack and Wall in the 1960s. It is to be noted that the GCT applies primarily to pain sensations, but can also apply to other exteroceptive and proprioceptive afferents.

According to Melzack and Wall, the neurons of the substantia gelatinosa of Rolando are able, like a "gate" being opened or closed, to facilitate or block the flow of pain impulses depending on their level of excitation. The neurons of the substantia gelatinosa have an inhibitory function whereby, when they are activated by large-diameter Aβ fibers, they "close the gate" i.e., the activated inhibitory neuron exerts its inhibitory action and does not let the impulse through. Conversely, when the neurons are inhibited by small-diameter Aδ and C fibers, they "open the gate" i.e., the blocked inhibitory neuron no longer exerts its impeding action and lets the impulse through. The "gate" is a control system that prevents excessively intense pain sensations from disabling the sensory neural network, or, alternatively, that allows perceived pain to be reduced or even annulled.

Intense nociceptive stimulation activates the neurons of the substantia gelatinosa of Rolando, which inhibit direct pain afferents on their way to the neurons of lamina V, thus excluding the circuit.

Lamina V, as mentioned, contains the neurons of origin of the spinothalamic tract. These neurons are of two types:

- Wide-range neurons, which respond to low intensity thermal, irritant, and mechanical stimuli applied to the skin, increase their firing rate as the stimuli increase in intensity, have a very wide receptive field, and respond to a wide range of different stimuli.
- High-threshold neurons, activated only by noxious mechanical stimuli, to which they respond with rapidly depleting discharges, signaling a change in the intensity of a sensation and not merely its presence. Stimulation must be sufficiently intense for activation to occur. These neurons have a receptive field only slightly larger than that of peripheral neurons, and respond to a single type of nocicep-

tive stimulus. High-threshold neurons therefore have properties opposite to those of wide-range neurons, in that they respond to only one type of stimulus, and only when it is sufficiently intense. They signal, quite precisely, the location of the stimulation, and then return to their rest condition.

Wide-range neurons and high-threshold neurons are somewhat complementary to one another. The former respond only to low-intensity painful and potentially painful stimuli, generally alerting the nervous system but not locating or classifying the stimulus. The latter are activated only by intensely painful stimuli and have the function of identifying the position and quality of a stimulus that has already been perceived. These are the neurons of origin of the large spinothalamic tract. They can be divided into the anterior and lateral spinothalamic tracts. When these neurons decussate at the spinal cord level of origin, they ascend towards the brain stem and thalamus, where the next synaptic stations are located.

Spinobulbar fibers are an important component of the spinothalamic tract. These fibers enter the medullary reticular formation, whose neurons are organized into various small, numerous nuclei; they send excitatory fibers to the substantia gelatinosa, and, most significantly, transmit protopathic information to all the regions of the central nervous system.

Most of the fibers of the spinothalamic tract reach the thalamus, where consciousness of protopathic and pain information arises and where, together with the spinal lemniscus, this information is integrated with epicritic information. The spinothalamic tract and the spinal lemniscus are thus two highly evolved sensory systems that complement one another in achieving conscious awareness. The widespread and extremely versatile spinothalamic system appears to convey rapid and selective awareness of nociceptive information. The spinal lemniscus appears to be responsible for discriminative and exploratory sensitivity. The combination of the characteristics of these two systems provides the CNS with a sophisticated means of gathering and optimally analyzing information from the external (and internal) environments

HYPOTHESIS OF A NEURONAL MODULATION MECHANISM INDUCED BY NEUROMUSCULAR TAPING

The skin receives various types of stimuli (mechanical, thermal, and pain), which are recognized through the activation of specific receptors (mechanoreceptors, proprioceptors, thermoreceptors, and nociceptors).

Mechanoreceptors respond to increases in perpendicular pressure (Merkel disks), to changes in mechanical force applied and to its direction (Meissner's corpuscles), to mechanical deformations in a plane tangent to the skin surface (Ruffini corpuscles), to very small movements (up to 10 μm in length), and to variations in very rapid movements (up to 400 Hz) (Vater-Pacini corpuscles).

Proprioceptors function as transducers. Modified by the stretching of tendons or contraction of muscles, they transform the changes in length to which they are subjected into nerve impulses that are transmitted to the spinal cord or brainstem along high-velocity conductive nerve fibers. Nociceptors, on the other hand, are activated by algogenic substances coming from injured tissues, from the vascular district, or from the nerve fibers themselves, while thermoreceptors respond to changes in the temperature of the external and internal environment.

Gate control theory provides a model for interpreting molecular activation of nociceptors and also a basis for interpreting the mechanism of action of the other types of sensitivity (pro-

topathic). The function of the gate is to modulate afferent stimuli. This function is based on the interaction of and reciprocal modulation among nociceptive and non-nociceptive nerve fibers. This interaction involves both the small-caliber pain fibers (types Aδ and C) and the large-caliber, non-pain fibers (type Aβ). These fibers converge at the level of the substantia gelatinosa of the posterior horn of the spinal cord where various types of sensation are recognized.

Lamina II (substantia gelatinosa of Rolando) neurons exert an inhibitory action on the afferents to the spinothalamic tract, which is responsible for conveying protopathic information to a higher level. If the Aβ fibers carry non-pain stimuli, they activate the inhibitory neurons, which thus block the transmission of any pain signals to the thalamus and the cerebral cortex. In this configuration, the gate is "closed" and no pain is felt. If the Aδ or C fibers transmit pain impulses instead, they inhibit the inhibitory neurons, which then cannot block the transmission of pain signals to the thalamus and the cerebral cortex. In this configuration, the gate is "open" and pain is perceived.

Most information passing via the spinothalamic tract converges on the posterior nucleus of the thalamus together with a small part coming from the medial lemniscus. The posterior nucleus of the thalamus responds to pain impulses and has bilateral receptive fields that are not somatotopically organized. Another thalamic nucleus involved in the discriminative aspects of pain is the ventral posterolateral nucleus, which projects to the somatosensory cortex. Thus, while the intralaminar nuclei of the thalamus respond in a similar way to those of the posterior group, they are also involved in the affective and autonomic, "arousal" responses associated with pain. These are innervated by the spinoreticular thalamic system, and have extensive projections to subcortical sites, the frontal lobe, and the limbic system.

Ultimately, if a pain stimulus and a mechanical stimulus, like that produced by NeuroMuscular Taping, are transmitted simultaneously, the transmission of the pain stimulus will be attenuated as a result of the excitatory action exerted by the Aβ fibers on the inhibitory neurons of the substantia gelatinosa of Rolando.

Our hypothesis is that NeuroMuscular Taping exerts interference activity on the neurons of the posterior horns of the spinal cord, depolarizing them and preventing them from sending pain impulses. It may therefore be possible to discuss neuromodulation induced by NeuroMuscular Taping.

3

Types of Application

NeuroMuscular Taping applied with the eccentric technique produces a lengthening stimulus on both the skin and subcutaneous layers. This stimulus increases skin elasticity and restores normal extension of muscles and tendons as it performs a decompressive action. In combination with the influence exerted by skin folds on joints and on muscle and tendon paths, the tape's decompressive action increases extension of muscle tissue, connective fascia and skin, thereby reducing their congestion and normalizing response and functioning (Figs. 3.1-3.3). Decompressive stimulus increases interstitial spaces, reduces skin and subcutaneous tissue compression, and enables normal blood and lymphatic circulation to be restored.

Concentric NeuroMuscular Taping, on the other hand, produces a shortening stimulus at both cutaneous and subcutaneous levels with a compressive action. This stimulus increases the contraction of the skin, muscles, and tendons yet it reduces blood and lymph flow.

Given that NeuroMuscular Taping is essentially nothing more than direct skin stimulation, correct application is based on thorough knowledge and understanding of the tegumentary apparatus (skin and subcutaneous tissues) and of its complex role in the control and coordination of body movement.

SKIN THICKNESS AND ELASTICITY

Skin thickness varies according to gender, ethnicity, body region and the level of mechanical stress to which the skin is subjected. Thick-

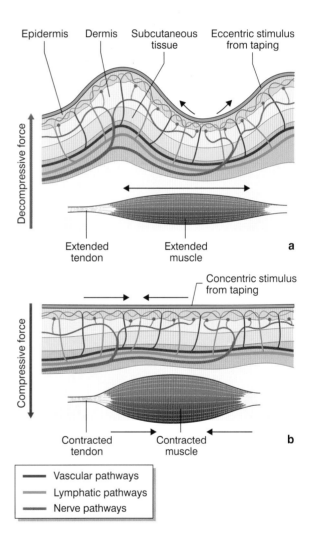

Figure 3.1 Decompressive force (a) and compressive force (b). When tape is applied using the decompressive technique (a), it delivers an indirect eccentric stimulus to the underlying muscle. It also produces a decompressive force that increases the space between the skin and the underlying tissues. Tape applied using the compressive technique (b), on the other hand, delivers a concentric stimulus that favors muscle contraction and reduces the space between the skin and the underlying tissues.

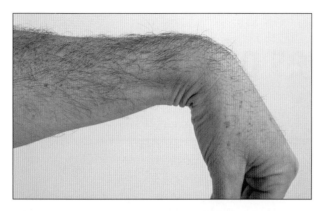

Figure 3.2 When the wrist is flexed, the skin on the dorsal aspect stretches, while that on the palmar as pect forms folds. In this way, the space between the skin and the underlying tissues is reduced on the-dorsal aspect but increased on the palmar aspect.

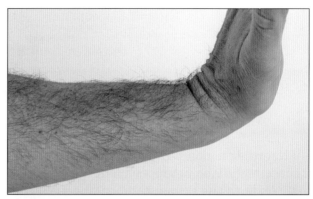

Figure 3.3 Conversely, when the wrist is extended it is the skin on the palmar surface that is stretched, reducing the subcutaneous space, while the skin on the dorsal aspect forms folds, generating a decompressive force that increases the subcutaneous space.

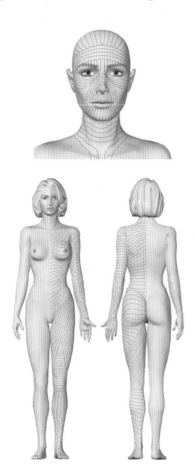

Figure 3.4 Langer's lines. These lines define the directions along which the skin has least elasticity and deformability.

ness ranges from 0.5 to 2 mm, but in some areas it can be as great as 4 to 5 mm. In general, the skin is thinner on flexor than on extensor aspects of the body. It is thicker in males and in the dorsolateral areas (of the head, neck, and trunk), tending to become thinner towards the ventral areas (abdomen, groin, and distal extremities of the limbs). It is thicker (4 mm) in the posterior cervical region, on the palms of the hands, and the soles of the feet. However, it is very thin (0.5 mm) in other areas, namely the eyelids, the foreskin and labia minora, and the external auditory meatus.

Skin is very elastic, with good strength and distensibility. A 3 × 100 mm strip of skin can sustain up to 10 kg, stretching by up to 50%. However, skin elasticity is not uniform all over the body, being greater in the extensor (convex) areas of a joint, over the front of the knee, and behind the elbow, for example, whereas it is less elastic at the sides or back of a joint. Despite its remarkable resistance and good elasticity, excessive and prolonged stretching of the skin – resulting from pregnancy or weight changes – can cause partial tearing of the three-dimensional connective tissue fiber lattice of the dermis, resulting in unattractive internal scars, commonly called stretch marks.

As noted above, the skin is not uniformly elastic and distensible, i.e., its tension, both at rest and in motion, is not the same in all directions. Skin tension depends on the collagen and elastic fiber organization of the dermis and is greater in one direction and less in the perpendicular direction. Specifically, the elastic fibers are not completely relaxed, but in tension. This state-of-rest tension is oriented differently in different regions of the body. Accordingly, there exist trajectories along which tension is greater, with corresponding trajectories of lesser tension perpendicular to these. Hence, a round wound tends to deform into an oval shape.

It follows that lines of skin tension can be mapped on the surface of the body. Also known as cleavage lines or *Langer's lines*, after the Austrian pathologist who identified them at the start of the nineteenth century, these define the directions along which the skin is least elastic and most resistant to deformation (Fig. 3.4). Surgeons should take these lines into consideration, since incisions should, as far as possible, be made along the dominant axes of tension in order to prevent the formation of unsightly scars and to ensure good cosmetic results, reducing the tension on the wound as it is sutured.

An application of elastic adhesive tape onto the skin should also take these lines of minimum cutaneous elasticity, i.e., Langer's lines, into account. In general, a path perpendicular to these lines should be followed in order to exploit the direction of greater elasticity of the skin and thus accentuate the skin-folding effect. However, Langer's lines alone do not provide sufficient information to guide tape placement. Indeed, NMT affects other structures beyond the skin, producing decompression of the cutaneous structure and of the proximate subcutaneous tissue.

Although it is bound to the deeper layers by means of the hypodermis, the skin's elasticity and deformability offers degrees of mobility that allow it be raised into folds, sometimes large ones. This mobility contributes to keeping joints in their axes through facilitating joint movement while limiting joint excursion.

In some regions of the body, the structure of the dermis and hypodermis is such that the skin adheres firmly to underlying tissue, preventing it from being lifted into folds. These areas, where it is not possible to give the skin "a pinch," are the anterior margin of the tibia, the iliac crest, the groin area, the sacral region, the shoulder at the acromion, the scalp, the soles of the feet, and the palms of the hands (Figs. 3.5-3.8).

The outer surface of the skin is varied in the arrangement and emphasis of its irregularities. On the volar surfaces of the fingertips, for example, each individual's skin displays *dermatoglyphs* (fingerprints), unique genetically determined patterns of grooves and ridges that form

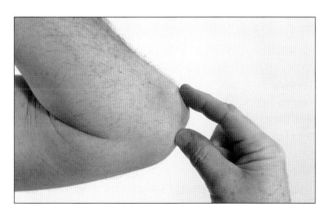

Figure 3.5 When the elbow is flexed, the dorsal skin is stretched and cannot be lifted.

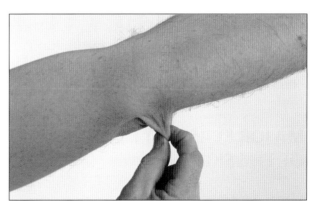

Figure 3.6 When the elbow is extended, the dorsal skin is relaxed and can be lifted.

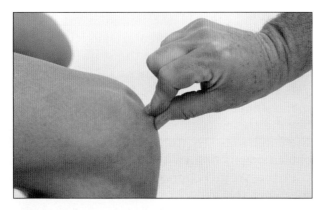

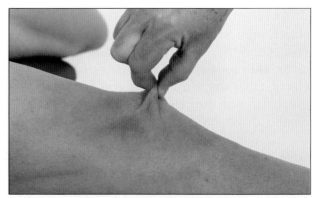

Figure 3.7 When the knee is flexed, the anterior skin is stretched and cannot be lifted.

Figure 3.8 When the knee is extended, the anterior skin is relaxed and can be lifted.

in the third month of fetal development and remain unchanged throughout life.

The *fingerprints* everyone leaves behind on the surfaces of objects they touch with their fingertips are due to deposits of microscopic drops of sweat from the pore openings neatly arranged along the ridges between the grooves of the fingerprints. *Creases* are grooves that form as a result of muscle and joint movements (temporary creases) or are due to the adherence of skin to superficial fascia of the body (permanent creases). *Movement creases* are due to muscle contraction and are perpendicular to the direction of the underlying muscle fibers. As we age, these creases become more prominent as a result of ongoing mechanical stress, becoming deeper and permanent, like the "lines" on the palm of the hand. Deep grooves are typical of the glabrous skin of the knees and elbows. *Wrinkles* or *age lines* are permanent skin furrows of variable depth, appearing as the skin loses elasticity with age.

MAJOR ELASTICITY LINES OF THE SKIN

In addition to Langer's lines, other maps of skin elasticity exist, such as Kraissl's lines, which mainly refer to lines on the face. Kraissl's

lines are different from Langer's lines, because the former were identified on living subjects and not on cadavers.

It is these lines of greater elasticity, rather than those of least elasticity, that are of particular interest to NeuroMuscular Taping. This is because by following areas of greater cutaneous elasticity and accentuating the skin folds, it is possible to create decompression both at skin level and at subcutaneous level.

A basic rule for correct application of NeuroMuscular Taping is to follow the *Major Elasticity Lines* of the skin (MELs) with the tape. Partly through research, but mainly through observing results obtained after tape applications, suitable maps of these lines have been developed (Fig. 3.9). These Major Elasticity Lines of the skin have been derived from studying the body in movement and the dynamics of movement coordination. With the exception of some joint correction applications, maximum therapeutic benefit will be obtained by following these lines when applying tape with either decompressive or compressive methods.

Generally, skin elasticity lines follow the paths of superficial muscle fibers, though not in all cases, such as, for example, over the rhomboid minor, the rhomboid major and the masseter muscles. Skin elasticity reflects movement around joints. The skin becomes more elastic in a longitudinal direction as it approaches a joint.

NEUROMUSCULAR TAPING from Theory to Practice

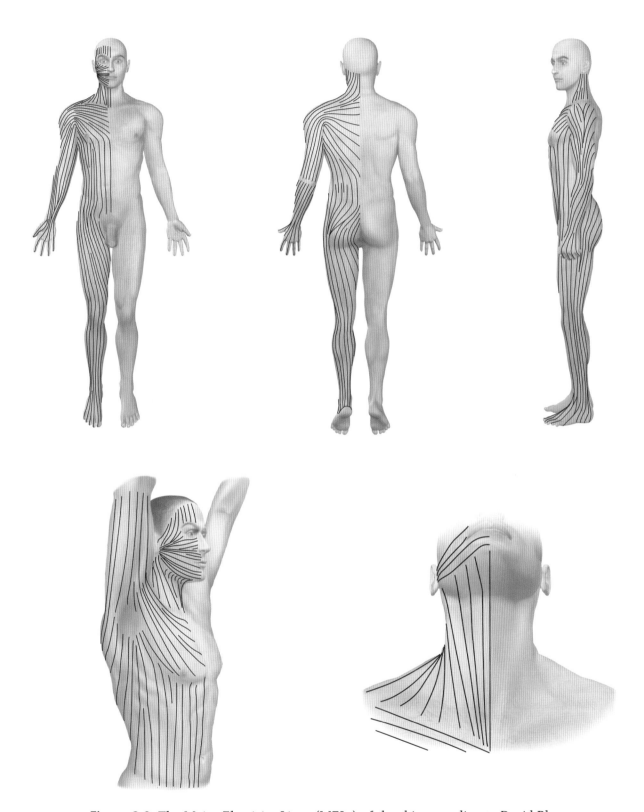

Figure 3.9 The Major Elasticity Lines (MELs) of the skin according to David Blow.

This happens, for example, at the front of the knee. Conversely, it becomes less elastic longitudinally in the middle of a limb, for example on the anterior margin of the tibia.

These lines are not fixed, unidirectional lines, but have a *Range of Elastic Action* (REA), which has been studied in order to obtain information about how the skin is able to promote coordination of movement. The REA goes from 0° to 25° to 45° relative to the longitudinal axis (Fig. 3.10). For example, the skin covering the dorsal aspect of the metacarpophalangeal joint of the index finger is elastic in the longitudinal direction only. This is because the joint moves only in flexion-extension. This skin therefore has an REA of 0°. The REA of the skin on the anterior aspect of the knee is 25°; the skin there accordingly permits a greater range of motion of up to 25°, enabling the full range of flexion and extension in this large joint. Similarly, the REA of skin on the back of the neck over the cervical vertebrae is 45°; here the skin allows for an increased range of up to 45°, enabling the neck joints to flex, extend and rotate the head.

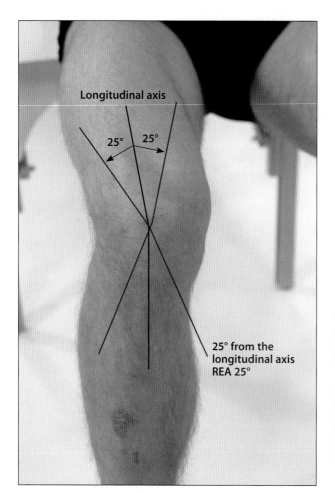
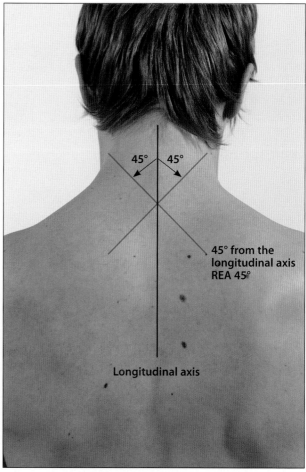

Figure 3.10 Range of Elastic Action (REA) according to David Blow.

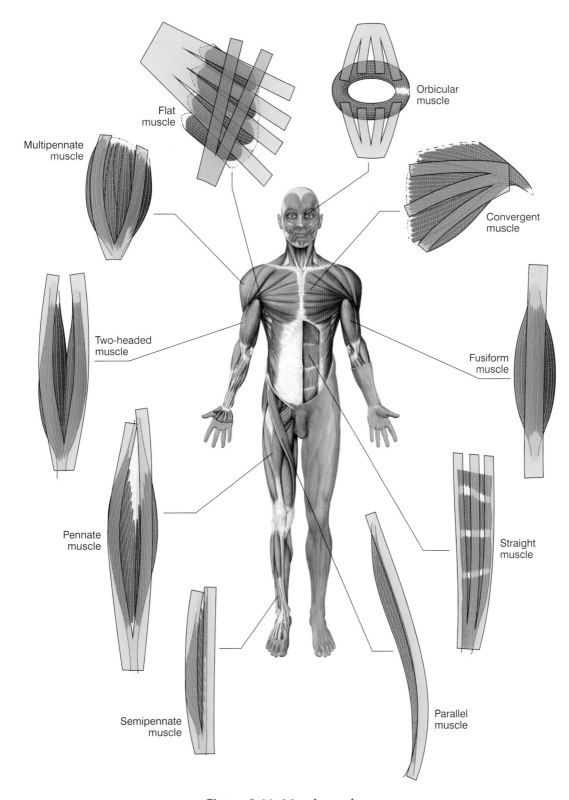

Figure 3.11 Muscles and tapes.

Cutting the tape

The shape of the tape will depend on the area to be treated and the type of application.

The tape used has to be as long as the muscle being treated with an additional several centimeters to serve as the base (starting) anchor and tail (finishing) anchor (Fig. 3.11). It is important to take care that the anchors do not encroach on the paths of other muscles, the lymphatic or vascular pathways, areas of joint closure in the axillary, inguinal, clavicular, sternocleidomastoid, or trapezius regions. Even where they have been properly applied without any tension, over-long tape anchors can lead to excessive compression.

Several of the tape cuts used in NeuroMuscular Taping are shown below.

I-shaped cut

For application over the muscle belly
(e.g. rectus abdominis, flexor hallucis brevis)

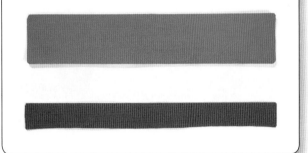

Y-shaped cut

For application around the muscle belly
(e.g. biceps brachii, gastrocnemius, descending part of the trapezius)

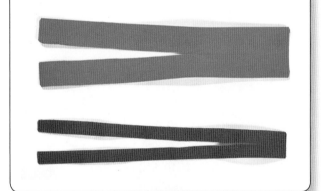

W-shaped cut

For distribution over the muscle belly
(e.g. pectoralis major)

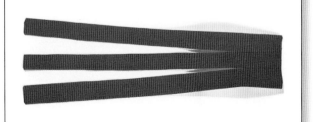

X-shaped cut

The center of the tape is applied over a fixed point and the strips are applied over the muscle belly.
(E.g., for rhomboid minor and rhomboid major, the center of the tape is fixed over the fourth thoracic vertebra.)

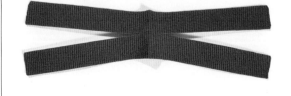

Fan-shaped cut with four strips

Draining application
(e.g., for anterior neck drainage)

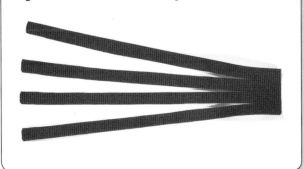

Fan-shaped cut with five strips

Draining application
(e.g., for adhesive capsulitis or frozen shoulder)

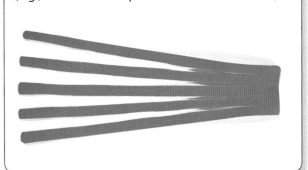

Combined Y- and I-shaped cut

Decompressive application
(e.g., for the calcaneal tendon, Achilles tendon, or gastrocnemius)

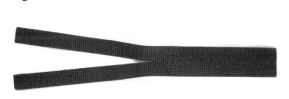

Combined Y- and fan-shaped cut

Decompressive application
(e.g., for the calcaneal spur)

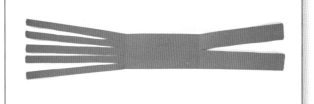

Preparing the Tape

Preparing the fan with five strips

Step 1

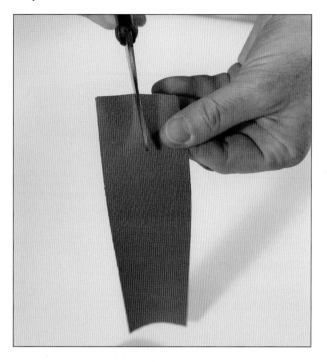

Step 2

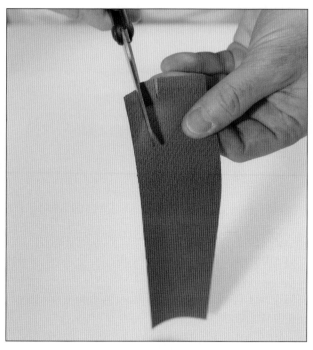

Step 3

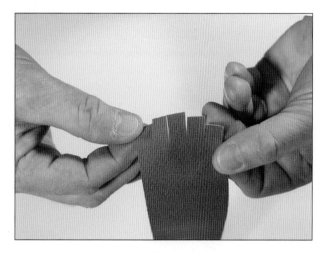

Step 4

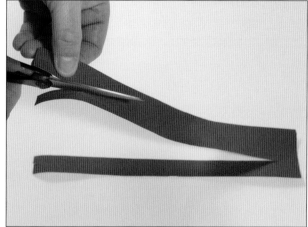

NEUROMUSCULAR TAPING from Theory to Practice

Preparing the Tape

Preparing a single-hole cut

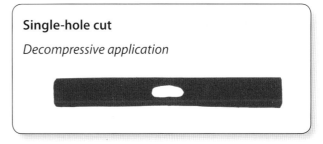

Single-hole cut

Decompressive application

Step 1

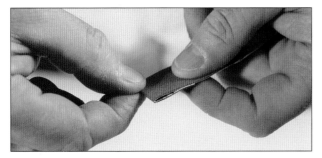

Step 2

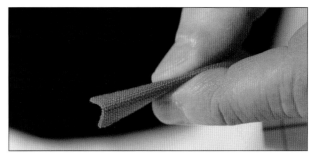

Step 3

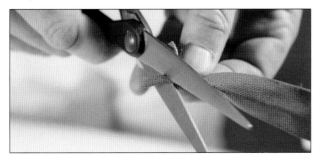

Step 4

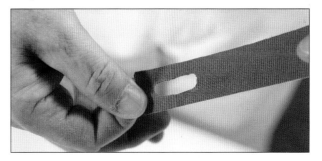

Preparing a two- or three-hole cut

Decompressive application
(e.g., for carpal tunnel syndrome)

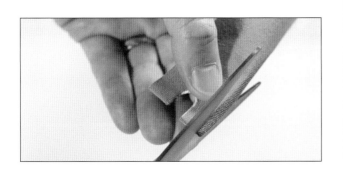

One-, two- and three-hole cuts

Functional applications

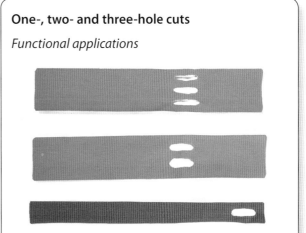

Separating the tape from its backing paper

For better tape adhesion, pay attention to how the cotton tape is separated from its backing paper. Refrain from touching the adhesive to ensure that the tape adheres properly to the patient's skin for the required amount of time. The backing paper should therefore be removed starting from one end by folding the paper back. In this way, the end tape can be held at the place where the paper is folded over. Then break the paper liner by pulling the sides in opposite directions.

In some cases it is possible to tear the paper backing in the middle of the tape and to remove it starting from this point. It is suggested that you fold the paper back in order to avoid touching the adhesive.

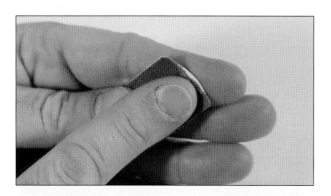
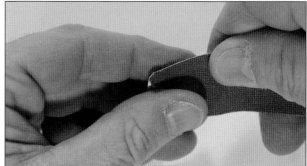

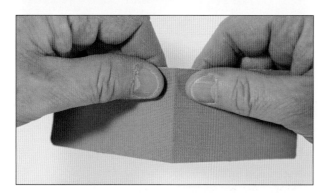
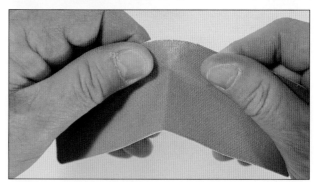

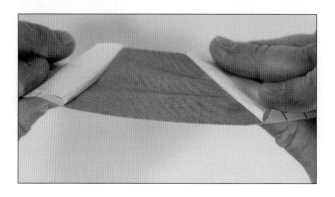

Preparation of the body area to be treated

The patient's skin must be dry, clean, and free of oil, creams, and ointments. The tape is applied directly to the skin and good adherence is essential for it to be effective. If creams, ointments, or lotions have been applied, e.g., massage cream or gel for ultrasound, the skin should be cleaned with alcohol or washed with soap and water before proceeding with Neuro-Muscular Taping. The operator's hands must also be clean and dry.

However, be aware that frequent use of alcohol for cleaning can cause dry or irritated skin.

Following sports, the patient should take a shower to remove any sweat before applying the tape. If the tape is to be in place during sporting activity it should be applied one hour beforehand. Use a spray adhesive to improve the adhesion as needed.

It is also a good idea to shave any body hair to promote adhesion. In this case it is best to avoid using a normal razor, as this could irritate the skin. Alternatively, shave the area several hours before applying the tape, or use an electric razor.

If the skin is irritated or has moles, abrasions, unhealed scars, or signs of skin allergy, taping the affected area is discouraged. Scar tissues from burns must be completely healed before taping.

If the patient reports itchiness in the area where the tape has been applied, it must be removed. Nevertheless, take care to not mistake an increase in blood flow for skin irritation. In fact, itching that is felt immediately after application, and which may last for ten to twenty minutes, is a sign of increased blood flow. In this case, the tape is working and so should be left in place.

Patient's age

NeuroMuscular Taping can be used on people of all ages, from infants to the elderly.

In cases of obstetric torticollis, for example, a very narrow tape less than 1 cm in width is applied, using the decompressive technique, over the path of the descending part of the trapezius and over the sternocleidomastoid in two separate applications.

With elderly patients, special attention should be paid to the condition of the skin, which may be easily irritated. Despite the lack of elasticity and a reduction in the amount of connective tissue between the dermis and the epidermis in elderly patients, NeuroMuscular Taping yields excellent results.

Duration and number of applications

The duration of application varies. Tape can remain in place from several hours to several days, up to a maximum of ten days.

In acute conditions, where the patient's condition is evolving, tape is applied for short periods. In cases of trauma-induced edema, for example, tape should be reapplied daily in order to obtain the maximum draining effect. When the aim is to maintain achieved results, applications can stay in place for seven to ten days.

However, basic taping has a duration of three to four days.

The number of applications is unlimited. As NeuroMuscular Taping is a therapeutic tool, particularly useful in rehabilitation, the number of applications will depend on the progress of therapy.

In situations such as multiple sclerosis and other progressive degenerative diseases, the use of the technique can continue indefinitely until the patient's symptoms, and consequently their quality of life, improve.

Tape application

Initial and final anchors must always be applied without imparting tension to that part of the tape. Before applying the initial anchor, the patient places their limb in position. If the patient is unable to achieve full mobilization, the therapist stretches the patient's skin away from the limb to be treated.

The tape must form closely spaced skin folds during movement. This is possible only if it adheres well to the skin. Rounding off the tape's edges to improve adherence is an effective technique.

External fixatives such as adhesive sprays can be used during sporting activities, but they are not generally recommended, as they may cause irritation.

Once applied, the tape is warmed by rubbing the palm of the hand along the direction of application. This activates the adhesive and improves adherence.

Tape removal

The tape must be removed gently and not torn off. Below are the correct methods for removing tape:
- Pull the tape in the opposite direction to that of hair growth while stretching the skin the other way.
- Lift it off by gently, working widthwise rather than lengthwise.
- Wet the tape with water before removing it (with children, in particular, moistening of tape with water or oil before removal is recommended).
- Where possible, it is recommended that the tape be removed while taking a shower.

Patients may wash, shower, and swim without concern, as the tape will not lose its adhesive properties. Afterwards, however, it is a good idea to dry the tape using a hair dryer, dabbing it first with a dry towel. It is nevertheless always best to check that the tape is still adhering well. On average, a tape will maintain adherence for three to four days.

> NOTE: The therapeutic and rehabilitative outcomes of NeuroMuscular Taping depend on the method of application used, not on the color of the tape.

Contraindications

NeuroMuscular Taping is a minimally invasive, non-pharmacological technique that does not cause adverse reactions, with the possible exception of skin irritation in particularly sensitive patients. Even this problem can be considerably reduced by using a good quality adhesive that does not contain alcohol.

The tape must always be applied by qualified personnel. If it is applied incorrectly due to poor knowledge of the technique or incorrect diagnosis, NeuroMuscular Taping can worsen the patient's symptoms. Proper application, on the other hand, causes symptoms such as pain and immobility to improve rapidly.

The tape used is not a sterile medical device and must therefore not be applied on or near infected areas.

NeuroMuscular Taping improves blood circulation and lymphatic drainage and may therefore be contraindicated in the following conditions:
- Acute thrombosis
- Cancer and metastases
- Phlebitis
- Acute congestion in association with diabetes
- Current infection
- Acute trauma from severe muscle injury and tendonitis
- The immediate post-operative period
- Wounds, infections, or skin ulceration
- Edema in cardiac failure

General Principles for Application

NeuroMuscular Taping provides local stimulus to the area where it is applied. In patients who have undergone knee replacement surgery, for example, tape cannot be applied on the front of the knee until the wound has completely healed. Instead, it can be applied postoperatively in the quadriceps femoris region, the popliteal region, and on the calf in order to avoid blood congestion, to decompress the muscles, to improve drainage, and to prevent retraction of the muscle fibers due to immobilization.

Pregnancy is not considered a contraindication. It is possible to perform treatments to relieve sciatica, back pain, and inguinal hernias. However, any applications (decompressive or compressive) on the abdomen should be avoided during pregnancy.

Decompressive NeuroMuscular Taping gives excellent results in the treatment of fibrocystic breast conditions.

NeuroMuscular Taping is a rehabilitation therapy and its implementation should proceed through the following therapeutic steps:
- Diagnosis and assessment of the clinical picture
- Establishment of the clinical objective
- Therapeutic treatment
- Consolidation of rehabilitation.

As indicated in previous chapters, the tape can only be used to stimulate the skin in one of two ways, compressive or decompressive (Fig. 3.12). The choice depends on the patient's condition, diagnosis, clinical picture, rehabilitation goal, and the target area of the treatment. For example, if a muscle is contracted or retracted following a period of immobilization, the tape must be applied using the decompressive tech-

nique. If the muscle is hypotonic it is useful to use the compressive technique to improve its contraction.

However, it is important to bear in mind that tape applied using the latter technique (compressive) can be left in place for a limited time only. Because it exerts compressive stimulation, a compressive application can reduce the blood supply and lead to cramps.

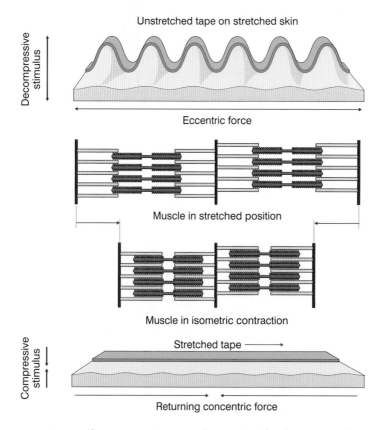

Figure 3.12 Decompressive and compressive stimulation. In the first case, the tape, tending to return to its original length, delivers an eccentric, decompressive stimulus. In the second, tending to shorten, it delivers a stimulus that is concentric and compressive.

Decompressive Technique

With this technique, the tape is applied without tension to stretched skin.

When applying the decompressive technique to the deltoid, for example, it is necessary to stretch the skin overlying the muscle itself. The tape anchor, which is placed in a neutral position, must be distal to the muscle insertion. One strip of the tape is applied over the anterior fibers of the deltoid (clavicular portion) and the other over the posterior fibers (spinal portion).

The tail ends of the tape finish at the origin of the muscle. During flexion and extension of the muscle, skin folds are seen that are accentuated by the presence of the tape. These folds cause decompressive stimulation.

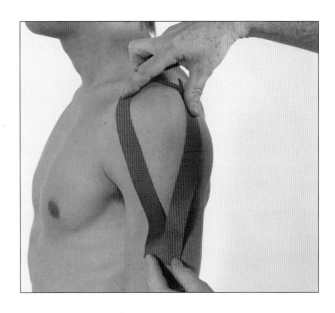

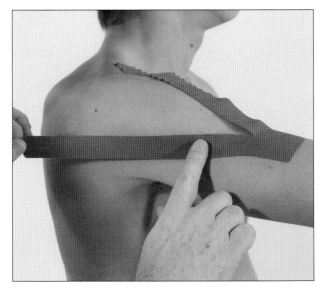

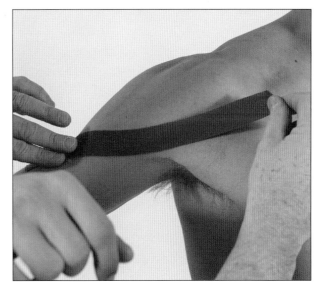

NOTE: All muscle applications described in this manual from Chapter 4 onwards are performed using the decompressive technique.

Compressive Technique

With this technique, the tape is applied to skin during slight isometric contraction of the underlying muscle.

The tension of the tape can range from zero to 25%. In general, tension is applied when treating muscles with a long belly (e.g., the biceps brachii).

Working on the deltoid again, but this time using the compressive technique, the muscle must be contracted in order to shorten the skin.

The tape anchor, which is placed in a neutral position, must be distal to the muscle insertion. One strip of the tape is applied with 0% tension over the anterior fibers of the deltoid and the other over the posterior fibers. The tail ends of the tape end at the origin of the muscle.

During muscle flexion and extension, note the absence of folds in the skin and the tautness of the tape. It is the taut and compact tape that produces the compression stimulus.

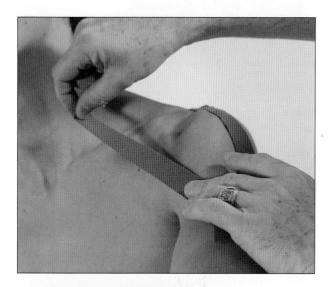

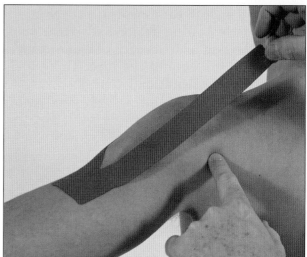

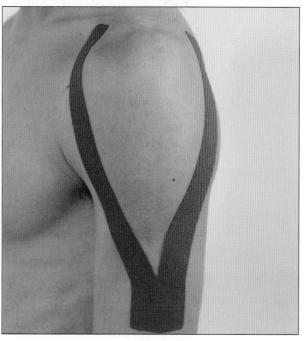

NOTE: The compressive technique should not be used on muscles around the neck that have a connection with the spinal column, such as the trapezius muscles and the spinal muscles.

Decompressive and Compressive Techniques

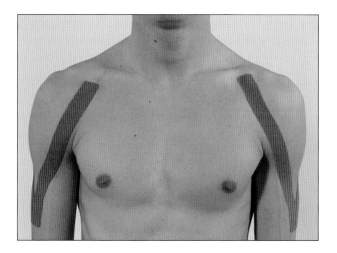

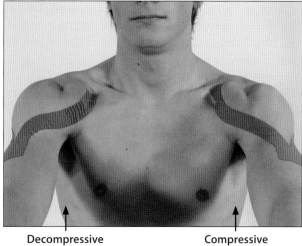

Decompressive   Compressive

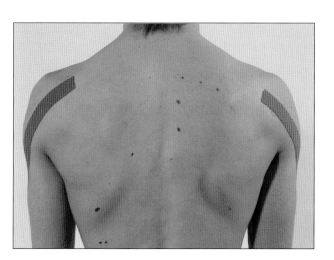

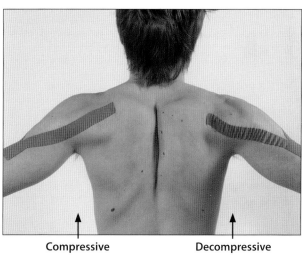

Compressive   Decompressive

BASIC CONCEPTS OF THE CORRECTION TECHNIQUE

Using NeuroMuscular Taping, with either the decompressive or the compressive method, the elasticity of the tape can be exploited to attain different types of stimulation in order to achieve different correction objectives.

The main areas of intervention are:
1. Muscular
2. Ligament/tendon
3. Joint decompression
4. Joint compression
5. Lymphatic
6. To create decompression
7. Functional

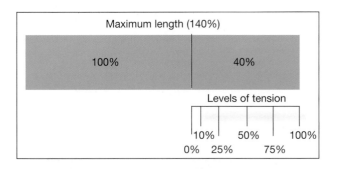

Table 3.1 Tape tension

Tension	Percentage (%)
No tension	0
Very slight	10-15
Slight	25
Moderate	50
Strong	75
Maximum (never used)	100

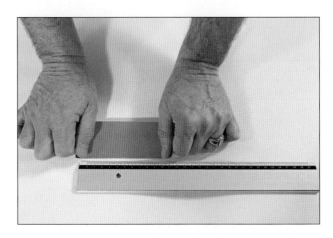

0% tape tension.

Table 3.2 Tension applied to tape by correction technique

Type of correction	Percentage (%)
Muscular	0-25
Ligament/tendon	25-50-75
Joint decompression	0
Joint compression	50
Lymphatic	0
To create decompression	0-25
Functional	0-25

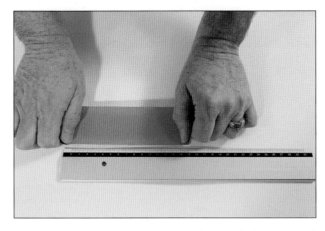

Maximum extension is to 40% beyond the original length.

MUSCLES

The muscles of the musculoskeletal system consist of striated skeletal muscle tissue, which is also found in some organs of the digestive and respiratory systems (tongue, soft palate, pharynx, larynx, esophagus, and rectum). The skeletal muscles, which number around 370, are organs made up of bundles of (voluntary) striated muscle fibers supported and held together by loose connective tissue that is rich in blood vessels and nerve ramifications. Every muscle is attached to a bone or another muscle by means of tendons and aponeuroses, formed by bundles of collagen connective tissue and elastic fibers. These arise in turn from the muscle connective tissue support structure and extend beyond the muscle. Muscles have various shapes; they may be elongated and fusiform, with one or more bellies, flattened and laminar, ribbon-like or circular (sphincter muscles). Muscles sometimes have two or more muscle bellies. Examples of this include the biceps brachii, the triceps brachii, and the quadriceps femoris muscles, which have a tendon of origin at one end and, two, three, or four tendons of insertion at the other. In other cases, the tendon runs through the muscle, with the short muscle fibers arranged obliquely to it, like the barbs of a feather. These muscles are accordingly termed pennate muscles.

The voluntary muscles also include, in the face and neck, the mimic muscles, which are connected, at least on one end, to the dermis and move the skin of the face, enabling facial expression (mimic movements).

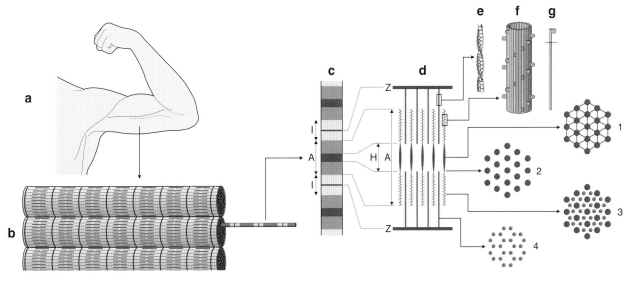

Figure 3.13 Diagram of the organization of skeletal muscle at the macroscopic (the muscle), microscopic (fiber cells, with their characteristic cross-striation), and submicroscopic levels (myofibril, formed by two types of myofilaments): **a**) triceps brachii, **b**) striated muscle fibers, **c**) myofibril, **d**) structure of the sarcomere. The positions of the A and I bands, the H zone, and the Z lines are shown, as are the arrangements of the thick and thin myofilaments. **e**) Magnification of a thin filament showing the structure of the actin molecule. **f**) Structure of a thick filament. **g**) Myosin molecule. The dotted line indicates the site of cleavage following treatment with trypsin. The part in beige is the light meromyosin, the part in gray is the connecting segment, and the part in blue is the myosin head. The connecting segment and the head form the heavy meromyosin. **1-4**) Cross-sections of the sarcomere showing the arrangement of the myofilaments at the level of the M line and the site of anchorage of the thick filaments (**1**), the H zone, which contains only thick filaments (**2**), the A band, where the thick and thin filaments interdigitate (**3**), and the I band, which contains only thin filaments (**4**).

The structure of muscle

Striated skeletal muscle tissue is composed of supracellular elements resulting from the fusion of multiple primary cells and from mitosis not followed by separation of the daughter cells. For this reason, each of these elements has many nuclei located beneath the plasma membrane or sarcolemma. Known as muscle fibers, these are cylindrical in shape, with a diameter

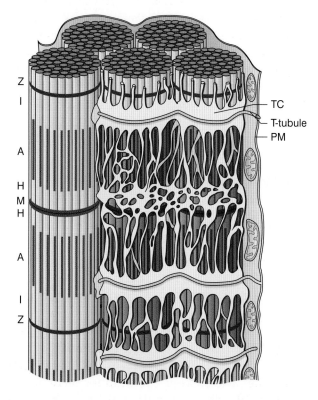

Figure 3.14 Three-dimensional schematic representation of the sarcoplasmic reticulum of a striated skeletal muscle fiber (mammal). The reticulum surrounding each myofibril is made up of longitudinal tubules that anastomose at the level of the H band of the sarcomere and dilate, at the junction between the I and A bands, into terminal cisternae (TCs). Between each pair of TCs is a T-tubule (T). The T and the two TCs form a triad. T-tubules are invaginations of the plasma membrane (PM).

of 10 to 100 µm and are as long as the muscle itself (ranging in length from a few millimeters to over 30 cm) (Fig. 3.13).

Muscle fibers have abundant smooth endoplasmic reticulum (sarcoplasmic reticulum), formed in part by canaliculi, which are invaginations of the sarcolemma and in part by cisternae (Fig. 3.14). The cytoplasm (sarcoplasm) contains molecules of contractile proteins organized into filaments (*myofilaments*), which in turn form bundles of *myofibrils*, all oriented parallel to the longitudinal axis of the fibers themselves. The contractile proteins are myosin, organized into thick myofilaments, and actin, troponin, and tropomyosin, organized into thin filaments. The myofibrils show a characteristic regular geometric arrangement, giving this tissue its typical striated appearance with alternating dark and light bands.

In skeletal muscle, a fine sheath of fibrillar connective tissue called the *endomysium* surrounds each fiber. Muscle fibers are grouped into bundles or fascicles, each of which is also surrounded by a thin layer of connective tissue, the *perimysium*. Finally, a denser external connective tissue layer called the *epimysium* surrounds the entire muscle. Running through the connective tissue that forms the muscle supporting structure are nerves and blood vessels that provide nourishment to the muscle fibers. The organization of the fibers making up the connective tissue allows reciprocal sliding of the muscle fascicles and, when required, their partial and independent contraction.

The body or belly of the muscle is richly vascularized, flexible and expandable up to a certain limit. Beyond this limit it offers considerable resistance to traction. Even in the resting state, muscle fibers maintain a basal level of contraction, called *muscle tone*, which keeps the muscle ready to be activated (i.e., to contract) in response to the arrival of a nerve impulse.

On the basis of their structural, ultrastructural, and biochemical properties, muscle fibers are divided into three basic types.

The *red fibers* are also known as *type I slow*

fibers or *slow oxidation* (SO) *fibers*. They are red because they are rich in the oxygen-binding protein myoglobin and contain many mitochondria and a dense network of capillary vessels. They are resistant to fatigue, which is why they are abundant in the muscles involved in maintaining posture. These fibers primarily utilize oxidative metabolism.

The white fibers (with low myoglobin content) are also known as *fast (type IIb)* or *fast-twitch glycolytic (FTG) fibers*. These have a glycolytic metabolism, which means that they use the anaerobic splitting of glycogen to produce the energy they need. During contraction, they acquire an oxygen deficit and as a result, they cannot work for long and are susceptible to fatigue.

The intermediate fibers are also called *fast (type IIa) fibers* or *fast-twitch oxidative (FTO) fibers*. These have characteristics intermediate between those of the other two types. They are resistant to fatigue but are able to produce greater levels of force than slow fibers.

Each muscle usually contains all three types of fibers, but in varying proportions. Slow fibers normally occupy the innermost part of the muscle, which is more extensively vascularized, whereas fast fibers, not resistant to fatigue, occupy the more superficial regions, being less richly vascularized. For example, postural muscles, such as the soleus, are principally (80–90%) made up of slow fibers, while oculomotor muscles (extrinsic muscles of the eyeball) and calf muscles used for walking are made up almost entirely of fast fibers. The vastus lateralis of the thigh is relatively rich in intermediate fibers.

Tendons and aponeuroses

Voluntary (or skeletal) muscles are inserted onto bones by means of *tendons*. If the muscles are flat or wide, they are attached to bones, and to each other, by means of *aponeuroses*. Tendons and aponeuroses are highly resistant structures formed of dense fibrillar connective tissue arranged in parallel bundles. These are cords, or laminae, of collagen fibers that are oriented in the direction of the muscle fibers with little amorphous extracellular matrix. They also contain elastic fibers, which enable slight elongation of the tendon, necessary to distribute tension in the event of sudden and rapid contraction of the muscle; these elastic fibers also serve to restore the tendon to its original length after the end of the stimulus. The *muscle-tendon junction* is the zone at the end of the muscle where muscle connective tissue (endomysium, perimysium and epimysium), responsible for ensuring muscle tissue support and trophism, continues beyond the ends of the muscle fibers to become a tendon (or aponeurosis). Tendons and aponeuroses are not attached to the surface of the bone, but are directly continuous with the connective tissue fibers of the periosteum.

Motor unit

Every muscle fiber is innervated by just one motor neuron, while a single motor neuron can innervate a number of muscle fibers. A set of muscle fibers innervated by the same motor neuron, and therefore contracting at the same time in response to an impulse conveyed along the axon of that neuron, is termed a *motor unit* (Fig. 3.15). The motor unit is the smallest functional muscle unit. The lower its innervation ratio (i.e., the smaller the number of fibers innervated by the motor neuron), the better the muscle is able to progressively and accurately gradate its workload. If a motor neuron innervates two thousand muscle fibers, as in the case with a large muscle such as the quadriceps femoris or an extensive one like the latissimus dorsi, the degree of refinement of the muscle activity will be minimal. But if the motor neuron innervates only a dozen or so muscle fibers, as in the case of the small muscles that move the eyeball or the fingers, the muscle will work in a

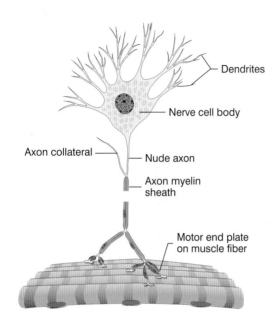

- Dendrites
- Nerve cell body
- Axon collateral
- Nude axon
- Axon myelin sheath
- Motor end plate on muscle fiber

Figure 3.15 Diagram of a motor unit. From the top down are shown the motor neuron body, the axon (or axis cylinder), and the furcation of the motor fiber, which forms synapses at the motor end plates of all the muscle fibers it innervates.

much more refined and precise way. Generally, a motor unit is proportional to muscle volume, meaning small muscles generate precise, fine motor movements while large ones are used to generate force.

Motor units typically comprise fibers with similar structural and biochemical properties, so the same muscle can contain, albeit in different proportions, fast motor units susceptible to fatigue, fast fatigue-resistant motor units, and slow fatigue-resistant motor units.

Motor units are influenced by the intensity of the signal traveling along the motor pathways, which are the bundles of axons that, in the CNS, carry motor commands from the telencephalon to the motor neurons of the brainstem and spinal cord. There are two motor pathways, the *pyramidal*, which begins in the telencephalon and descends without interruption to the motor neurons, and the *extrapyrami-*

dal pathway, which also begins in the telencephalon, but has intermediate stations along its course, some of which are under the control of the cerebellum.

Muscle work

A fundamental principle of muscle work is that muscles work when they contract (which does not necessarily mean that they shorten). The force thereby generated depends on the number, length, and orientation of a muscle's fibers.

In long muscles, the action of the muscle usually involves shortening, associated with tensile strength. Longitudinally oriented fibers provide a muscle with high-speed execution but little strength or resistance. Muscles with obliquely oriented fibers, on the other hand, perform limited movements. However, because these contain a large number of short fibers, they are able to generate considerable and prolonged force over their limited range of movement.

Muscles may be divided according to their function into flexors and extensors, adductors and abductors, pronators and supinators, and internal and external rotators, although these definitions actually refer to the movements accomplished. A muscle can furthermore be classified as agonist or antagonist depending on whether it promotes or opposes a particular movement. Muscles hardly ever work alone. To perform a movement, even a simple one, several agonist muscles are generally recruited simultaneously.

Muscle work is calculated as the resultant of weight lifted, or moved, and the extent of its movement in space. The unit of measurement is the kilogram-meter (kg-m). For example, the muscle work required to lift a 5 kg weight a distance of 2 m is 10 kg-m. Any task performed by a muscle entails energy expenditure, expressed in terms of oxygen consumption (ml/min) and also the consumption of glucose, or other metabolic substances needed for contraction, which are transported to the muscle tissue by blood. The oxygen consumption of a healthy adult at rest is 250 ml/minute, increasing with the amount of effort expended. With moderate exertion, the level of oxygen consumption increases up to threefold, and with heavy exertion, it can reach as much as four to eight times the at-rest level.

Muscle work (or contraction) is divided into isotonic (dynamic) and isometric (static). *Isotonic* or *dynamic contraction* results in shortening of the muscle, that is, a reduction of the distance between the origin and the insertion of the muscle. *Isometric* or *static work* does not involve muscle shortening but an increase of muscle tone.

JOINTS

Joints are categorized both by their morphology and according to their functional characteristics. They are divided into two groups:
- *Synarthroses* or *coarticulations*, which do not allow any movement or allow only very limited movement
- *Diarthroses* or *synovial joints*, which allow more or less extensive movement of the two bones forming the joint

Synarthroses have little relevance to the purposes of this text. They are therefore described only briefly for the sake of completeness.

Synarthroses are joints in which two or more bones are fixed firmly together by means of connective tissue. In *syndesmoses* (e.g., the sutures of the skull), the bony elements are united by fibrous connective tissue. In *synchondroses* (e.g., between the first rib and sternum), the connecting tissue is hyaline cartilage. In *symphyses*, connection is made with fibrous cartilage. Examples of symphyses include the fusion between the two bones of the pubis and the intervertebral discs and fusion between the vertebral bodies. In the latter case, the movements of the spine are due to the particular structure of the discs and the summation of all the small movements allowable between one vertebra and another.

Diarthroses are joints that enable movements that are more or less extensive, as the two or more articulating bones are not in contact with one another. To keep them close but not touching, the articular bone ends are held together by a fibrous sleeve, or *joint capsule*, containing *synovial fluid*, which has a lubricating and trophic function. The articular surfaces, again covered with hyaline cartilage, may be concave, convex, flat, or shaped like a pulley, with one surface having a concave shape and the other a complementary convex one. Diarthroses, or synovial joints, are classified according to the shape of the articular surfaces, which determine the type and range of motion they enable.

When the two articular surfaces are not perfectly complementary, there may be one or more discs of fibrous cartilage, called *menisci*, between them. The menisci of the knee, between the femur and tibia, are particularly well known. In other synovial joints, when one of the surfaces is not sufficiently concave, the articular surface is completed by a *labrum* or ring in order to ensure a good joint fit. This is seen, for example, in the articulation of the scapula and the humerus (the shoulder joint or glenohumeral joint).

The joint capsule is a fibrous sleeve that surrounds the two articular heads and is fixed at a certain distance from the articular surfaces directly on the periosteum of the bones. The capsule forms a joint cavity containing synovial fluid. This serves as a lubricant, facilitates sliding (without rubbing) of the articular surfaces and also has a trophic effect on the articular cartilage.

Synovial fluid is a clear, colorless, plasma-derived viscous fluid, rich in protein and hyaluronic acid. This fluid is constantly renewed by the *synovial membrane* that lines the inside of the joint capsule. The joint heads are lubricated by synovial fluid in different ways. When the joint is at rest or subjected to a light load, hydrostatic or hydrodynamic lubrication occurs. With increasing loads, the type of lubrication changes, becoming elastodynamic, hydrostatic, and self-pressurized.

Apart from the distinction between articular head shapes, diarthroses can also be characterized on the basis of the number of axes around which movement is allowed. This gives rise to the following categories:

- *Uniaxial diarthroses* are characterized by movement around a single axis, as in the case of hinge (ginglymus) joints (elbow joint, between the humerus and the radius), pivot joints (elbow and wrist joints, between the radius and the ulna), and double condyles (knee joint, between the femur and the tibia).
- *Biaxial diarthroses* are characterized by movement around two mutually orthogonal axes.

They have two degrees of motion, one greater and one lesser, as in the condyles (e.g., the wrist joint, between the radius and ulna and the hand).

- *Triaxial diarthroses* are characterized by movement around three mutually orthogonal axes, having three degrees of motion. They are highly mobile ball-and-socket joints (enarthrosis) that include the shoulder joint between the scapula and humerus, and the hip (coxofermoral) joint between the hip and the femur.

Accessory organs such as ligaments (bands of fibrous connective tissue) are important elements in highly mobile joints. Ligaments, which contain more elastic fibers than tendons do, help to keep the bones together and, being well supplied with proprioceptors, warn of danger situations, such as when the joint is being subjected to excessive or inappropriate stress.

MUSCLE CORRECTION TECHNIQUE

Muscle correction technique, in both its compressive and decompressive forms, has a number of different applications. It can be used to restore correct muscle tension, facilitate muscle extension and normalize elasticity and muscle tone; it can reduce muscle fatigue, correct joint alignment, increase muscle contraction, or reduce excessive relaxation of a muscle (Fig. 3.16).

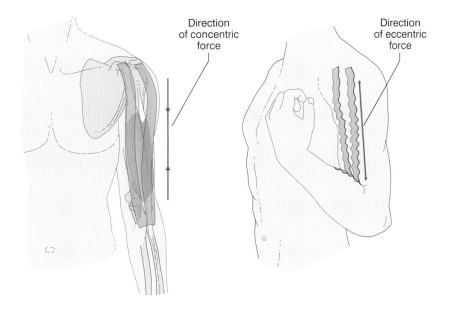

Direction of concentric force

Direction of eccentric force

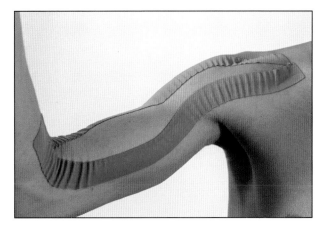

Figure 3.16 An application of the decompressive muscle correction technique (biceps brachii): when the patient flexes the elbow, the folds that form in the tape and skin generate an eccentric (lengthening) stimulus.

NOTE: For different muscle applications, see later chapters.

LIGAMENT AND TENDON CORRECTION TECHNIQUE

This technique is used to deliver either a compressive or decompressive stimulus over the path of a tendon or ligament in order to provide support. When using the compressive technique, the tape is applied over the ligament or tendon with moderate to strong tension (25-50-75%). Maximum tension (100%) must not be applied, as the excessive stimulus would impede movement and reduce the joint's range of motion and the coordination of muscle, tendon, and joint movements.

With the decompressive technique, the tape is applied without tension over the course of the tendon, with the tendon stretched.

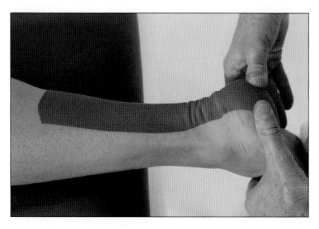

Compressive application.

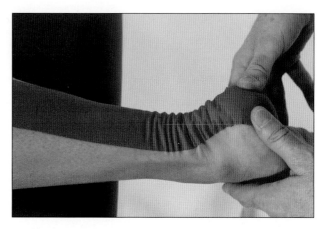

Decompressive application.

Application - Achilles Tendon

Compressive technique

TAPE SPECIFICATIONS

- 1 tape
- Width 5 cm (2")
- Length 20-25 cm (8-10")
- I-shaped

CLINICAL APPLICATIONS

- For motor activity, to increase the explosiveness of movement

TAPE APPLICATION

1. Apply the base anchor (5 cm long) to the heel, keeping the foot aligned with the leg and at right angles to it.

2. With tension applied (25–50–75%), position the tape over the calcaneal (Achilles) tendon as far as its insertion.

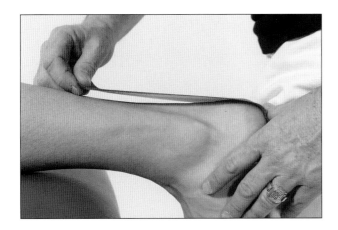
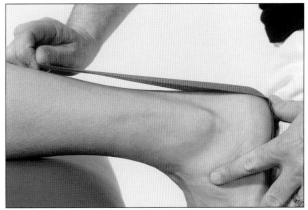
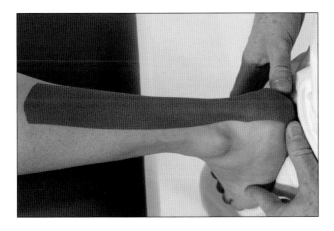
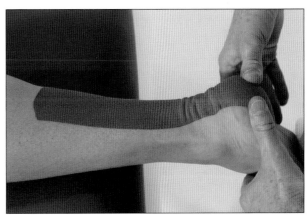

Application - Achilles Tendon

Decompressive technique

TAPE SPECIFICATIONS

- 1 tape
- Width 5 cm (2")
- Length 25-30 cm (10-12")
- I-shaped

CLINICAL APPLICATIONS

- Paratenonitis
- Improve Achilles tendon elasticity
- Achilles tendinosis

TAPE APPLICATION

1. Apply the base anchor (5 cm long) to the heel, keeping the foot aligned with the leg and at right angles to it.

2. With the foot dorsiflexed, apply the tape, without tension, over the Achilles tendon as far as its insertion.

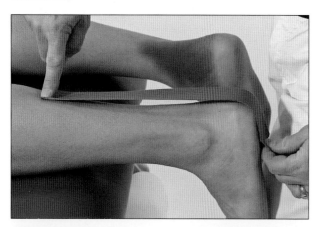
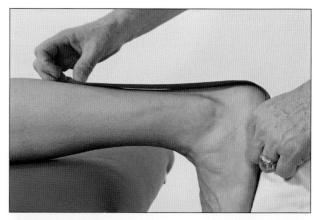
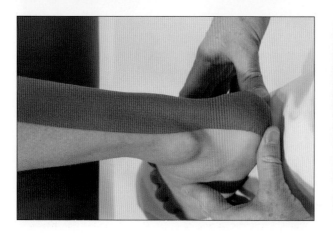
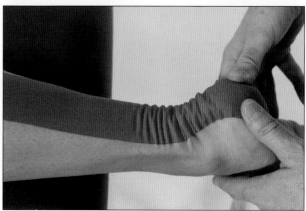

Application - Tibial Collateral Ligament (Medial)

TAPE SPECIFICATIONS

- 1 tape
- Width 2.5 cm (1")
- Length 25 cm (10")
- I-shaped

CLINICAL APPLICATIONS

- Medial collateral ligament injury
- Postsurgical knee rehabilitation
- Lateral (peripheral) knee stabilization

TAPE APPLICATION

1. The patient stands with knee extended and weight evenly distributed on both feet.

2. Starting with a lower base anchor, apply the tape with 25–50% tension over the course of the tibial collateral ligament.

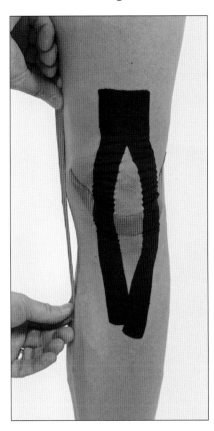 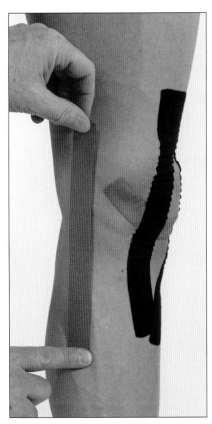 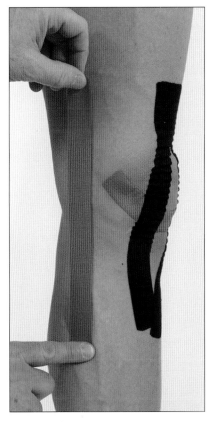

NOTE: The photographs refer to taping of the tibial collateral ligament as part of a functional knee application.

With this technique, as with the previous one, the folds that are formed on the tape and skin produce decompression of the tissue and as a result increase the space between the skin and underlying bone (Figs. 3.17–3.19).

Unlike the previous case, however, here the target of the application is a joint and not a specific painful point.

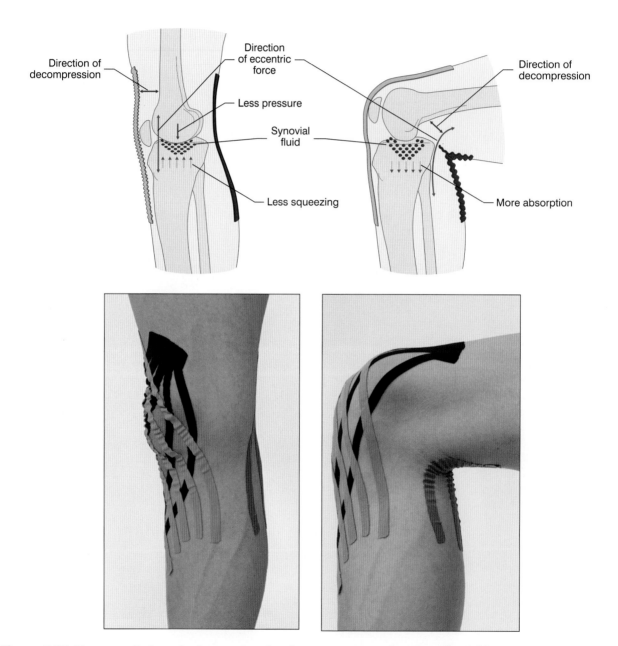

Figure 3.17 Tapes applied to the knee using the decompressive technique. The folds generate an eccentric (lengthening) and a decompressive stimulus simultaneously; this increases the spaces between the skin and the underlying bone surface and affected joint itself. The alternation of tape folding and tape stretching caused by the patient's movements also facilitates extraction and absorption of synovial fluid by the joint cartilage.

Decompressive Joint Correction Technique

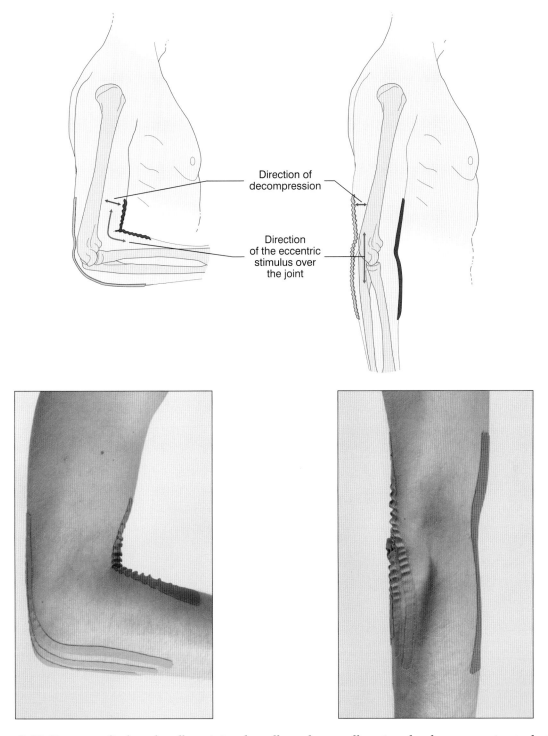

Direction of decompression

Direction of the eccentric stimulus over the joint

Figure 3.18 Tapes applied to the elbow joint dorsally and ventrally using the decompressive technique.

Decompressive Joint Correction Technique

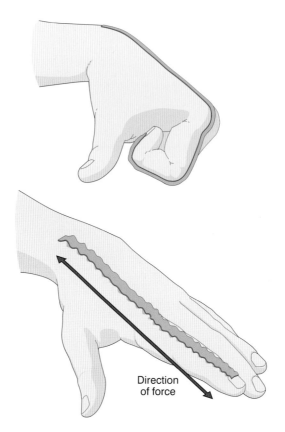

Direction of force

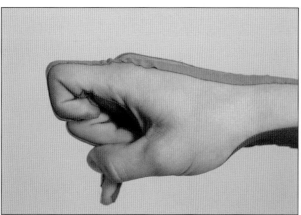
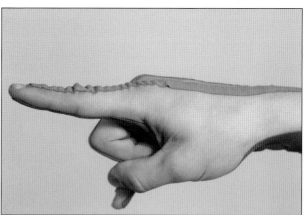

Figure 3.19 Decompressive tapes applied to the carpometacarpal, metacarpophalangeal, and interphalangeal joints of the index finger.

NOTE: Because of its powerful capacity to create space and decompression, this technique is indicated in acute and functional phases, but is contraindicated during sporting activity, as it may increase joint instability.

Application - Elbow Joint

TAPE SPECIFICATIONS

- 1 tape
- Width 5 cm (2")
- Length 25 cm (10")
- Fan-shaped with five strips

CLINICAL APPLICATIONS

- Scars such as those resulting from surgically treated fractures
- Epicondylitis with generalized pain

TAPE APPLICATION

1. The patient's elbow is flexed and the hand is turned towards the shoulder.

2. Apply the strips of tape close together and without tension, starting from the triceps brachii.

3. Folds appear on the skin when the elbow is extended.

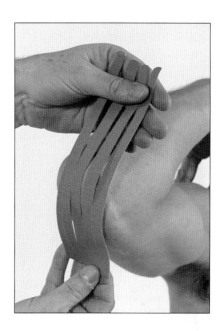

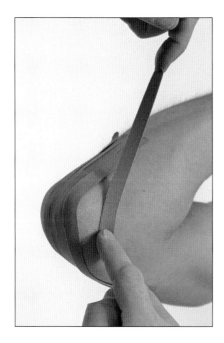

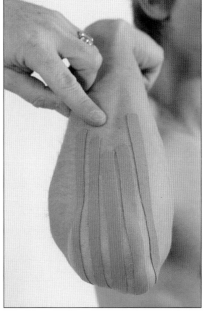

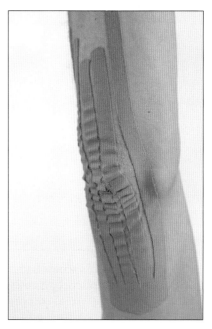

Application - Shoulder Joint

TAPE SPECIFICATIONS

- 2 tapes
- Width 5 cm (2")
- Length 25 cm (10")
- Fan-shaped with five strips

CLINICAL APPLICATIONS

- Symptomatic joint stiffness
- Subacromial/deltoid bursitis
- Post-surgical shoulder
- Primary and secondary adhesive capsulitis

TAPE APPLICATION

1. The anterior fan is applied with the patient's arm held extended and abducted at 90°. The base anchor is positioned below the clavicle and the three lower tape tails are applied over the shoulder and along the biceps brachii. The patient then lowers the arm to 45° abduction and the therapist applies the two upper strips of tape.

2. The posterior fan is applied with the patient's arm forward flexed to 90°. Position the anchor below the scapular spine and proceed with the application on the posterior aspect of the arm following the same procedure as for the anterior fan.

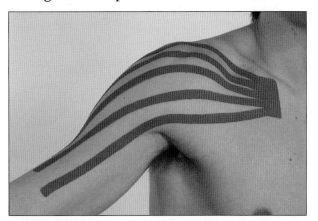
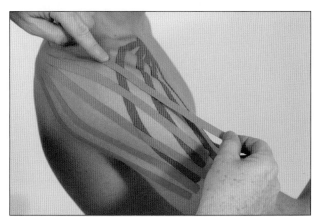
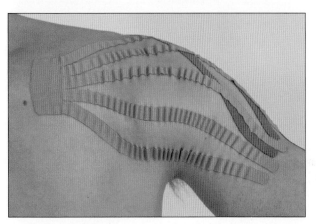
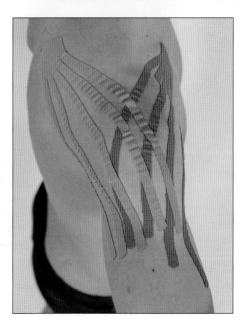

NOTE: If joint movement improves, the tape should be reapplied to prevent the existing tape from giving rise to compression.

Application - Knee Joint

TAPE SPECIFICATIONS

- 2 tapes
- Width 5 cm (2")
- Length 30 cm (12")
- Fan-shaped with five strips

CLINICAL APPLICATIONS

- Gonarthrosis
- Rheumatoid arthritis
- Post-surgical rehabilitation

TAPE APPLICATION

1. Apply the base of the first fan 1 cm laterally to the center-line of the quadriceps femoris, so that the middle of the central strip of tape will lie over the center of the patella, or knee-cap.

2. Wrap the lateral strip, without tension, around the anterolateral aspect of the knee before taking it down vertically. Apply the next strip around the lateral margin of the patella.

3. Apply the medial strip, without tension, over the anteromedial aspect of the knee and then downward vertically. Apply the next strip around the medial margin of the patella.

4. Finally, the central strip is applied over the center of the patella.

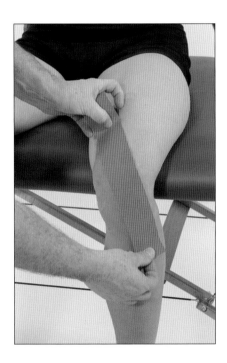
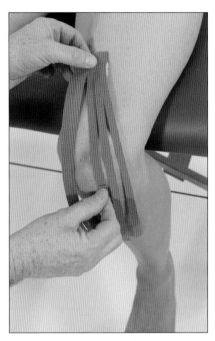
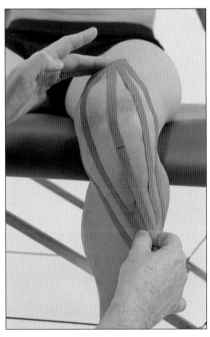
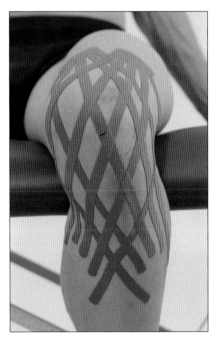

JOINT CORRECTION TECHNIQUE: COMPRESSIVE METHOD

Use the tape's stretching capacity on the surface of the skin to provide a joint-positioning stimulus.

The degree of stimulus is determined by traction and the amount of tension applied to the tape.

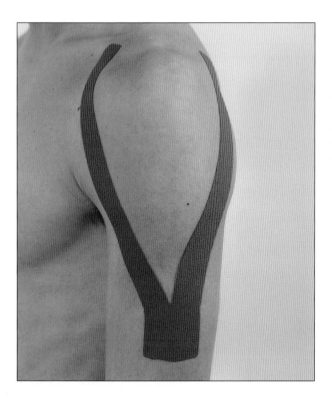

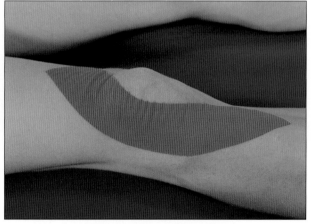

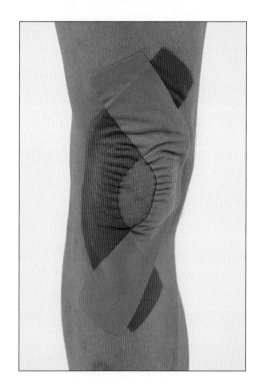

NOTE: In joint correction, a tape tension of 50% is used.

I-Shaped Application - Dynamic

Patella axis correction

TAPE SPECIFICATIONS

- 1 tape
- Width 5 cm (2")
- Length 25-30 cm (10-12")
- I-shaped

CLINICAL APPLICATIONS

- Lateral patellar instability

TAPE APPLICATION

1. Remove the paper in the middle of the tape and apply a third of its width over the patella.

2. With the patient flexing the knee to 90°, apply the tape in a half-moon shape at 50% tension.

3. Extension of the leg causes wrinkles to appear, while flexing it increases the degree of compression in the lateromedial direction.

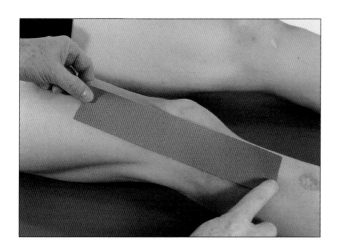
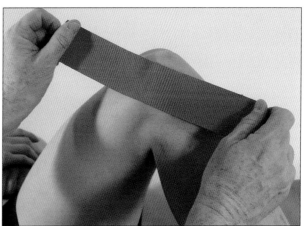
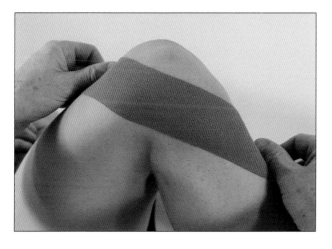
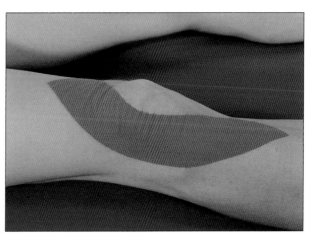

I-Shaped Application - Combined Dynamic

Patella axis stablization

TAPE SPECIFICATIONS

- 2 tapes
- Width 5 cm (2")
- Length 25-30 cm (10-12")
- I-shaped

CLINICAL APPLICATIONS

- Patellar instability

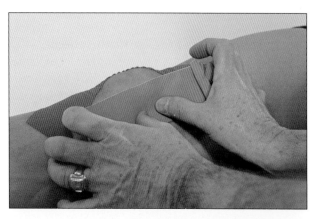

TAPE APPLICATION

1. The first half moon is applied following the same procedure as for patella axis correction; the second is then applied in the same way.

2. These two half moons, one internal and the other external, globally stabilize the patella. The two tapes run over the lateral and medial margins of the patella.

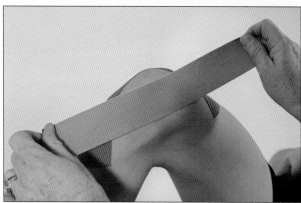

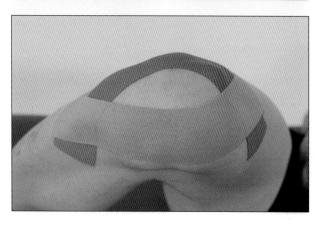

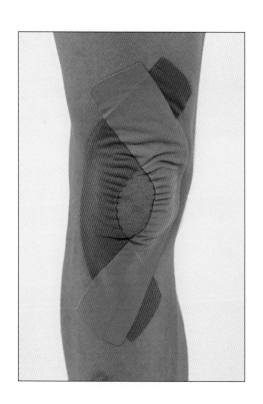

I-Shaped Application - Static

Lifting stabilization of the head of the humerus

TAPE SPECIFICATIONS

- 2 tapes
- Width 5 cm (2")
- Length 20-25 cm (8-10")
- I-shaped

CLINICAL APPLICATIONS

- Post-traumatic shoulder instability

TAPE APPLICATION

1. Stabilize the shoulder by placing the patient in a neutral position with the arm along the patient's side and the elbow flexed. Starting at the middle of a length of tape, remove the backing paper as far as 1 cm from each end. Then position the tape with the midpoint over the acromion and, with 50% tension, draw it downwards and apply it anteriorly and posteriorly. Apply the two ends without tension.

2. Also apply the second tape with 50% tension. Place the midpoint below the head of the humerus and then apply the tape in such a way as to impart a transverse and upward direction to the fibers of the deltoid. Apply the ends without tension.

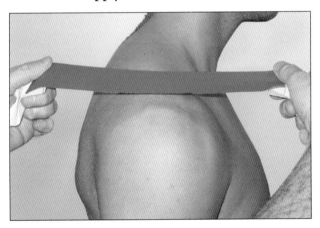
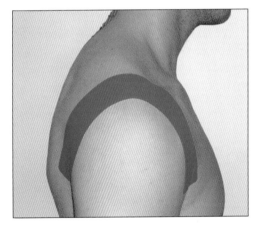

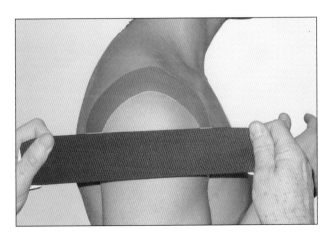
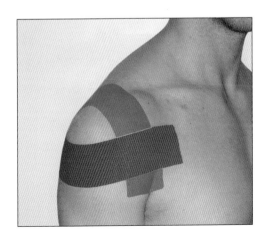

Y-Shaped Application - Static (Pulled Technique)

Patella and knee joint axis correction

TAPE SPECIFICATIONS

- 1 tape
- Width 5 cm (2")
- Length 25 cm (10")
- Anchor 5 cm (2")
- Y-shaped

CLINICAL APPLICATIONS

- Correction of the patellofemoral joint axis

TAPE APPLICATION

1. Position the base of the tape laterally or medially to the patella (laterally in the case of medial patellar instability associated with varus knee, medially if the instability is lateral and associated with valgus knee). Position the tail of the tape on the posterior margin of the tibial or fibular collateral ligament without extending it to the back of the knee (popliteal area).

2. After removing the backing paper, place the tape on the patella.

3. With one hand, hold the base of the tape firmly and push the patella in the direction of the base of the Y. With the other hand, apply the tape strips with 50% tension around the upper and lower margins of the patella. The two tails should converge towards the opposite side of the knee, but not overlap.

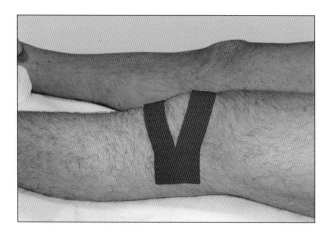
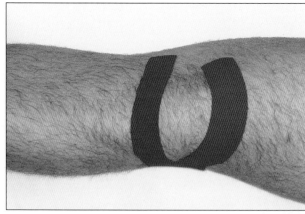

Y-Shaped Application - Static

Shoulder positioned forwards

TAPE SPECIFICATIONS

- 1 tape
- Width 5 cm (2")
- Length 20 cm (8")
- Y-shaped

TAPE APPLICATION

1. The patient holds the arm abducted and externally rotated. Once the base anchor has been positioned at the center of the scapula, apply the tape with 50% tension and fix it frontally.

Correction with the deltoid contracted

1. The patient contracts the muscle to impart greater stability. Position the tape, without tension, over the anterior fibers (clavicular section) with the arm slightly flexed, and over the posterior fibers (spinal section) with the arm slightly extended.

CLINICAL APPLICATIONS

- Correction of the axis of the shoulder in external rotation

NOTE: To be used during physical activity to lend stability to the shoulder in external rotation.

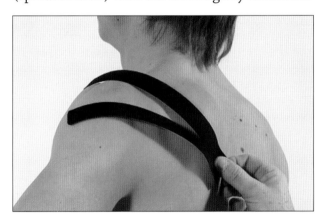
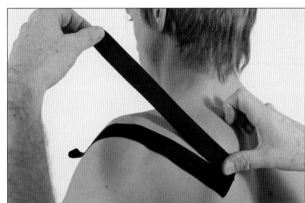
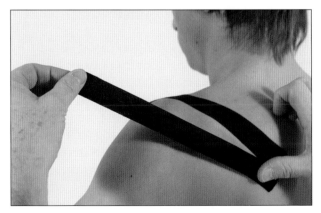
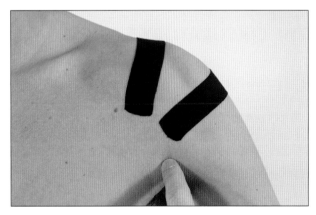

For a more detailed description of the application ➡ page 337

LYMPHATIC TAPING

When a tape is applied using the decompressive method over congested areas and in line with lymphatic pathways, it will normalize hydrostatic and osmotic pressure. A suitable dress of pressure on blood and lymphatic vessels favors blood circulation and lymphatic drainage. By lifting the skin, the tape increases the size of interstitial spaces, promotes improved circulation and fluid absorption, and reduces subcutaneous pressure. The tape continues to promote drainage over the entire period of application. To ensure optimal treatment of lymphatic edema, manual lymphatic drainage may be performed before tape application, or normal lymphatic drainage may be carried out over the tape.

The technique used will depend on the clinical picture. It is possible to treat:
- Edema with good lymph node function
- Edema with inadequate lymph node function
- Scar tissue
- Post-surgical edema and cicatrizing tissue
- Post-traumatic edema.

> NOTE: For lymphatic correction, the tape is cut in a fan shape and applied with 0% tension.

THE CIRCULATORY SYSTEM

The circulatory system is a complex system of channels – the *blood vessels* – carrying blood, which performs numerous functions that may be summarized as follows:
- Transportation of oxygen, nutrients and hormones and their distribution throughout the organism
- Removal of the products of cell catabolism, such as carbon dioxide and lactic acid
- Maintenance of constant body temperature
- Maintenance of homeostasis of body fluids

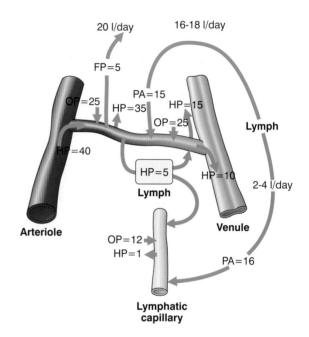

Figure 3.20 Diagram of the exchanges that take place at the level of the capillaries between the blood and the interstitial lymph as a result of the play of the hydrostatic pressure of the liquid (**HP**) and the osmotic pressure of the proteins (**OP**). The values are expressed in mmHg. **FP**: Filtration pressure. **PA**: Pressure of absorption.

- Contribution to immune processes through transporting phagocytic cells (granulocytes), immunocompetent cells (lymphocytes), and antibodies

Blood is kept circulating in blood vessels by the ceaseless pumping activity of the heart. Situated in the thorax, the heart is a hollow muscular organ that is divided into two non-communicating halves, right and left, and connected with the periphery (everything that lies outside of the heart itself) by means of arteries and veins. The vessels carrying blood away from the heart are called arteries, while those carrying blood to the heart are called veins. Blood rich in O_2 is termed *arterial blood* whereas blood rich in CO_2 is called *venous blood*.

Blood vessels are thinner the further away

they are from the heart. The vessels connecting arteries and veins are called *capillaries*.

Arterial blood is pumped from the left side of the heart into the aorta, which, through its branches, distributes it to all the organs. In the interstitial spaces of connective tissue between the organs, arteries become capillaries and release O_2 and metabolites into the extracellular matrix (interstitial lymph fluid). Here, the arterial blood, picking up CO_2 and catabolites, becomes venous blood and passes into the venous capillaries and then into the veins, which return it to the right side of the heart. From here, the venous blood is driven through the pulmonary arteries to the lungs, where the CO_2 is exchanged for O_2. The oxygen-enriched blood is then returned to the left side of the heart, which sends it to the organs via the aorta.

Because of the thickness of their walls, arteries and veins are impermeable; they serve only to transport blood. Capillaries originate at the ends of the small arteries (arterioles). Capillaries have a small diameter (10 µm on average) and extremely thin walls (0.5 µm on average). These thin walls, almost exclusively made up of endothelium, are permeable to the passage of O_2, CO_2, water, mineral salts and organic substances in both directions (Fig. 3.20). These exchanges occur in the interstitial spaces and in the lungs. The physical and chemical composition of the blood is thus altered during these exchanges.

The capillaries form extensive networks throughout the body. They give rise to venules which, converging, form increasingly large veins, which return the blood to the heart. In

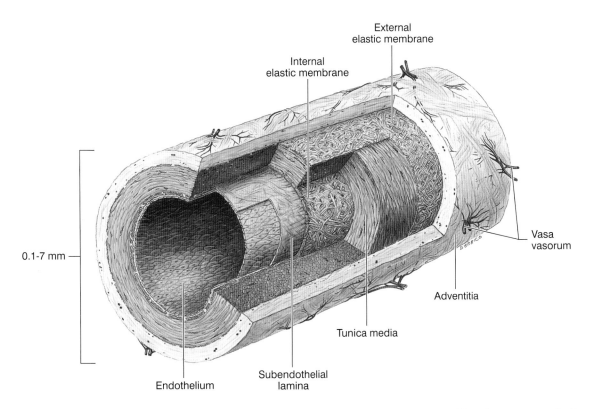

External elastic membrane

Internal elastic membrane

0.1-7 mm

Vasa vasorum

Adventitia

Tunica media

Subendothelial lamina

Endothelium

Figure 3.21 Three-dimensional representation of a muscular artery. The vessel has been cut in different planes to show its structural organization. **Light pink** represents the endothelium; **blue** represents the elastic membranes, internal and external; **dark pink** represents the muscle cells of the tunica media and **gray** represents the adventitial connective tissue.

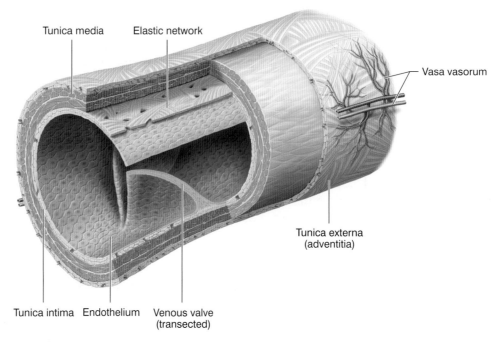

Tunica media   Elastic network

Vasa vasorum

Tunica externa
(adventitia)

Tunica intima   Endothelium   Venous valve
(transected)

Figure 3.22 Structure of a **propulsive vein**. The tunica media of propulsive veins is formed by smooth muscle. This structure allows the vein to contract and facilitate the distal propulsion of the blood.

the connective tissue, cells present in the blood may, if necessary, pass from the blood to the surrounding connective tissue, thereby opening a path between two neighboring endothelial cells. This is precisely what white blood cells, especially lymphocytes, do. These immune cells escape from the capillaries in order to move to the sites where they are needed to fight the microorganisms that constantly assail us.

The structure and diameter of capillaries may change depending on functional requirements. When at rest or when functional activity is minimal, many capillaries constrict to reduce or prevent the passage of blood. In fact, it is estimated that only 25% of the capillary network works constantly. When the functional requirements of an organ increase, its capillaries are re-opened and blood flow is restored to meet the increased requirements.

There are also continuous capillaries equipped with muscle cells. These are found in

organs that need a continuous blood supply, such as nervous tissue and muscle tissue, where the endothelium forms an unbroken sheet.

Arteries and veins differ from each other both structurally and functionally. Arteries have thicker walls, which are elastic in large arteries such as the aorta and muscular in medium and small arteries, which actively pump blood (Figs. 3.21 and 3.22). Veins have swallow's-nest-shaped valves not present in arteries to prevent backflow and to resist the effects of gravity on blood flow. Veins are more readily depressible and dilatable. They are strongly anchored to surrounding connective tissues, where their transport function is connected with body movement. Veins are also more numerous than arteries, and the volume of the venous system is actually twice that of the arterial system. Finally, the pressure of blood inside the veins is lower than in the arteries.

THE LYMPHATIC SYSTEM

The lymphatic system is part of the circulatory system. It is a one-way drainage system leading from the periphery towards the center. It carries fluid from the interstitial spaces of the organs to the blood vessels (Figs. 3.23–3.26). As we have seen, the blood system, via the capillaries (i.e., in the interstitial spaces of the organs), yields part of its blood plasma, or lymph. This, however, is not entirely recovered by the capillaries on the venous side, and the portion not recovered is taken up by the lymphatic system, which enriches it with various materials, particularly proteins, and returns it to the veins.

If lymph drainage of the tissues is absent or insufficient, a gradual build-up of interstitial fluids and their components occurs. This pathological condition is called *edema* or *lymphedema*, and it is characterized by an increase in volume of the interstitium.

In normal functional conditions, the concentration gradient ensures that plasma fluids containing oxygen, proteins and other blood-borne materials extravasate from the arterial capillaries into the interstitial space. The same passive mechanism of concentration difference causes a large proportion of these fluids, now containing CO_2, to be recovered by hematic capillaries on the venous side. The remaining portion is conveyed to the lymphatic capillaries: tiny dead-end vessels present in large numbers in the loose connective tissue of all organs. Lymphatic capillaries are permeable to macromolecules and make an essential contribution to the maintenance of interstitial hydrostatic and osmotic pressure. Due to the high permeability of these capillaries, the composition of lymph is practically the same as that of interstitial fluids, but its pressure is lower than that of plasma.

Lymphatic vessels can be divided into two main types (Fig. 3.27):
- *Lymphatic capillaries* are those that have a high absorption capacity and remove fluid and proteins from the interstitium. These capillaries

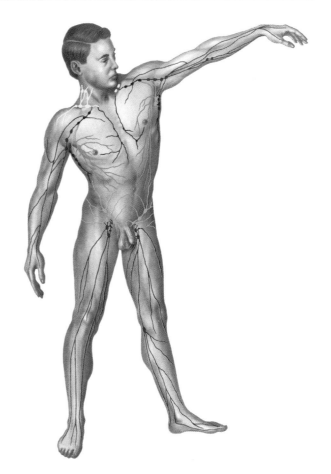

Figure 3.23 Schematic representation of some lymph centers or lymph node groups and the superficial territories of their tributaries. In **yellow**, the superficial and deep cervical lymph nodes; in **red**, the humeral (or lateral) axillary lymph nodes and the inferior superficial inguinal lymph nodes; in **green**, the pectoral (or anterior) axillary lymph nodes; in **blue**, the central axillary lymph nodes and the superomedial and superolateral superficial inguinal lymph nodes; in **black**, the parasternal lymph nodes and the subscapular (or posterior) axillary lymph nodes; and in **purple**, the apical axillary lymph nodes and the subclavian trunk.

arise as thin cylindrical dead-end channels in the extracellular matrix of connective tissue and they continue branching out to form a dense lymphatic network distributed superficially and deeply in the body's various organs and structures.

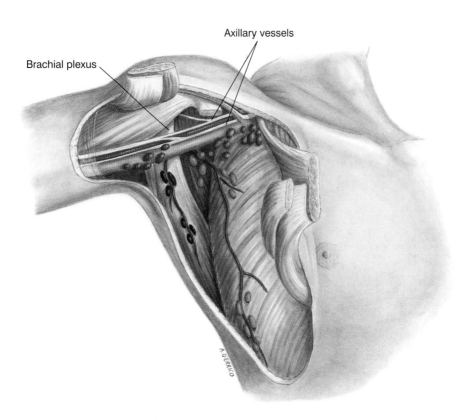

Brachial plexus

Axillary vessels

Figure 3.24 General organization of the axillary lymph nodes. In **red**, the humeral (or lateral) axillary lymph nodes; in **black**, the subscapular (or posterior) axillary lymph nodes; in **green**, the pectoral (or anterior) axillary lymph nodes; in **blue**, the central axillary lymph nodes; and in **purple**, the apical axillary lymph nodes.

– *Conducting lymphatic vessels* are larger in size and are divided into pre-collecting lymphatic vessels (which contain valves) and post-lymph-node collectors. The capillary network flows into the former and these discharge in turn into pre-lymph node collectors, which transport the lymph to regional lymph nodes. These, in turn, lead to the post-lymph node collectors (fewer in number than the afferent collectors), which take the lymph to the major lymphatic trunks and the lymphatic ducts. All organs and structures in the body are equipped with an interstitial lymphatic drainage system.

The most common form of lymphatic capillary is cylindrical, having an average diameter of 10–60 μm. The endothelial cells forming the one thin layer of its wall are flat, with numerous invaginations and cytoplasmic vesicles oriented towards both the luminal and the basal surfaces. The basal surface is in extensive contact with the extracellular connective tissue matrix. The suction pump action of the lymphatic capillary is due in part to the concentration difference between the outside and inside of the capillary itself, but also to the body movements that widen it and squeeze it. By reducing the pressure inside the capillary, temporary dilation causes a palpable suction effect from the interstitium towards the inside of the capillary. Because the lymphatic system is a low-pressure system in which the

Circulatory/Lymphatic Correction Technique

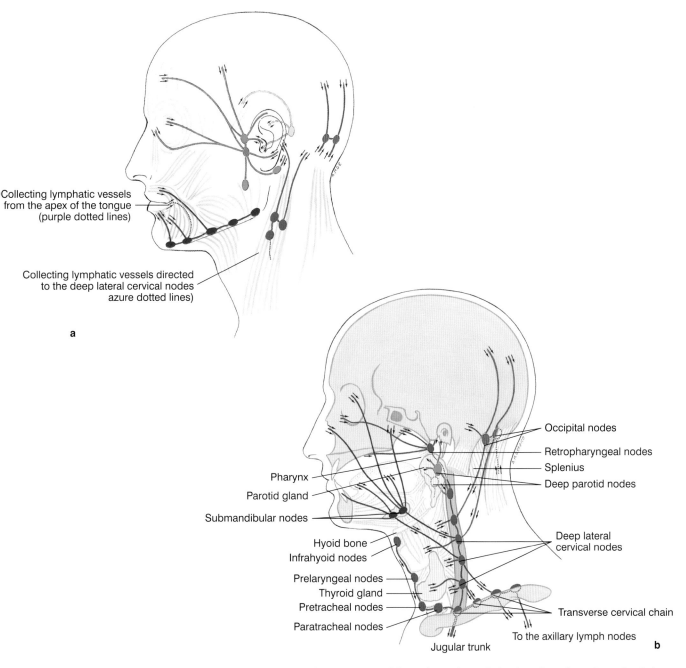

Collecting lymphatic vessels from the apex of the tongue (purple dotted lines)

Collecting lymphatic vessels directed to the deep lateral cervical nodes azure dotted lines)

a

Occipital nodes
Retropharyngeal nodes
Splenius
Deep parotid nodes

Pharynx
Parotid gland
Submandibular nodes

Deep lateral cervical nodes

Hyoid bone
Infrahyoid nodes
Prelaryngeal nodes
Thyroid gland
Pretracheal nodes
Paratracheal nodes

Transverse cervical chain
To the axillary lymph nodes
Jugular trunk

b

Figure 3.25 a) Schematic representation of the superficial lymph nodes of the head and neck and of the territories of their tributaries. In **orange**, the occipital lymph nodes; in **azure**, the superficial lateral cervical lymph nodes; in **yellow**, the mastoid (or posterior auricular) lymph nodes; in **green**, the preauricular and infra-auricular lymph nodes, and in **purple**, the submental lymph nodes. The **arrows** indicate the direction of lymphatic flow. **b)** Schematic representation of the deep lymph nodes of the head and neck. The different colors identify the various groups, the territories of their tributaries, and their lymphatic drainage pathways. All the lymph nodes in the region belong to the lateral deep cervical lymph nodes, whose efferent vessels form the jugular trunk. The **arrows** indicate the direction of lymphatic flow.

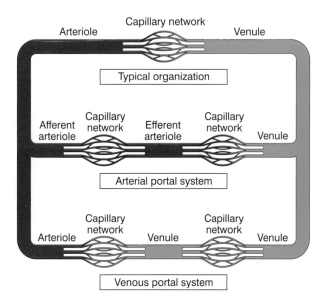

Figure 3.26 Schematic representation of the portal systems.

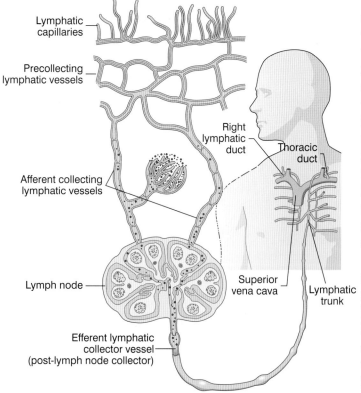

Figure 3.27 The lymphatic vessels, from capillaries to the lymphatic ducts.

lymph flows slowly, the propulsive force required to move it along is not great.

As indicated above, the main mechanism of lymph propulsion is dynamic. The compression and decompression caused by body movements perform a physiological pump-like action. Thus, there may be:

– External compression of the lymphatic vessels induced by bodily movements such as muscle contractions
– External compression of the lymphatic vessels caused by arterial pulsation of the blood vessels that accompany the lymphatic vessels, particularly in skeletal muscle
– Spontaneous contractile activity of lymphatic vessels which have muscle in their walls
– Changes in interstitial pressure that affect lymph formation pressure
– Respiratory movements

Compression action, especially expansion, of lymphatic capillaries is made possible by the anchorage of the basal side of the endothelial cells to the fibers of the extracellular matrix. These filaments are similar to elastin and they connect endothelial cells to the matrix collagen. Extremely sensitive to the forces in the interstitium, these fibers exert radial tension on the lymphatic capillaries, expanding them locally and causing re-absorption (Fig. 3.28). In higher vertebrates and humans, lymph is moved by the combined action of active and passive mechanisms, such as the muscle movement of contraction and relaxation.

The contractile activity of lymphatic vessels is peristaltic in nature. The swallow's-nest-shaped valves in the vessels prevent backflow of lymph during relaxation of the lymph wall. Progression of the lymph and the active propulsive action of lymphatic vessel walls differ depending on the area of the body in humans and are correlated to the pump action activated by body movement.

The improvement imparted to lymphatic drainage by NeuroMuscular Taping is based

Circulatory/Lymphatic Correction Technique

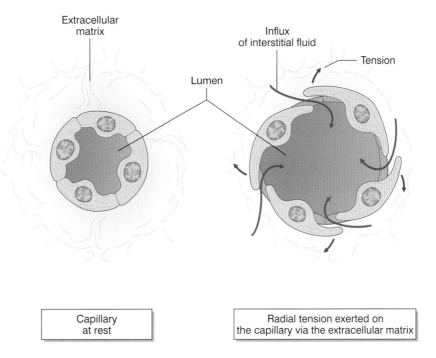

Extracellular
matrix

Influx
of interstitial fluid

Tension

Lumen

Capillary at rest

Radial tension exerted on the capillary via the extracellular matrix

Figure 3.28 The radial tension exerted by the anchoring filaments that secure the endothelial cells of the lymphatic capillary to the extracellular matrix causes dilation of the vessel and as a result the "suction" effect that underlies its capacity for absorption.

on the fact that the tape dynamically changes the decompression of lymphatic and blood vessels. The synergistic action between tape and body movement enhances the "pump effect" and therefore the relationship between circulation and lymphatic drainage.

Lymphatic Application - Back of the Hand

Application of tape to the back of the hand to improve lymphatic drainage and blood vascularization in the hand

TAPE SPECIFICATIONS

- 1 tape
- Width 5 cm (2")
- Length 25 cm (10")
- Fan-shaped with four or five strips

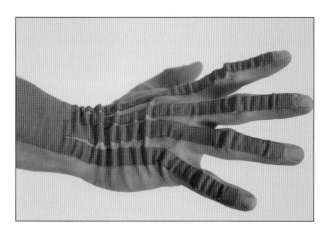

CLINICAL APPLICATIONS

- Edema of the back of the hand
- Hemiplegic hand
- Immobilization of a hand following a fracture or surgery

TAPE APPLICATION

1. With the patient's hand flexed and clenched in a fist, apply the strips of tape, without tension, over the back of the fingers and hand and the posterior surface of the wrist.

2. When the hand is extended, skin folds appear. These increase the interstitial spaces, facilitating lymphatic drainage.

Lymphatic Application - Knee

Doubled anterior fans - Application of tape to the knee to improve lymphatic drainage and blood vascularization in the knee

TAPE SPECIFICATIONS

- 2 tapes
- Width 5 cm (2")
- Length 30 cm (12")
- Fan-shaped with five strips

CLINICAL APPLICATIONS

- Generalized pain in the knee
- Anterior drainage of the knee
- Post-acute phase following surgery
- Gonarthrosis

TAPE APPLICATION

1. With the patient seated with knee flexed to 110°, apply the base anchor of the first fan to the thigh, laterally to the central line of the quadriceps femoris.

2. Without imparting tension, wrap the strips of tape around the front of the joint.

3. Place the base anchor of the second fan on the medial half of the thigh and also wrap the strips around the front of the joint, crossing over those of the first fan.

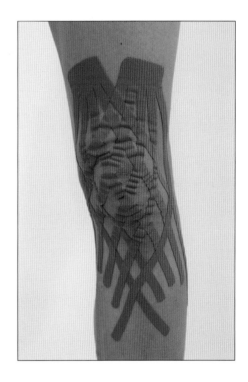

Lymphatic Application - Knee

Posterior fan - Application of tape to the knee to improve lymphatic drainage and blood supply to the knee

TAPE SPECIFICATIONS

- 1 tape
- Width 5 cm (2")
- Length 25 cm (10")
- Fan-shaped with five strips

CLINICAL APPLICATIONS

- Generalized pain in the knee
- Posterior drainage of the knee
- Post-acute phase following surgery
- Gonarthrosis

TAPE APPLICATION

1. With the patient standing with knee extended, apply the tape anchor behind the thigh, positioning it so that the middle portion of the tape is at the back of the knee.

2. Without imparting tension, apply the strips of tape over the back of the knee.

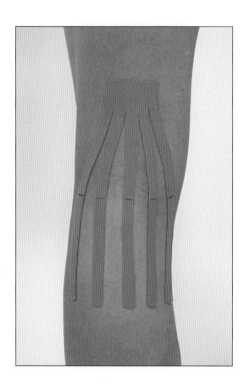

Plantar fan

TAPE SPECIFICATIONS

- 2 tapes
- Width 5 cm (2")
- Length 20-30 cm (8-12")
- Fan-shaped with five strips

CLINICAL APPLICATIONS

- Drainage of the foot
- Plantar fasciitis (plantar application)

TAPE APPLICATION

1. Apply the 20 cm plantar fan with the patient prone, knee flexed to 90°, and ankle dorsiflexed. Place the tape anchor on the heel and, without imparting tension to the tape, apply the strips along each metatarsal bone as far as the tip of each toe held in extension.

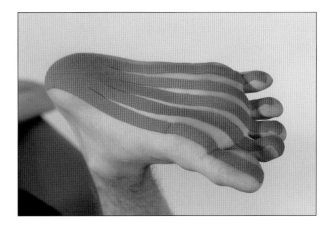

Lymphatic Application - Anterior Neck

TAPE SPECIFICATIONS

- 1 tape
- Width 5 cm (2")
- Length 20-25 cm (8-10")
- Fan-shaped with five strips

CLINICAL APPLICATIONS

- Anterior congestion of the neck

TAPE APPLICATION

1. With the patient's head held in the extended position, apply the tape anchor 5 cm below the manubrium of the sternum.

2. Apply the five strips around the trachea without imparting tension.

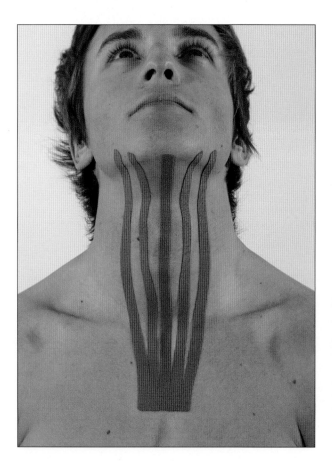
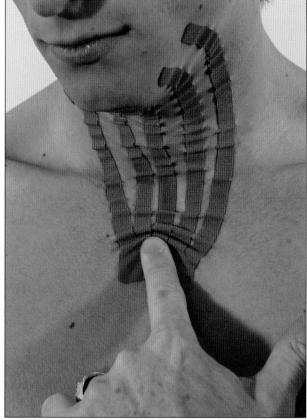

Lymphatic Application - Arm

TAPE SPECIFICATIONS

- 1 tape
- Width 5 cm (2")
- Length 35-45 cm (14-18")
- Fan-shaped with five strips

CLINICAL APPLICATIONS

- To promote drainage of the arm

TAPE APPLICATION

1. With the patient's arm extended and abducted through 90°, apply the tape anchor 5-10 cm medially to the axillary angle.

2. Apply the first three strips of tape over the course of the biceps brachii, starting with the lowest one.

3. With the patient lowering the abducted arm to 45°, apply the last two strips of tape. Thereafter, on flexing the arm, skin folds will appear.

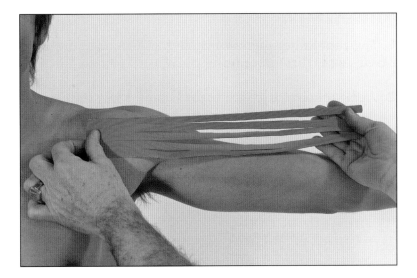

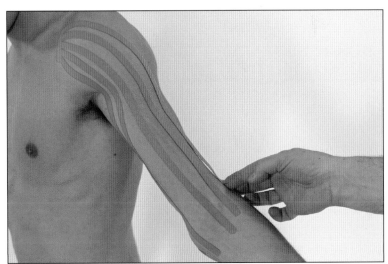

Lymphatic Application - Achilles Tendon

TAPE SPECIFICATIONS

- 1 tape
- Width 5 cm (2")
- Length 20 cm (8")
- Fan-shaped with five strips

CLINICAL APPLICATIONS

- Post-surgical drainage
- Tendinopathies of the Achilles tendon

TAPE APPLICATION

1. The patient lies prone with the foot extended over the end of the table and the ankle dorsi-flexed. Apply the anchor below the muscle-tendon junction of the gastrocnemius.

2. Without imparting tension to the tape, apply the external strips behind the malleoli, the middle strips to the lateral and medial margins of the calcaneal tendon (Achilles tendon), and the central strip along the middle of the tendon.

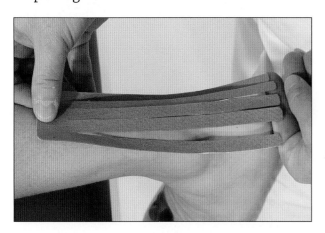 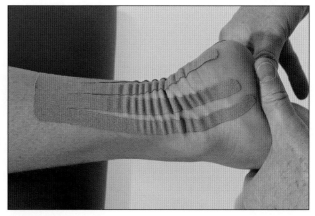

NOTE: The tape can be applied to the tendon alone or it can be forked and applied around the triceps surae muscle. If the tape is applied in an I-shaped form, its action is deep, i.e., it works on the tendon. If it is applied in a Y-shaped form it works at medium depth, and if it is applied in a fan-shaped form, the level of its action is superficial.

CORRECTION TECHNIQUE FOR CREATING DECOMPRESSION

With this technique, the skin above the painful and inflamed area is lifted to reduce hypersensitivity of the receptors. Four variants of this technique are used, in all of which the tape is usually applied with a tension of 0-25%. In the first variant, the skin is lifted before the tape is positioned. In the second and third variants, tape with a hole in it and tape applied in a star shape are used. In the fourth variant, the skin has to be stretched in the opposite direction.

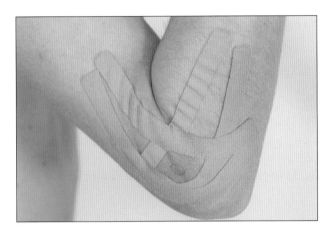

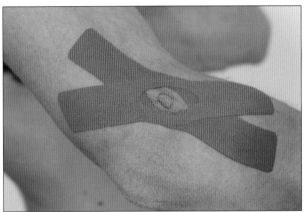

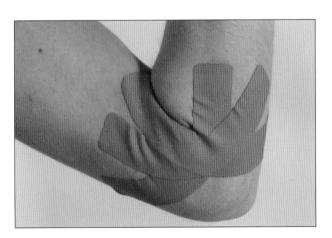

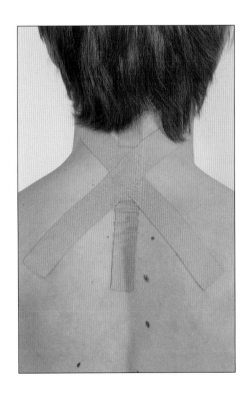

NOTE: To make this presentation complete, several applications to the elbow and neck of the first three techniques are illustrated here. However, these techniques are gradually being abandoned: due to their compressive nature, they have not been found to be particularly effective.

Skin Gathering Technique

TAPE SPECIFICATIONS

- 2 tapes
- Width 2.5 cm (1")
- Length 15 cm (6")
- Y-shaped

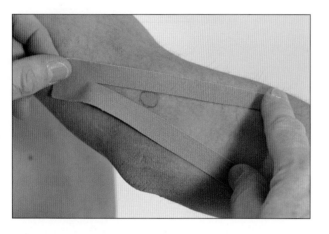

CLINICAL APPLICATIONS

- Pain at a precise point (trigger point type pain)

TAPE APPLICATION

1. The tape, without tension or with 25% tension, is placed on the skin around the painful point.

2. The skin overlying this point is raised manually during application of the strips of tape.

3. Two tapes are applied around the point.

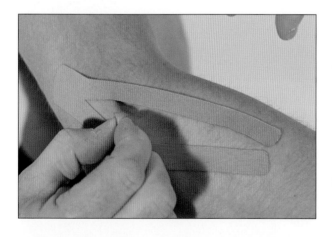

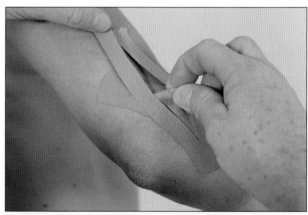

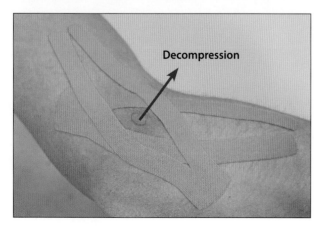

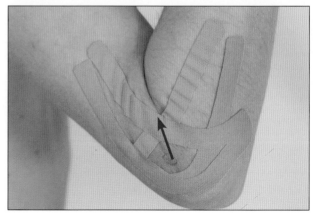

Hole Technique

TAPE SPECIFICATIONS

- 2 tapes
- Width 2.5 cm (1")
- Length 15 cm (6")
- I-shaped with a central hole

TAPE APPLICATION

1. Without tension, or with 25% tension, position the tape with the hole around the painful point.

2. Raise the skin overlying this point manually during application of the tape.

3. Apply two tapes around the point.

CLINICAL APPLICATIONS

- Epicondylitis

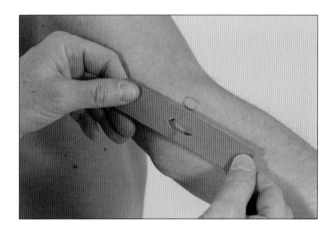

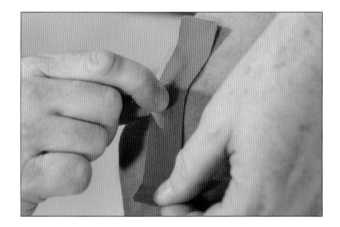

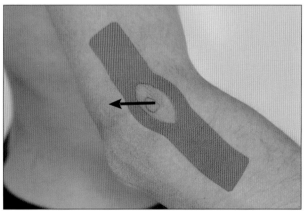

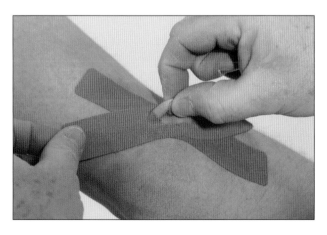

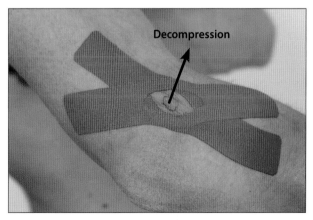

Crossover Technique

TAPE SPECIFICATIONS

- 3 tapes
- Width 2.5 cm (1")
- Length 15 cm (6")
- I-shaped

CLINICAL APPLICATIONS

- Epicondylitis in the post-acute phase

TAPE APPLICATION

1. Apply the tape with 25% tension over the painful part.

2. Apply three tapes, overlapping each other.

3. The crossover technique lends stability to the elbow and the use of several tapes supports the movement of the lateral epicondyle. Please note that this technique should not be used in cases of epicondylitis except in the post-acute phase.

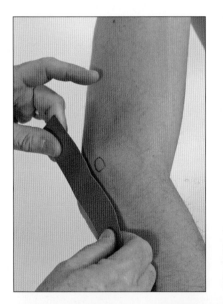 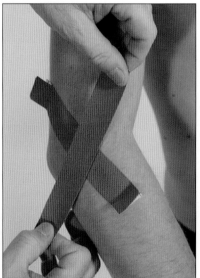 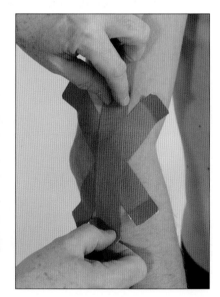

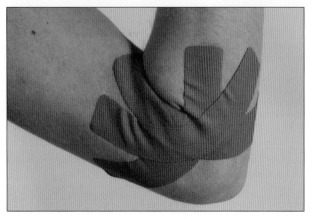

> NOTE: This technique is falling into disuse, because overlapping layers of tape produce compression, increasing pain and inflammation.

Skin Traction Technique

TAPE SPECIFICATIONS

- Width 2.5 cm (1")
- Length 25 cm (10")
- I-shaped

TAPE APPLICATION

1. Anchor the tape 5 cm proximally to the painful point.

2. The arm should be held supinated in the ulnar flexion position.

3. Pull the patient's skin in the proximal direction.

4. Apply the tape, without tension, over the course of the extensor muscles of the wrist and thumb. When the muscles contract, the tape creates decompression.

CLINICAL APPLICATIONS

- Acute epicondylitis

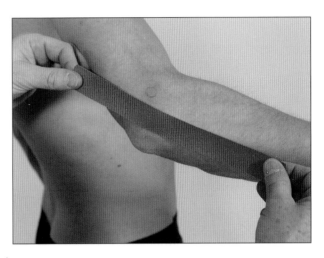

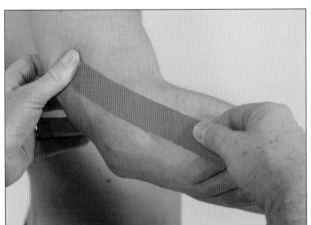

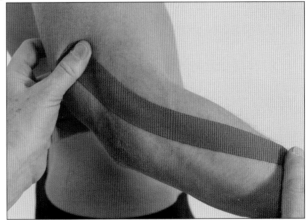

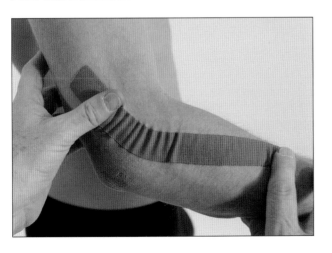

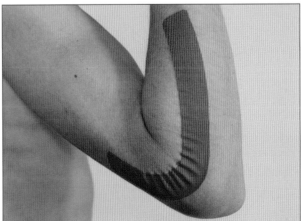

FUNCTIONAL CORRECTION TECHNIQUE

The functional correction technique is used when it is necessary to provide a functional stimulus or when movement is to be limited or facilitated. The tape is applied with tension ranging from 0 to 25%.

The joint is placed in the corrective or desired position. The tape anchors are then placed without tension and the tape is applied with the necessary tension.

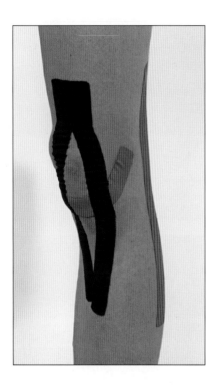

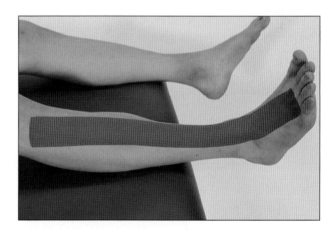

NOTE: Unlike traditional bandaging, this technique imparts a slight correction through light stimuli that are maintained around the clock. The aim is to exploit the action of the tape in conjunction with body mobility. Excessively strong and protracted stimulation (compression) can lead to muscle function imbalances.

Functional Application - Knee Joint

This is the functional stage in treatment of the knee joint, and it is a more specific application than the more general double-fan. Its purpose is to facilitate the sliding of the patella, guiding it in knee flexion and extension movements.

TAPE SPECIFICATIONS

- 1 tape
- Width 2.5 cm (1")
- Length 20-25 cm (8-10")
- I-shaped

- 1 tape
- Width 5 cm (2")
- Length 30 cm (12")
- Y-shaped with anchor 5 cm (2")

- 2 tapes (to obtain stabilization at the level of the tibial and fibular collateral ligaments)
- Width 2.5 cm (1")
- Length 20-25 cm (8-10")
- I-shaped

CLINICAL APPLICATIONS

- During resumption of sporting activity
- Functional stage following surgery
- Gonarthrosis

TAPE APPLICATION

1. With the knee flexed to 90°, apply the tape with 25% tension around the lower edge of the patella and then on both sides of the patella, keeping the tension constant.

2. Apply the 30 cm tape to the thigh, anchoring it so that the fork begins 6 cm above the upper edge of the patella. With the knee flexed to 110°, apply the tape without tension. The medial strip is made to outline the medial edge of the patella and end on the front of the tibia, while the lateral strip is made to outline the lateral edge of the patella before ending in the same point as the medial strip.

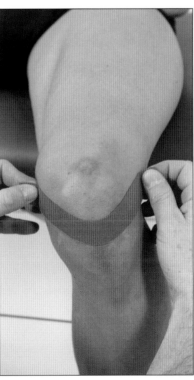
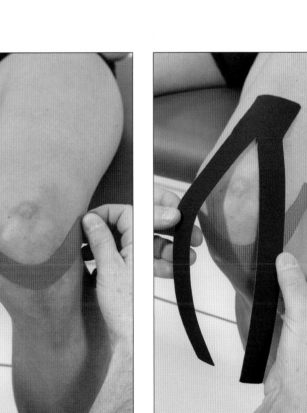

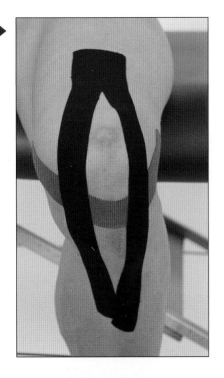

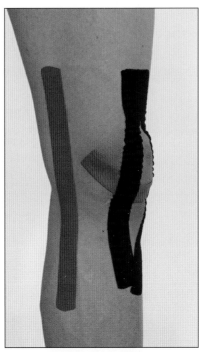

3. For application of tape at the level of the tibial and fibular collateral ligaments, the patient stands with knee extended, without rotation, with weight evenly distributed on both legs. Because the tape is applied with 25% or 50% tension, the anchor has to be positioned lower down so that the middle of the tape coincides with the joint fissure.

4. Place the tape anchor for the tibial collateral ligament at the same height as the one for the fibular collateral ligament.

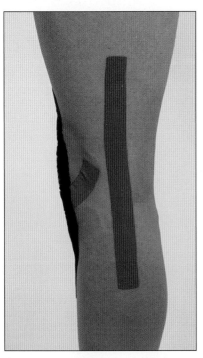

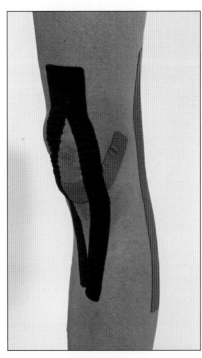

Functional Application - Supinated Equinovarus Foot

TAPE SPECIFICATIONS

- 1 tape
- Width 5 cm (2")
- Length 40 cm (16")
- I-shaped

CLINICAL APPLICATIONS

- Supinated equinovarus foot

TAPE APPLICATION

1. With the patient supine, place the foot in the corrected position and apply a tape from the bases of the second to fifth toes to the head of the fibula, so that the strip creates a bridge.

2. Apply the tape without tension and use the open hand to stroke it down onto the skin. This will cause the tape to adhere to the leg and the top of the foot, starting with the instep.

3. The tension on the tape increases to 25% when it adheres to the skin.

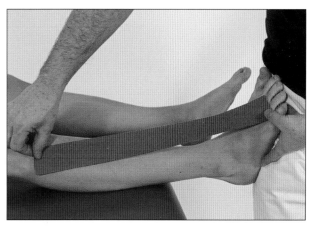

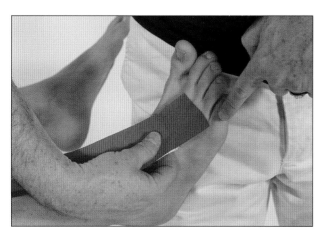

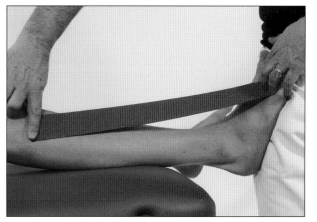

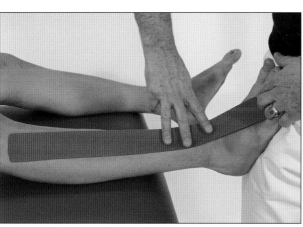

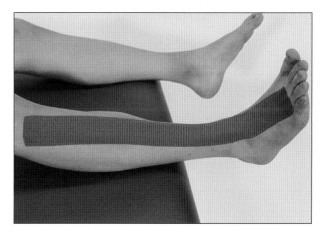

4

Head and Neck

- **Occipitofrontalis**
- **Orbicularis oculi**
- **Temporalis**
- **Masseter**
- **Lateral pterygoid**
- **Longus capitis, longus colli, sternohyoid and thyrohyoid**

- **Scalenus anterior**
- **Scalenus posterior**
- **Longissimus capitis, semispinalis capitis and semispinalis cervicis**
- **Splenius capitis**
- **Splenius cervicis**
- **Sternocleidomastoid**

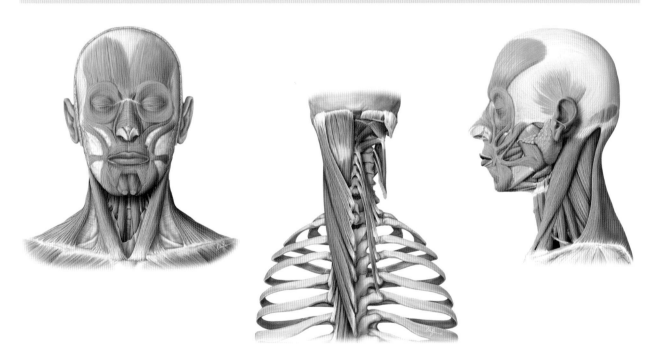

The following chapters (4-8) describe basic muscular applications that can be used individually or in combination. Applications for each individual muscle described use decompression, that is, the application of eccentric stimulus to the skin overlying the path of the muscle being treated. Decompression is considered the basic NeuroMuscular Taping application. Decompression improves the elasticity of muscle tissue, connective tissue and skin, normalizing their response and counteracting muscle retraction. Only in some situations, and only for certain muscle groups, might a compressive (or concentric) stimulus be appropriate.

OCCIPITOFRONTALIS

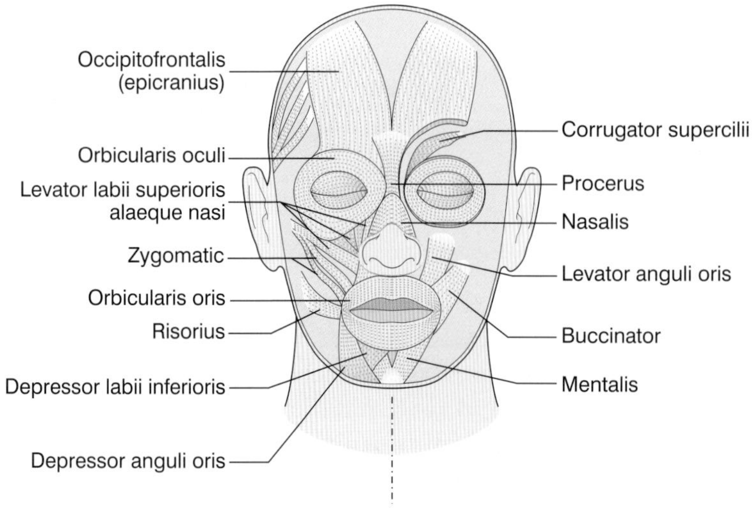
Occipitofrontalis
(epicranius)
Orbicularis oculi
Levator labii superioris
alaeque nasi
Zygomatic
Orbicularis oris
Risorius
Depressor labii inferioris
Depressor anguli oris
Corrugator supercilii
Procerus
Nasalis
Levator anguli oris
Buccinator
Mentalis

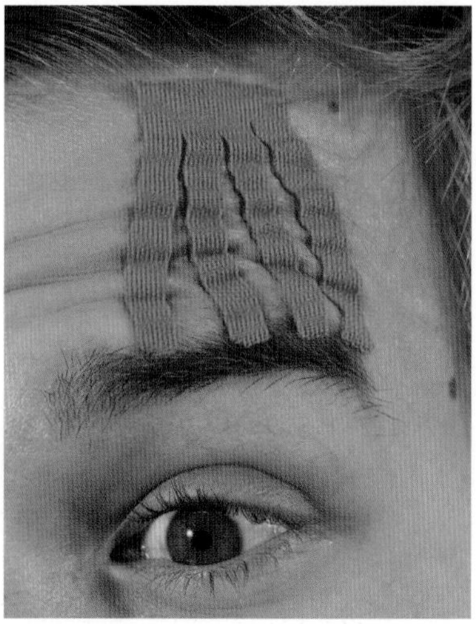

M. occipitofrontalis (Latin)

Origin

- *Frontal belly*: anterior margin of the galea aponeurotica, or epicranial aponeurosis
- *Occipital belly*: superior nuchal line

Insertion

- *Frontal belly*: deep surface of the skin above the eyes and glabellar region
- *Occipital belly*: posterior margin of the galea aponeurotica

Innervation: facial nerve [VII]

Action: acting from above or origin, the frontal belly raises the eyebrows and wrinkles the skin of the forehead horizontally. Acting from below, it moves the scalp forwards. The occipital belly retracts the scalp.

CLINICAL APPLICATIONS

- Headache
- Pain behind the eye and in the eyebrow and eyelid region
- Pain in the frontal bone region
- Ophthalmoparesis

Combined Applications

- Orbicularis oculi ➡ page 104
- Rhomboid major ➡ page 148
- Rhomboid minor ➡ page 146
- Semispinalis capitis ➡ page 122
- Sternocleidomastoid ➡ page 131
- Descending part of the trapezius ➡ page 136

TAPE SPECIFICATIONS

- 1 tape
- Width 2.5 cm (1")
- Length 5 cm (2")
- Anchor 1 cm (0.37")
- Fan-shaped with four strips

To facilitate application, the tape can be cut into individual strips without an anchor.

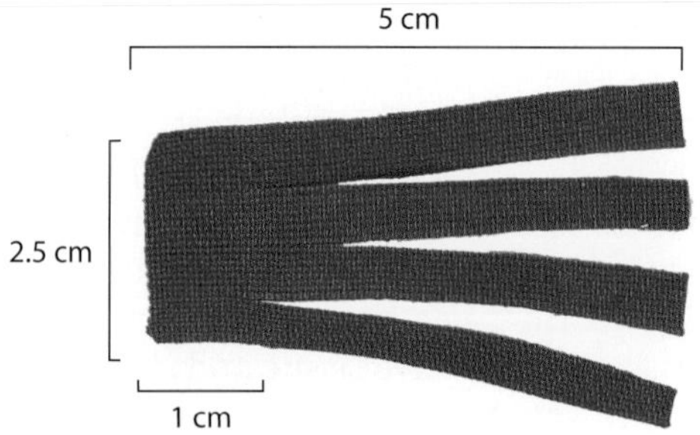
5 cm
2.5 cm
1 cm

Occipitofrontalis - Tape Application

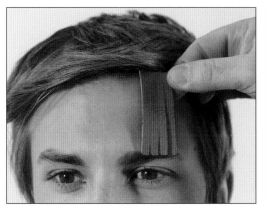 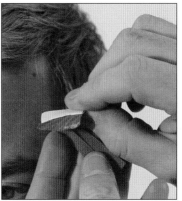 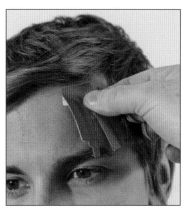

📏 From the hairline to the eyebrow

🧍 Face relaxed

1. Apply the base of the fan to the forehead, at the hairline.

2. Stretch the patient's skin using thumb and forefinger.

3. The tape is applied, without tension, as far as the eyebrow; distribute the strips across the forehead, taking care not to stretch the tape when applying.

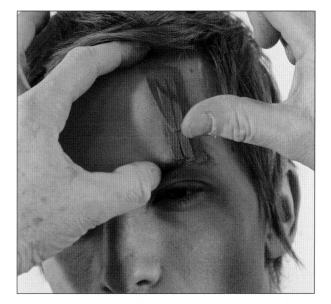

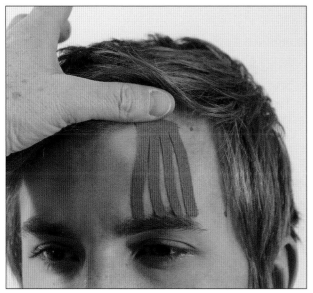 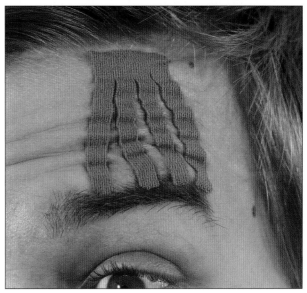

ORBICULARIS OCULI

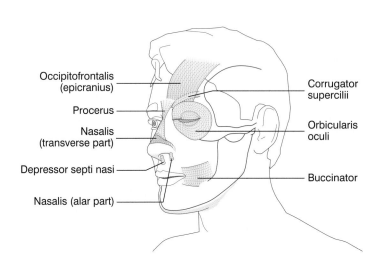

Occipitofrontalis (epicranius)
Procerus
Nasalis (transverse part)
Depressor septi nasi
Nasalis (alar part)
Corrugator supercilii
Orbicularis oculi
Buccinator

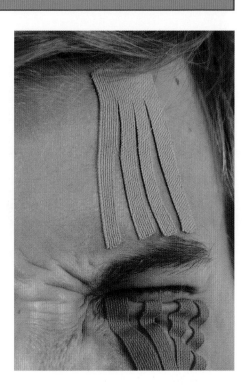

M. orbicularis oculi (Latin)

Origin
- *Orbital part*: upper margin of the medial palpebral ligament; medial third of the supraorbital margin
- *Palpebral part*: medial palpebral ligament
- *Deep part (lacrimal part)*: posterior lacrimal crest

Insertion
- *Orbital part*: lower margin of the medial palpebral ligament; medial third of the infraorbital margin; lacrimal sac
- *Palpebral part*: raphe palpebralis lateralis or lateral palpebral ligament
- *Deep part (lacrimal part)*: inserts with the palpebral portion of the muscle

Innervation: facial nerve [VII]

Action: closes the palpebral fissure; conveys the tears toward the inner corner of eye, dilates the lacrimal sac and facilitates the flow of tears.

CLINICAL APPLICATIONS

- Headaches
- Migraine
- Eyelid myoclonus
- Trigeminal neuralgia
- Drooping eyelid
- Eyelid paralysis

Combined Applications

- Semispinalis capitis ➡ page 122
- Sternocleidomastoid ➡ page 131
- Temporalis ➡ page 107
- Descending part of the trapezius ➡ page 136

Orbicularis Oculi - Tape Application

TAPE SPECIFICATIONS

Upper application
- 1 tape
- Width 2.5 cm (1")
- Length 5 cm (2")
- Anchor 1 cm (0.37")
- Fan-shaped with four strips

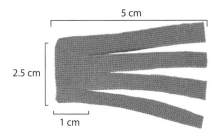

Lower application
- 1 tape
- Width 2.5 cm (1")
- Length 4 cm (1.6")
- Anchor 1 cm (0.37")
- Fan-shaped with four strips

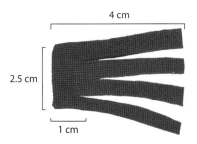

Lateral application
- 1 tape
- Width 2.5 cm (1")
- Length 5 cm (2")
- Anchor 1 cm (0.37")
- W-shaped

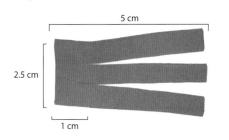

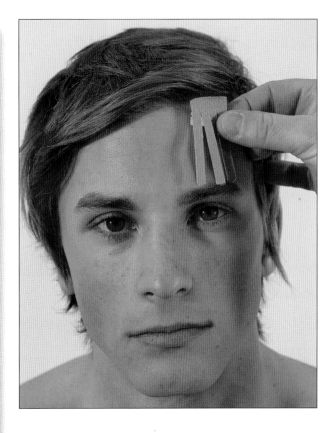

Upper application

🎗 From the hairline to the eyebrow

🧍 Face relaxed

1. Apply the base of the fan to the forehead, at the hairline.

2. Stretch the patient's skin using thumb and forefinger.

3. The tape is applied, with no tension, as far as the eyebrow; distribute the strips across the forehead, taking care not to stretch the tape during application.

Orbicularis Oculi - Tape Application

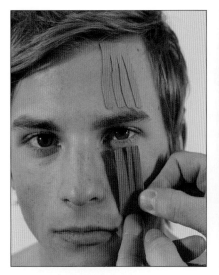 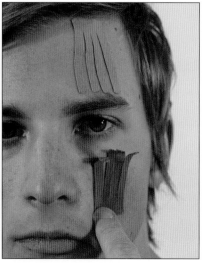 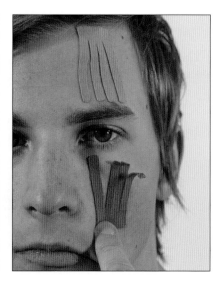

Lower application

🗘 From 1 cm above the corner of the mouth to 1 cm above the infraorbital margin

🕴 Face relaxed

1. Apply the base of the fan medially to the zygomatic process.

2. Pull the patient's skin downward.

3. The tape is applied, without tension, as far as the lower edge of the lower eyelid; distribute the strips of tape across the area; take care not to stretch the tape during application.

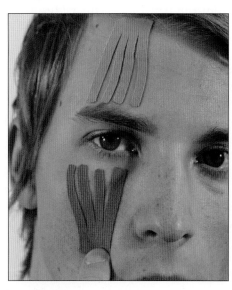 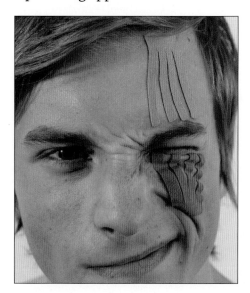

Lateral application

Use the same technique employed for the temporalis. ➡ page 107

NEUROMUSCULAR TAPING from Theory to Practice

TEMPORALIS

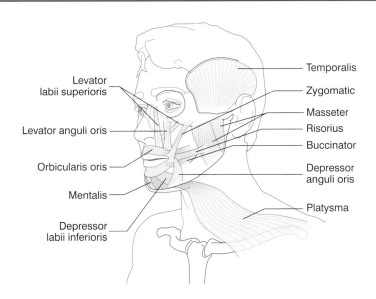

- Temporalis
- Zygomatic
- Masseter
- Risorius
- Buccinator
- Depressor anguli oris
- Platysma

- Levator labii superioris
- Levator anguli oris
- Orbicularis oris
- Mentalis
- Depressor labii inferioris

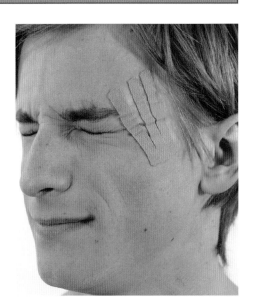

M. temporalis (Latin)

Origin: temporal fossa, including the parietal, temporal and frontal bones; deep surface of the temporal fascia

Insertion: coronoid process of the mandible; anterior margin of the ramus of the mandible

Innervation: deep temporal nerves (anterior and posterior), which are branches of the mandibular division [V3] of the trigeminal nerve [V]

Action: contributes to lateral movements, elevation and retraction of the mandible.

CLINICAL APPLICATIONS

- Headache
- Pain in the eyebrow
- Tooth hypersensitivity
- Facial paralysis
- Ophthalmoparesis
- Temporomandibular joint disorder
- Dental attrition

Combined Applications

- Masseter ➡ page 109
- Sternocleidomastoid ➡ page 131
- Descending part of the trapezius ➡ page 136

TAPE SPECIFICATIONS

- 1 tape
- Width 2.5 cm (1")
- Length 5 cm (2")
- Anchor 1 cm (0.37")
- W-shaped

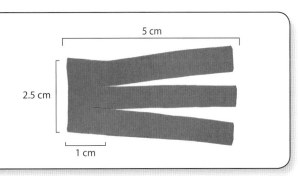

5 cm

2.5 cm

1 cm

Temporalis - Tape Application

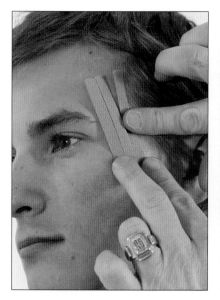 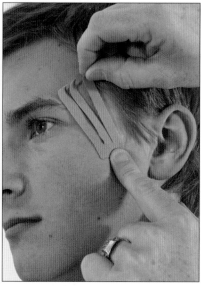 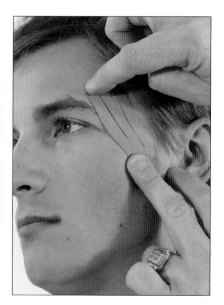

From 1 cm below the coronoid process of the mandible to the upper margin of the temporal fossa

Face relaxed

1. Apply the base below the coronoid process of the mandible.

2. Pull the patient's skin downward and toward the earlobe.

3. The tape is applied without tension as far as the hairline and temporal bone. In this way, skin folds form when the patient's eyes are closed.

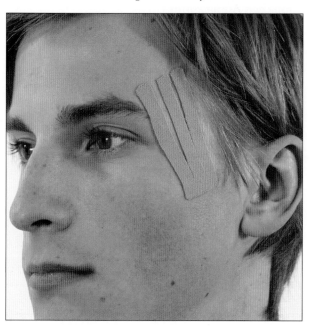 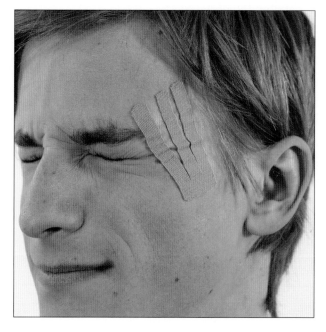

MASSETER

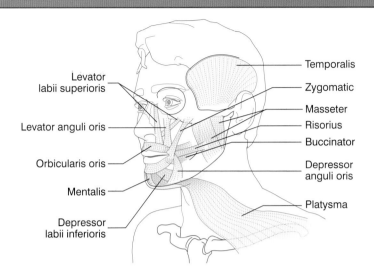

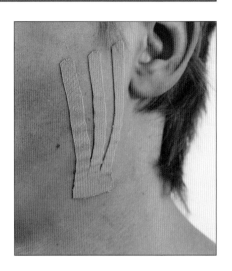

M. masseter (Latin)

Origin
- *Superficial part*: zygomatic process of the maxilla
- *Deep part*: deep surface of the zygomatic arch

Insertion
- *Superficial part*: angle and lower half of the lateral surface of the ramus of the mandible
- *Deep part*: upper part of the ramus of the mandible; coronoid process of the mandible

Innervation: trigeminal nerve [V]

Action: elevation, slight lateral deviation, protrusion and retrusion of the mandible

CLINICAL APPLICATIONS

- Tension headache/stress-induced headache
- Tooth pain
- Temporomandibular joint pain
- Ear pain
- Tinnitus
- Trismus (tight jaw clenching)

Combined applications

- Sternocleidomastoid ➥ page 131
- Temporalis ➥ page 107
- Descending part of the trapezius ➥ page 136

TAPE SPECIFICATIONS

Application 1
- 1 tape
- Width 2.5 cm (1")
- Length 10 cm (4")
- Anchor 1 cm (0.37")
- W-shaped

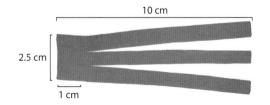

Application 2
- 1 tape
- Width 2.5 cm (1")
- Length 15 cm (6")
- Anchor 1 cm (0.37")
- Y-shaped or W-shaped

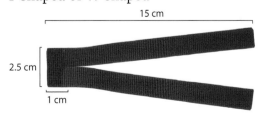

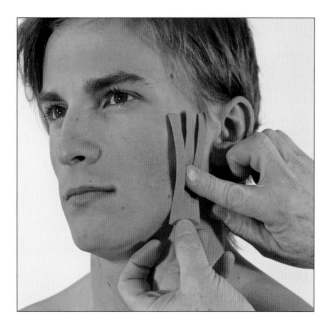
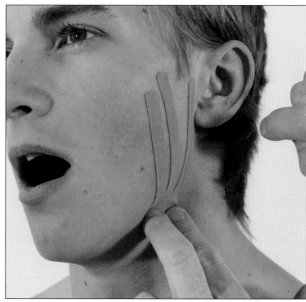

Application 1

📏 From 1 cm below the ramus of the mandible to 1 cm above the zygomatic process of the maxilla

🧍 Face relaxed

1. Apply the base of the tape below the ramus of the mandible.

2. Ask the patient to open their mouth and pull the skin downward.

3. The tape is applied without tension as far as the zygomatic process of the maxilla.

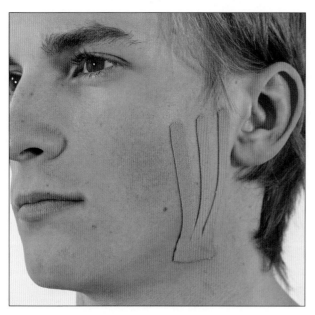
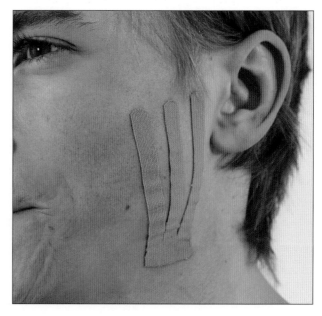

Masseter - Tape Application

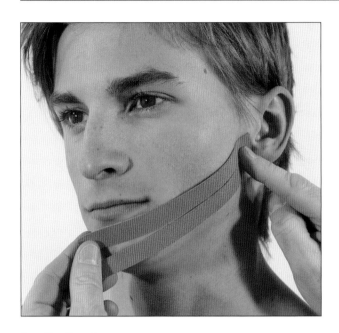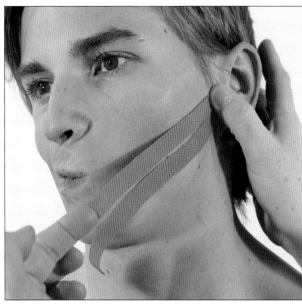

Application 2

📏 From the temporomandibular joint to 2 cm beyond the middle of the chin prominence (measurement taken with patient's face relaxed)

🧍 Twist the lip to the side opposite to that of the application

1. Apply the base of the tape to the angle of the jaw, just in front of the ear lobe.

2. Pull the skin toward the ear.

3. The tape is applied without tension up to the chin.

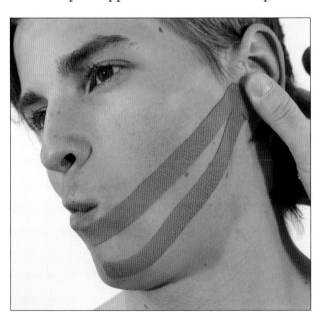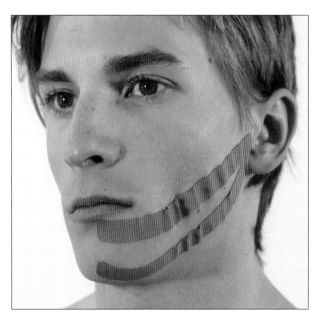

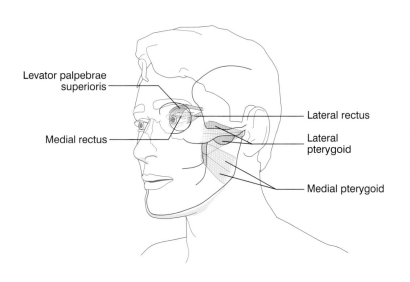

Levator palpebrae superioris

Medial rectus

Lateral rectus

Lateral pterygoid

Medial pterygoid

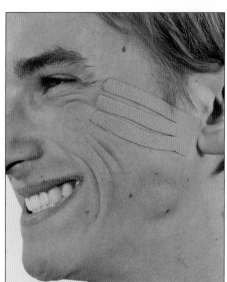

M. pterygoideus lateralis (Latin)

Origin
- *Upper head*: lower part and lateral surface of the greater wing of the sphenoid bone
- *Lower head*: lateral plate of the pterygoid process of the sphenoid bone

Insertion: temporomandibular joint capsule and disc; pterygoid fossa on the medial surface of the neck of the mandibular condyle

Innervation: trigeminal nerve [V]

Action: protrudes the mandible; opens the mouth; moves the mandible from side to side (as happens when chewing).

CLINICAL APPLICATIONS

- Reduced mouth opening
- Craniomandibular pain
- Trigeminal neuralgia
- Mastication problems
- Painful temporomandibular joint dysfunctions
- Tinnitus

Combined applications

- Masseter. Application 2 ➥ page 109
- Sternocleidomastoid ➥ page 131
- Descending part of the trapezius ➥ page 136

TAPE SPECIFICATIONS

- 1 tape
- Width 2.5 cm (1")
- Length 7 cm (2.75")
- Anchor 1 cm (0.37")
- W-shaped

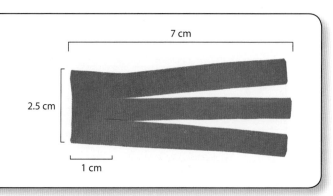

7 cm

2.5 cm

1 cm

Lateral Pterygoid - Tape Application

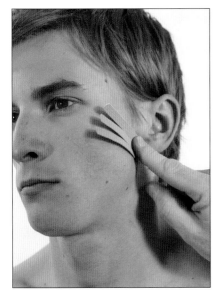 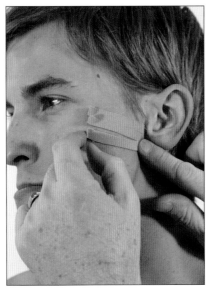 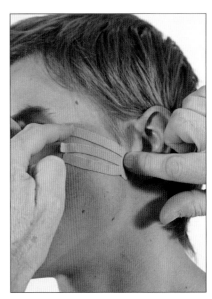

From the pterygoid process of the sphenoid bone to the lower lateral corner of the orbit

Face relaxed

1. Apply the base of the tape to the pterygoid process of the sphenoid bone.

2. Pull the patient's skin toward the ear.

3. The tape is applied with no tension as far as the lower lateral corner of the orbit. In this way, when the patient moves their lower jaw toward the side of the application, or raises the corners of the mouth (as when smiling), folds will form in the skin.

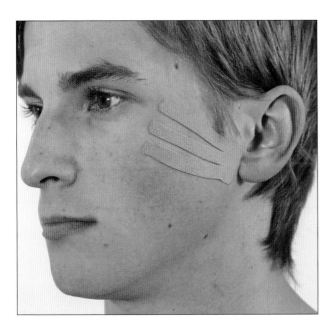 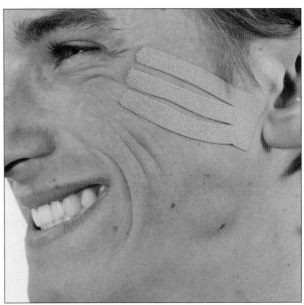

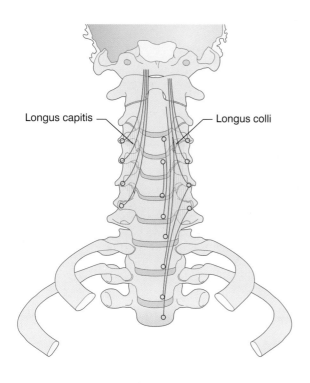

Longus capitis — Longus colli

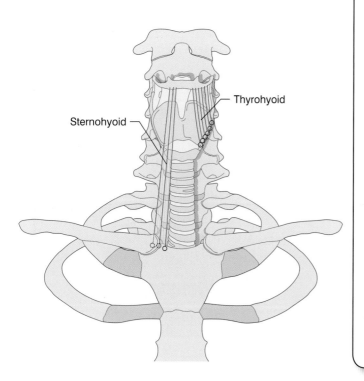

Sternohyoid — Thyrohyoid

M. longus capitis (Latin)

M. longus colli (Latin)

M. sternohyoideus (Latin)

M. thyrohyoideus (Latin)

Origin
- *Longus capitis*: anterior tubercles of the transverse processes of C3 to C6
- *Longus colli*
  - *Vertical part*: anterior surfaces of the vertebral bodies from T1 to T3 and from C5 to C7
  - *Superior oblique part*: anterior tubercles of the transverse processes from C3 to C5
  - *Inferior oblique part*: anterior surfaces of the vertebral bodies from T1 to T3
- *Sternohyoid*: upper and posterior aspect of the manubrium sterni; posterior surface of the medial end of the clavicle and posterior sternoclavicular ligament
- *Thyrohyoid*: oblique line of the thyroid cartilage

Insertion
- *Longus capitis*: basilar part of the occipital bone
- *Longus colli*
  - *Vertical part*: anterior sides of the vertebral bodies from C2 to C4
  - *Superior oblique part*: anterior tubercle of the atlas
  - *Inferior oblique part*: anterior tubercles of the transverse processes of C5 and C6
- *Sternohyoid*: medial part of the lower margin of the hyoid bone
- *Thyrohyoid*: lower margin of the body of the hyoid bone

Innervation: ansa cervicalis, C1-C3

Action: the long muscles of the head and neck work together to produce flexion of the cervical spine and lateral bending of the neck.

The sternohyoid and thyrohyoid muscles depress the hyoid bone and the larynx; they are active mainly in swallowing and coughing, neutralizing the thrust caused by the hyoid bone, which moves the head towards the cervical spine.

Anterior Neck Muscles

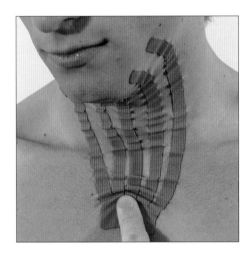

CLINICAL APPLICATIONS

- Compression of the vertebrae of the cervical spinal cord
- Sequelae of whiplash injury
- Facial drainage
- Symptomatic cervical herniation
- Thoracic outlet syndrome
- Acute torticollis

Combined Applications

- Semispinalis muscles of the head and neck ➡ page 122
- Descending part of the trapezius ➡ page 136

MUSCLE TEST

Patient: supine

Test: partial flexion (grade 2) or full flexion of the head and neck (grade 3) starting from the supine position, with the chin lowered (retracted, drawn toward the sternum) and the arms outstretched above the head

Pressure: the examiner applies pressure to the patient's forehead, in a posterior direction.

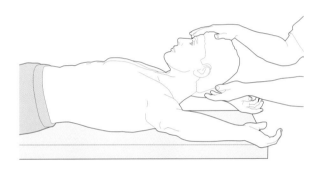

TAPE SPECIFICATIONS

Application 1
- 1 tape
- Width 5 cm (2")
- Length 25 cm (10")
- Anchor 2 cm (0.75")
- Fan-shaped with five strips

25 cm

5 cm

2 cm

Application 2
- 1 tape
- Width 5 cm (2")
- Length 25 cm (10")
- Anchor 2 cm (0.75")
- Fan-shaped with four strips

25 cm

5 cm

2 cm

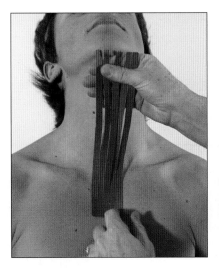
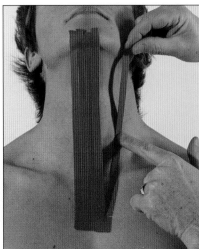
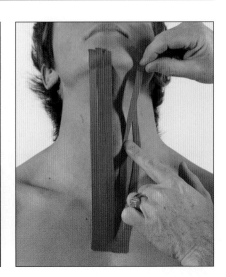

Application 1

🔖 From the chin to 5 cm beyond the sternoclavicular joint

👕 Head extended

1. Apply the base of the tape below the manubrium sterni.

2. For ease of application, the two internal strips should first be placed just inside the sternocleido-mastoid and taken over the lateral parts of the hyoid bone, as far as the mandible. Place the two external strips alongside them, as far as the mandible. Finally, position the central strip over the tracheal carina as far as the lower jaw. The skin will thus form folds when the patient returns their head to neutral position or flexes it. To activate the application, the skin must be pushed manually upward from the point of anchorage while the patient performs flexion and extension movements of the head.

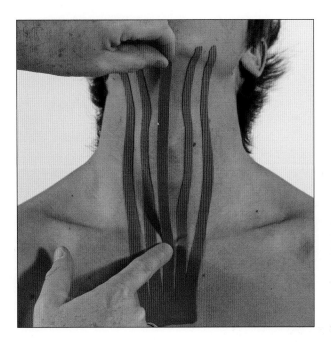
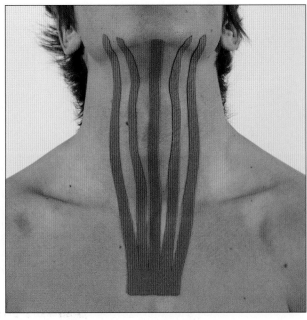

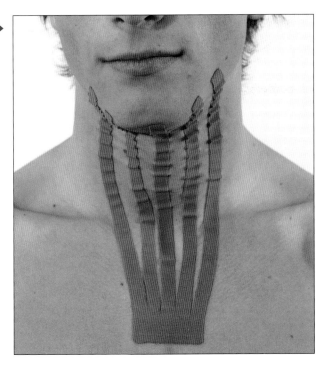

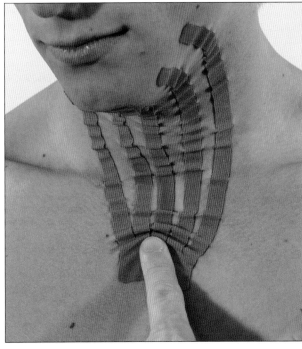

NOTE: For this application the tapes must always be positioned medially and symmetrically.

Application 2

1. The same technique can also be applied using a fan-shaped cut with four strips, omitting the central strip.

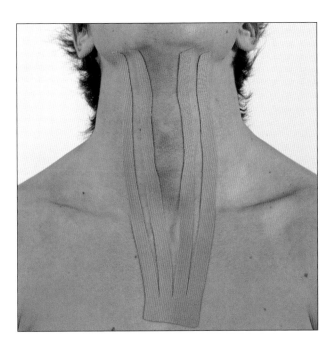

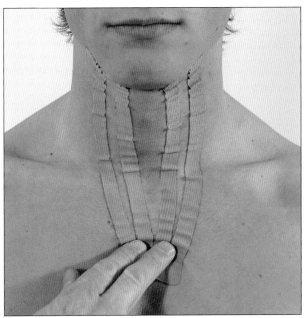

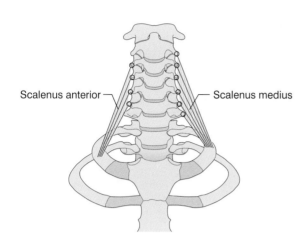

Scalenus anterior — Scalenus medius

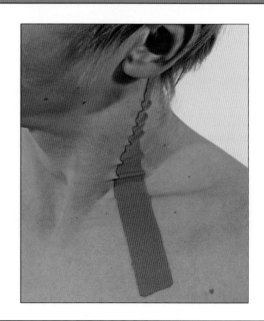

M. scalenus anterior (Latin)

Origin: anterior tubercles of the transverse processes of C3 to C6

Insertion: anterior scalene tubercle on the inner margin of the first rib (medial two-thirds)

Innervation: spinal nerves C4-C6

Action: the scalene muscles act unilaterally as lateral flexors and bilaterally as anterior flexors of the cervical spine. Concurrently, these muscles also greatly influence the respiratory muscles (during inhalation).

The involvement of the scalenus anterior may be detected during flexion and rotation of the neck toward the painful side, when it is possible to feel pain radiating from the third to fourth cervical vertebrae to the upper edge of the clavicle.

MUSCLE TEST

Patient: supine

Test: flexion of the head and neck starting from the supine position, with the chin lowered (retracted, drawn toward the sternum) and the arms outstretched above the head

Pressure: the examiner applies pressure on the patient's forehead, in a posterior direction.

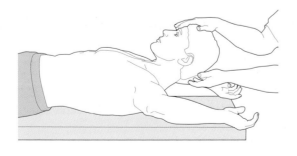

CLINICAL APPLICATIONS

- Whiplash
- Back, shoulder and arm pain
- Tongue and throat rehabilitation after oncology treatment and surgery
- Shoulder-girdle syndrome
- Brachial plexus syndrome
- Cervical spine syndrome
- Rib cage syndrome

Combined applications

- Deltoid ➡ page 161
- Triceps brachii ➡ page 180
- Descending part of the trapezius ➡ page 136

Scalenus Anterior - Tape Application

TAPE SPECIFICATIONS

- 2 tapes
- Width 1.25-2.5 cm (0.50-1")
- Length 15 cm (6")
- I-shaped

15 cm

2.5 cm

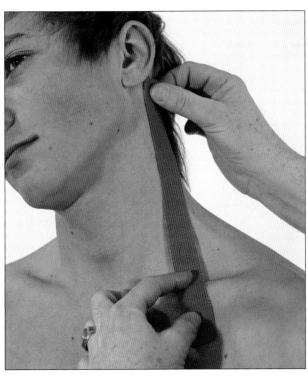

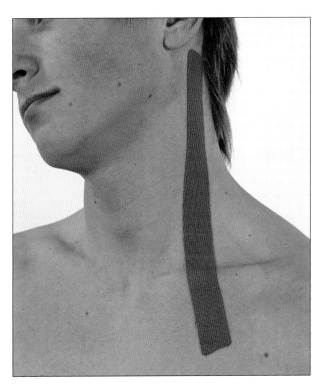

From the transverse process of C3 to 2 cm beyond the scalene tubercle on the inner margin of the first rib

Head tilted and rotated 30° in the direction opposite to the side of the application

1. Place the tape anchor below the tubercle of the anterior scalene muscle.

2. Apply the tape without tension and aligned with the origin of the scalenus anterior, when the muscle is at its point of maximum extension.

NOTE: As the scalene muscles influence posture (due to their connections with the spinal column), application of the tape must always be bilateral and symmetrical.

SCALENUS POSTERIOR

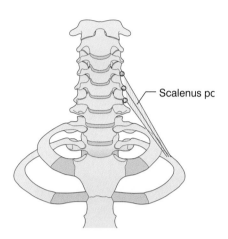

Scalenus pc

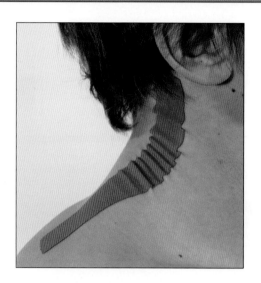

M. scalenus posterior (Latin)

Origin: posterior tubercles of the transverse processes from C4 to C6

Insertion: lateral surface of the second rib

Innervation: spinal nerves C3 to C7

Action: the scalene are a group of three pairs of muscles (scalenus anterior, scalenus medius and scalenus posterior) located in the neck on both sides of the spine. The scalenus anterior and scalenus medius muscles are responsible for eleva-

tion of the first rib and contralateral rotation of the neck, while the scalenus posterior is responsible for elevation of the second rib and ipsilateral rotation of the neck.

The scalene muscles act unilaterally as lateral flexors and bilaterally as anterior flexors of the cervical spine. These muscles also greatly influence the respiratory muscles (during inspiration).

Involvement of the scalenus posterior becomes apparent when pain irradiating from the middle cervical vertebrae is perceived at the top of the shoulder and the medial margin of the scapula.

MUSCLE TEST

Patient: supine

Test: flexion of the head and neck starting from the supine position, with the chin lowered and the arms outstretched above the head

Pressure: the examiner applies posterolateral pressure to the head, in the opposite direction to the side being examined.

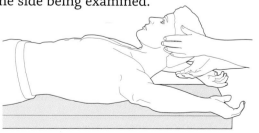

CLINICAL APPLICATIONS

- Whiplash
- Cervical sprains and strains
- Back, shoulder and arm pain
- Cervical disc herniation
- Tongue and throat oncological and surgical rehabilitation
- Shoulder-girdle syndrome
- Cervical spine syndrome
- Rib cage syndrome

Combined applications

- Deltoid ➡ page 161
- Rhomboid major ➡ page 148
- Rhomboid minor ➡ page 146
- Triceps brachii ➡ page 180

Scalenus Posterior - Tape Application

TAPE SPECIFICATIONS

- 2 tapes
- Width 1.25-2.5 cm (0.50-1")
- Length 15 cm (6")
- I-shaped and Y-shaped

15 cm

2.5 cm

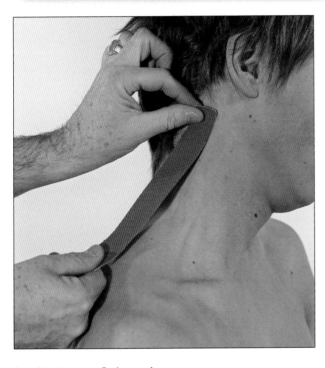
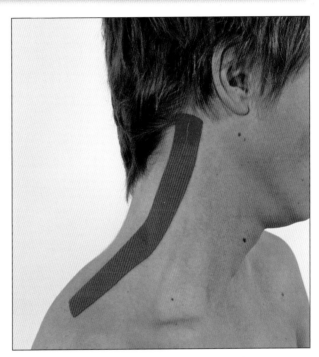

Application 1 - I-shaped

🔖 From the transverse process of C3 to 2 cm below the second rib

⚕ Neck rotated and tilted about 30° in the opposite direction to the muscle being treated

1. Apply the tape base below the second rib.

2. The patient flexes their neck slightly with gaze turned outward. Apply the tape without tension, aligned with the origin of the scalenus posterior, when the muscle is at its point of maximum extension.

Application 2 - Y-shaped

1. Apply the tape base below the second rib.

2. With no tension, apply the two strips so that they skirt the path of the muscle as far as its point of origin.

NOTE: As the scalene muscles influence posture, due to their connections with the spinal column, the application of the tape must always be bilateral and symmetrical.

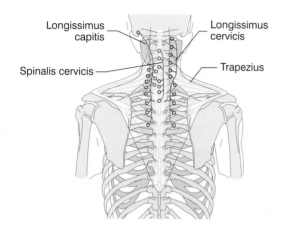

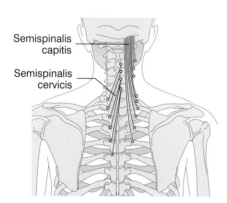

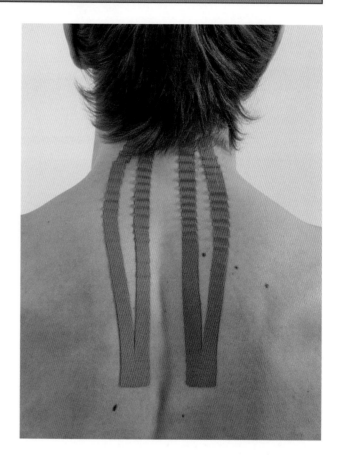

M. longissimus capitis (Latin)

M. semispinalis capitis (Latin)

M. semispinalis cervicis (Latin)

Origin
- *Longissimus capitis*: transverse processes of the first five thoracic vertebrae (T1-T5); articular processes of the last three cervical vertebrae (C5-C7)
- *Semispinalis capitis*: transverse processes of the last four cervical vertebrae and of the first six thoracic vertebrae (C4-C7 and T1-T6)
- *Semispinalis cervicis*: transverse processes of the first six thoracic vertebrae (T1-T6)

Insertion
- *Longissimus capitis*: mastoid process of the temporal bone
- *Semispinalis capitis*: between the superior and inferior nuchal lines of the occipital bone
- *Semispinalis cervicis*: spinous processes of the second to the fifth cervical vertebrae (C2-C5)

Innervation: posterior branches of the cervical and thoracic spinal nerves

Action
  Longissimus capitis: extends and bends the head laterally, it helps to maintain the physiological curvature of the thoracic and cervical spine in standing and sitting positions.

  Semispinalis capitis: the most powerful extensor of the head: it also assists in rotation of the head.

  Semispinalis cervicis: extends the cervical and thoracic segments of the spine and plays a role in contralateral rotation of the neck.

Posterior Neck Muscles

MUSCLE TEST

Patient: prone

Test: extension and rotation and lateral bending of the head, starting from the prone position

Pressure: apply pressure in an anterior direction on the head in front of the occipital bone.

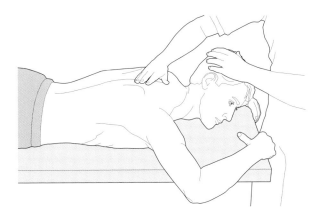

CLINICAL APPLICATIONS

- Headache
- Sequelae of whiplash injury
- Cervical disc disorder
- Suboccipital pain
- Symptomatic cervical disc herniation
- Limited rotation of the neck
- Reduced cervical flexion
- Neck pain and stiffness

Combined applications

- Pectoralis major ➥ page 152
- Sternocleidomastoid ➥ page 131
- Descending part of the trapezius ➥ page 136

TAPE SPECIFICATIONS

- 2 tapes
- Width 2.5 cm (1")
- Length 20-25 cm (8-10")
- Anchor 2 cm (0.75")
- Y-shaped

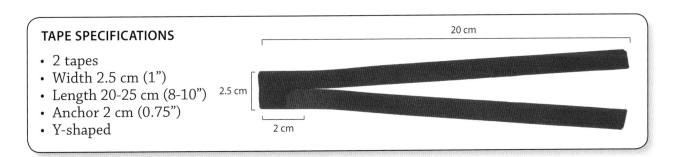

20 cm

2.5 cm

2 cm

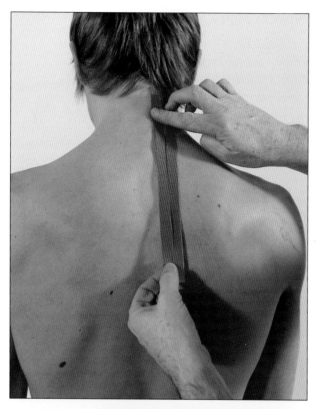
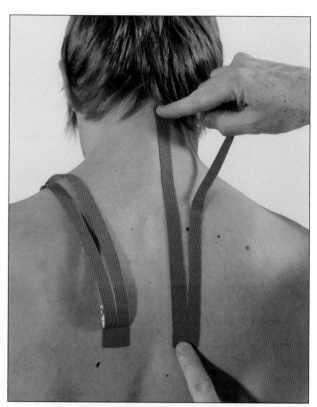
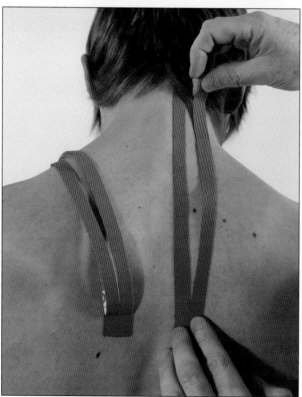
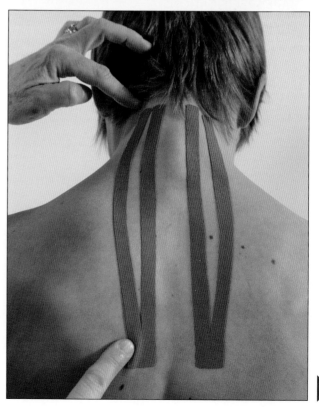

Posterior Neck Muscles - Tape Application

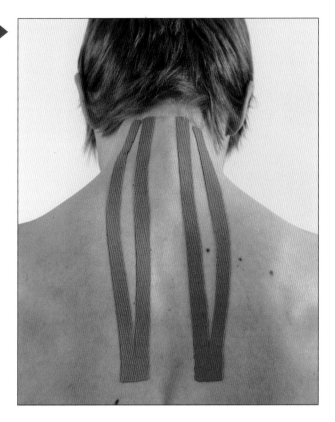 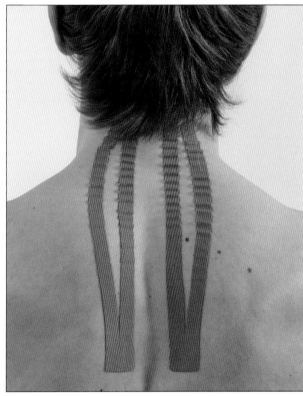

From the hairline in the occipital region to 2 cm beyond the sixth thoracic vertebra

The patient flexes their neck to 45° producing accentuated dorsal kyphosis

1. Apply the tape anchor just below the transverse process of the sixth thoracic vertebra.

2. Apply the medial strip with no tension parallel to the backbone, as far as the hairline.

3. With the patient's head flexed to 45°, apply the lateral strip without tension; this strip should diverge from the medial strip in the region of the seventh cervical vertebra before converging with it again as it nears the hairline.

NOTE: As the posterior muscles of the neck influence body posture, due to their connections with the spinal column, tape application must always be bilateral and symmetrical.

SPLENIUS CAPITIS

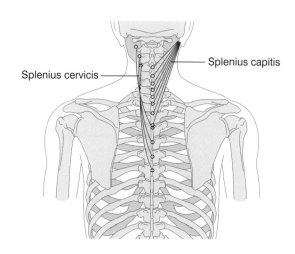

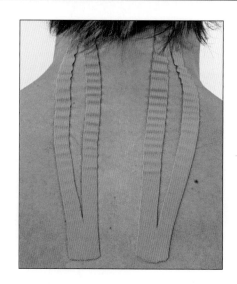

M. splenius capitis (Latin)

Origin: lower part of the nuchal ligament, spinous process of the C7 vertebra, spinous processes of the first 3-4 thoracic vertebrae

Insertion: mastoid process of the temporal bone and occipital bone and anterior two-thirds of superior nuchal line

Innervation: posterior branches of spinal nerves C2-C4

Action: when activated bilaterally, the splenius muscle, along with the other extensor muscles, produces extension of the neck and head; when activated monolaterally, it produces posterolateral extension of the neck and rotation of the head, always to the same side. Through its shortening, this muscle is often involved in torticollis, along with the sternocleidomastoid muscle of the opposite side.

CLINICAL APPLICATIONS

- Headache
- Sequelae of whiplash injury
- Post oncological and surgical neck rehabilitation
- Stiffness and limited ipsilateral rotation of the cervical spine
- Torticollis

Combined applications

- Levator scapulae ➡ page 141
- Masseter ➡ page 109
- Rhomboid major ➡ page 148
- Rhomboid minor ➡ page 146
- Splenius cervicis ➡ page 129
- Sternocleidomastoid ➡ page 131
- Trapezius ➡ page 136

MUSCLE TEST

Patient: prone

Test: extension and rotation or lateral bending of the head and neck with the face turned toward the side being examined

Pressure: the examiner applies pressure in an anterior direction on the head in front of the occipital bone.

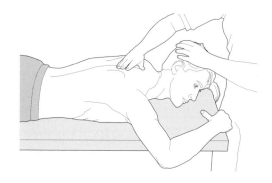

Splenius Capitis - Tape Application

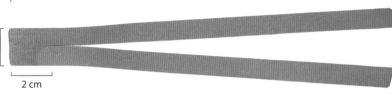
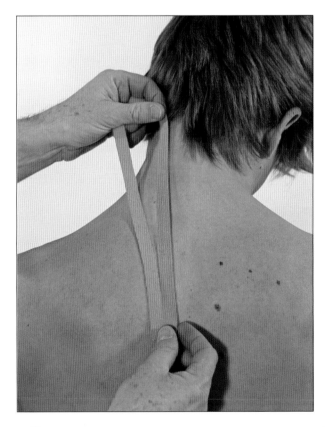

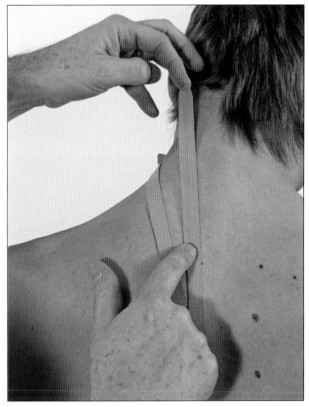

From the hairline at the level of the mastoid process of the temporal bone to 2 cm beyond the spinous process of the fourth thoracic vertebra

The patient flexes their neck to 45° and rotates their head away from the side of the muscle to be treated

1. Apply the base of the tape 2.5 cm below the spinous process of T4.

2. For ease of application, remove the protective backing paper from the strips of tape and place the strips medially along the descending part of the trapezius.

Splenius Capitis - Tape Application

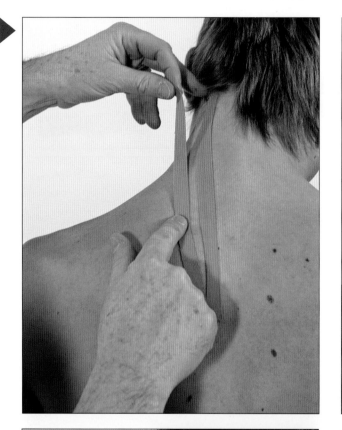

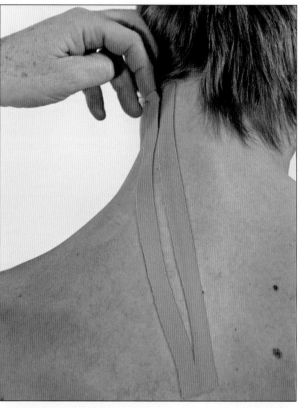

3. With the neck flexed at 45°, have the patient rotate their head in an opposite direction to the side being treated.

4. Apply the tape, without tension, in an upward and outward direction just below the mastoid process of the temporal bone.

5. Keeping the neck flexed, have the patient rotate their head in the other direction and apply the tape to the other side.

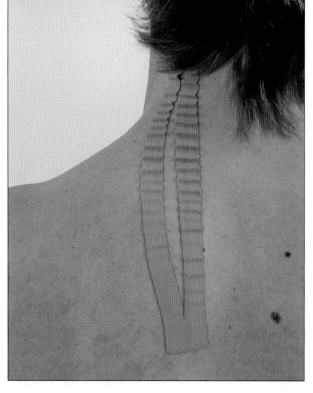

NOTE: As the splenius muscle, being connected with the vertebral column, influences body posture, tape application must always be bilateral and symmetrical.

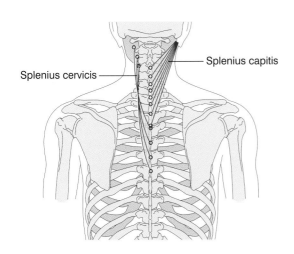

Splenius cervicis — Splenius capitis

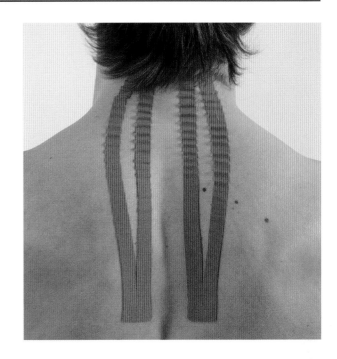

M. splenius cervicis (Latin)

Origin: spinous processes from T3 to T6

Insertion: posterior tubercles of transverse processes of the three upper cervical vertebrae

Innervation: lower cervical nerves

Action: when activated bilaterally, the splenius muscle, along with the other extensor muscles, produces extension of the neck and head. When activated monolaterally, it produces posterolateral extension of the neck and rotation of the head, always to the same side. Through its shortening, this muscle is always involved in torticollis, along with the sternocleidomastoid muscle of the opposite side.

CLINICAL APPLICATIONS

- Sequelae of whiplash injury
- Symptomatic cervical herniation
- Reduced neck rotation
- Neck stiffness
- Torticollis

Combined applications

- Sternocleidomastoid ➡ page 131

TAPE SPECIFICATIONS

- 2 tapes
- Width 2.5 cm (1")
- Length 25-35 cm (10-14")
- Anchor 2 cm (0.75")
- Y-shaped

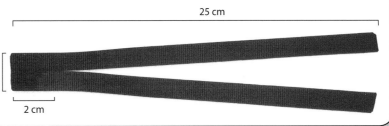

25 cm

2.5 cm

2 cm

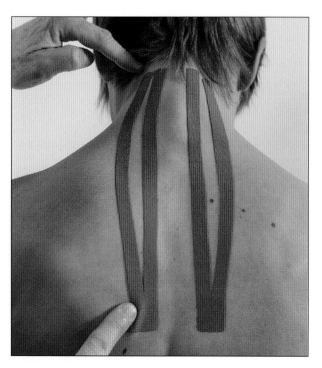

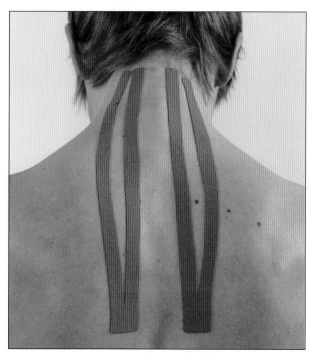

From the hairline to 2 cm beyond the transverse process of the sixth thoracic vertebra

The patient flexes their neck to 45° and rotates their head away from the side of the muscle to be treated

1. Apply the base of the tape just below the transverse process of the sixth thoracic vertebra.

2. For ease of application, remove the protective backing paper from the strips of tape and lay the strips medially along the descending part of the trapezius.

3. Apply the medial strip, without tension, skirting the course of the muscle in an upward direction toward the spinous process of C3.

4. Apply the lateral strip, maintaining some distance from the first before converging with it again at the level of the transverse process of C3.

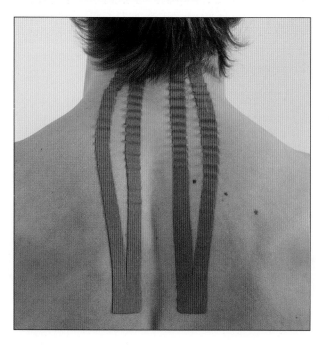

NOTE: As the splenius muscle, being connected with the vertebral column, influences body posture, the application of the tape must always be bilateral and symmetrical.

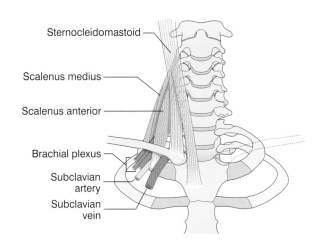

Sternocleidomastoid

Scalenus medius

Scalenus anterior

Brachial plexus

Subclavian artery

Subclavian vein

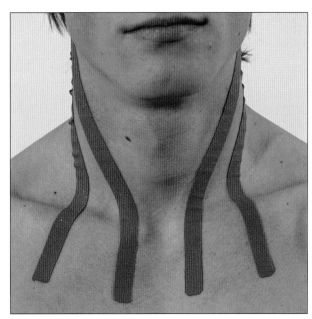

M. sternocleidomastoideus (Latin)

Origin
- *Sternal head*: anterior surface of the manubrium sterni
- *Clavicular head*: superior surface of the medial third of the clavicle

Insertion: mastoid process; lateral half of the superior nuchal line of the occipital bone

Innervation: accessory nerve and branches of the second and third cervical nerves C2-C3

Action: the sternocleidomastoid muscle helps to raise the sternum and clavicle. It has two points of origin and if one head of the muscle contracts, the cranium and mandible rotate toward the opposite side. Bilateral contraction of the muscle extends the head. The sternocleidomastoid muscle is also involved in breathing (deep breathing).

MUSCLE TEST

Patient: supine

Test: starting from the supine position with the arms outstretched above the head, execute anterolateral flexion of the neck with ipsilateral tilting and contralateral rotation of the head. Assess the two muscles separately.

Pressure: the examiner applies pressure, in a posterior oblique direction, to the temporal region of the head.

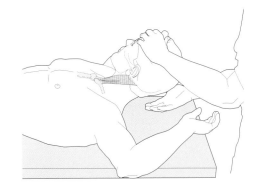

Sternocleidomastoid - Tape Application

CLINICAL APPLICATIONS

- Headache
- Sequelae of whiplash injury
- Brachial neuralgia
- Facial neuralgia
- Trigeminal neuralgia
- Post oncological and surgical throat rehabilitation
- Stiffness and limited rotation of the cervical spine

- Rib cage syndrome
- Costoclavicular symptoms
- Torticollis

Combined applications

- Levator scapulae ➥ page 141
- Splenius capitis ➥ page 126
- Descending part of the trapezius ➥ page 136

TAPE SPECIFICATIONS

- 2 tapes
- Width 2.5 cm (1")
- Length 25 cm (10")
- Anchor 1 cm (0.37")
- Y-shaped

25 cm

2.5 cm

1 cm

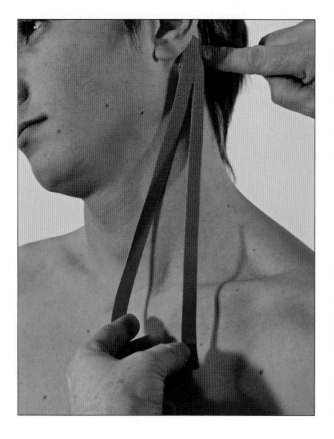
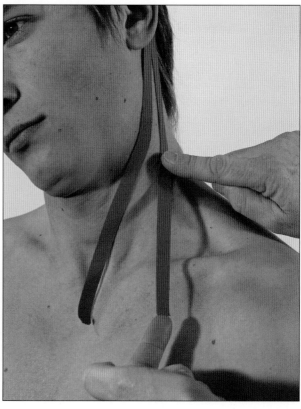

Sternocleidomastoid - Tape Application

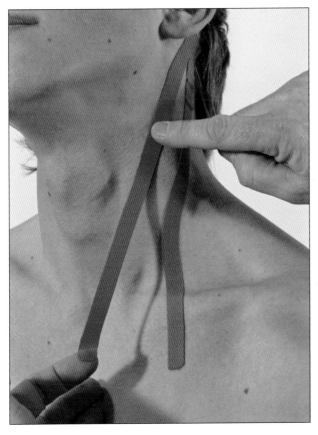 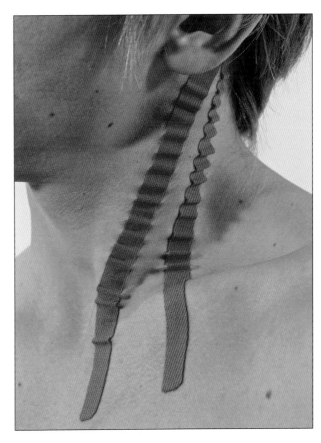

📏 From the mastoid process to 5 cm beyond the clavicle

🧍 Head slightly rotated toward the side of the application, extended and tilted to the opposite side

1. Apply the base of the tape 2.5 cm above the mastoid process, hairline permitting.

2. In this position, for ease of application, lay the ends of the tape beyond the clavicle. Apply the medial strip to the patient's skin along the muscle belly, ending beyond the anterior surface of the manubrium sterni.

3. Position the other strip of tape along the muscle belly ending beyond the medial third of the anterosuperior surface of the clavicle.

NOTE: As the sternocleidomastoid muscle, being connected with the spinal column, influences body posture, tape application must always be bilateral and symmetrical.

5

Shoulder and Shoulder Girdle

- Trapezius
- Levator scapulae
- Serratus anterior
- Rhomboid minor
- Rhomboid major
- Pectoralis major
- Pectoralis minor
- Latissimus dorsi

- Deltoid
- Supraspinatus
- Teres major
- Teres minor
- Infraspinatus
- Subscapularis
- Biceps brachii
- Triceps brachii

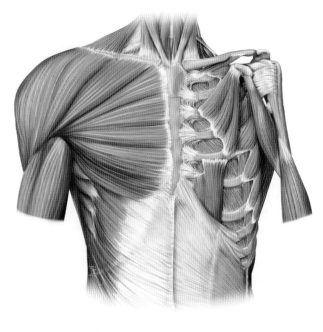

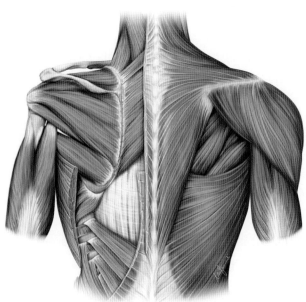

TRAPEZIUS

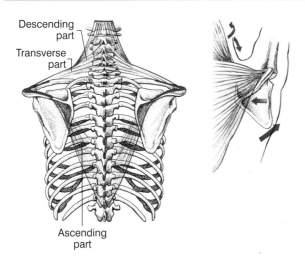

Descending part
Transverse part
Ascending part

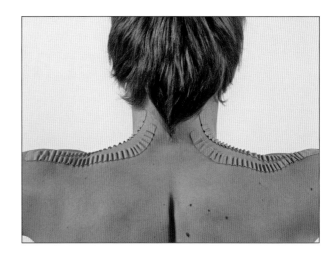

M. trapezius (Latin)

Origin
- *Descending part*:
  – External occipital protuberance
  – Medial third of the superior nuchal line of the occipital bone
  – Nuchal ligament
- *Transverse part*:
  – Posterior longitudinal ligament
  – Spinous processes and interspinous ligaments from the seventh cervical vertebra to the third thoracic vertebra
- *Ascending part*:
  – Supraspinous ligament
  – Spinous processes and interspinous ligaments from the third to the twelfth thoracic vertebrae

Insertion
- *Descending part*: posterior margin of the lateral third of the clavicle
- *Transverse part*: posterior margin of the spine of the scapula
- *Ascending part*: medial margin of the scapula at the point of origin of the spine

Innervation: spinal accessory nerve [XI] and branches of the cervical plexus (C2-C4)

Action: the trapezius has three regions: the descending, transverse and ascending parts.

The *descending part* comprises subsections of upper and lower fibers: the upper fibers assist in elevating the arm, while the lower fibers elevate the arm and at the same time rotate it upward and adduct it. Furthermore, when lifting objects, the upper fibers initially provide support to the distal clavicle and the acromion. The *transverse part* of the trapezius aids in adduction of the arm, while the *ascending part* aids in its rotation, lowering and adduction.

MUSCLE TEST

Patient: prone

Stabilization: not required of the examiner

Test of the transverse part: with the shoulder flexed at 90°, the scapula is adducted in neutral rotation and resistance is applied over the scapula.

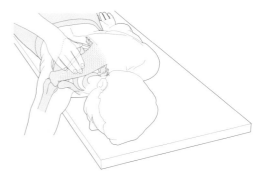

Trapezius

Test of the ascending part: the arm is raised and the patient's head is turned toward the side not being examined; the shoulder is abducted to 130° with resistance applied over the scapula in the direction of the depression.

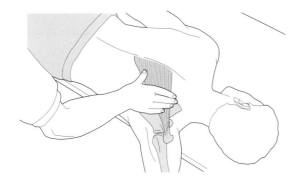

CLINICAL APPLICATIONS

- Stress-induced headache
- Whiplash injuries
- Symptomatic cervical disc herniation
- Neurological and motor shoulder rehabilitation
- Post-trauma and post-surgical shoulder rehabilitation
- Symptomatic shoulder stiffness
- Cervicobrachial syndrome

Combined Applications

- Adhesive capsulitis of the shoulder ➥ page 348
- Biceps brachii ➥ page 177
- Deltoid ➥ page 161
- Masseter ➥ page 109
- Sternocleidomastoid ➥ page 131

TAPE SPECIFICATIONS

Descending part
- 2 tapes
- Width 2.5 cm (1")
- Length 25 cm (10")
- Anchor 2 cm (0.75")
- Y-shaped

Transverse part
- 2 tapes
- Width 5 cm (2")
- Length 25 cm (10")
- Anchor 2 cm (0.75")
- W-shaped

Ascending part
- 2 tapes
- Width 5 cm (2")
- Length 30 cm (12")
- Anchor 2 cm (0.75")
- Y-shaped

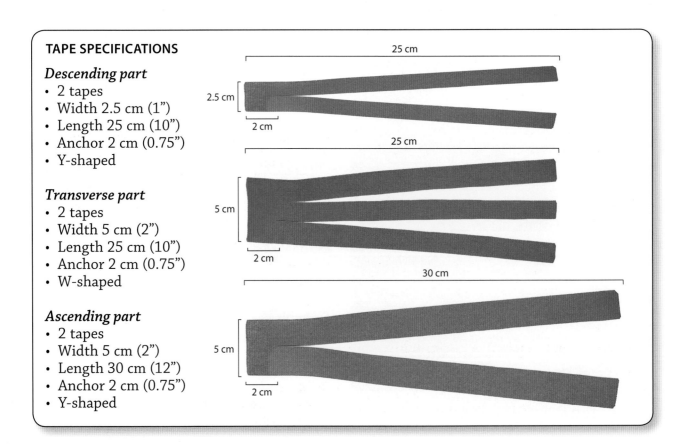

Descending Part of the Trapezius - Tape Application

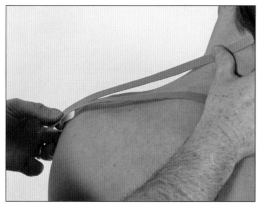
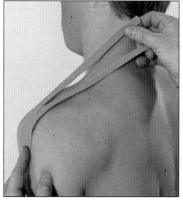
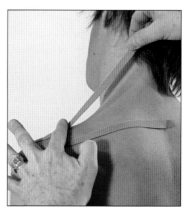

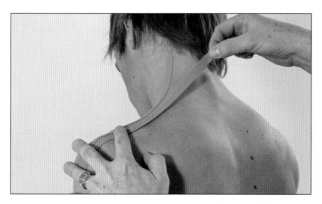

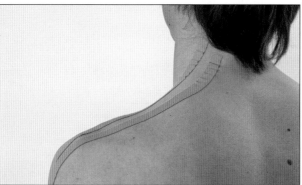

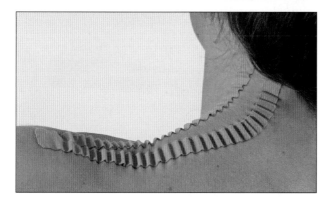

Descending part

- From 2.5 cm below the acromioclavicular joint to the hairline in the occipital region

- Head tilted away from the side of the application

1. Place the tape anchor 2.5 cm below the acromioclavicular joint.

2. For ease of application, remove the backing paper from the tape, except for the last 1.5 cm. First place one strip and then the other towards the scapula, following an oblique downward direction.

3. First fix the upper tape end, without applying tension, as far as the hairline, following the upper margin of the descending part of the trapezius.

4. Keeping the head tilted away from the application, the patient lowers their chin slightly and rotates the head to the same side (the side opposite to the application).

5. Apply the lower end of the tape without tension, outlining the posterior margin of the descending part of the trapezius.

6. Repeat the application, reversing the parameters, on the descending part of the trapezius on the opposite side.

Transverse Part of the Trapezius - Tape Application

Transverse part

📏 From the acromion along the spine of the scapula to 2 cm beyond the spinous processes of the upper thoracic vertebrae

🧍 Arm flexed to 90° and adducted, elbow flexed so as to touch the other shoulder with the hand

1. Place the base of the tape, which is cut in a W-shape, below the acromion.

2. Apply the tape, without tension, along the following paths:
- The upper strip along the upper margin of the scapula as far as the spinous process of C6
- The middle strip along the spine of the scapula as far as the spinous process of T1
- The lower strip below the spine of the scapula, curving downward toward the spinous process of T3.

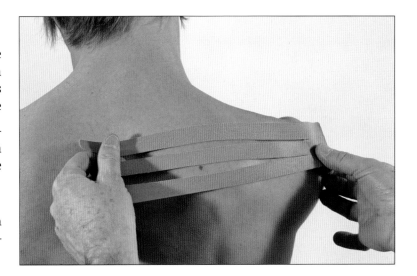

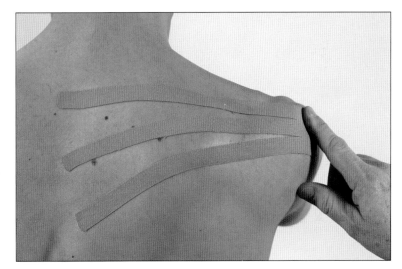

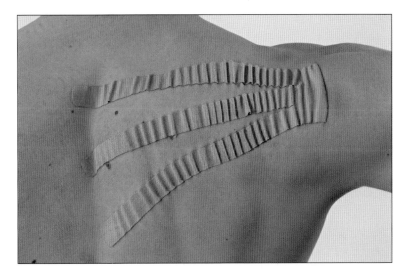

Ascending Part of the Trapezius - Tape Application

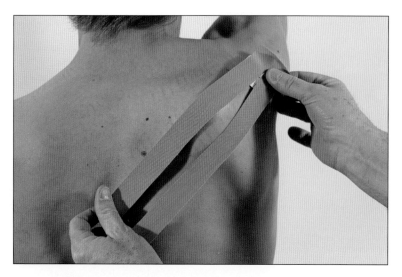

Ascending part

From the lateral end of the spine of the scapula to 2 cm beyond the spinous process of T12

Arm in full flexion and abduction, with associated slight medial rotation

1. Fix the tape anchor on the lateral border of the spine of the scapula.

2. Apply the tape, without tension, in the following way:
- The upper strip is applied below the spine of the scapula and then curves downward toward the spinous process of T7
- The lower strip is applied in the direction of the spinous process of T12, outlining the inferior margin of the ascending part of the trapezius.

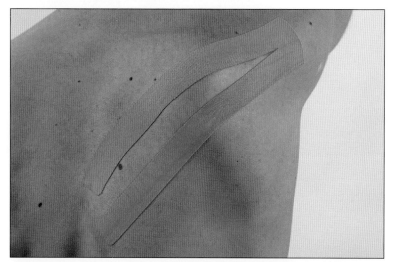

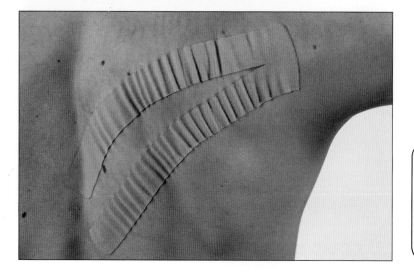

NOTE: As the trapezius muscle influences body posture, being connected with the spinal column, the application of the tape must always be bilateral and symmetrical.

LEVATOR SCAPULAE

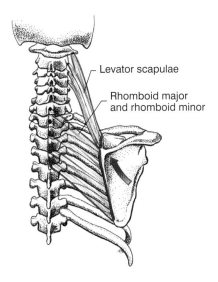

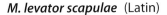
- Levator scapulae
- Rhomboid major and rhomboid minor

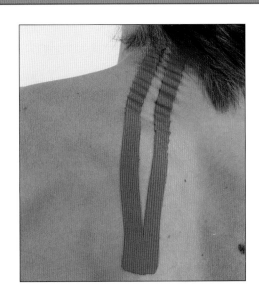

M. levator scapulae (Latin)

Origin: transverse processes of the first four cervical vertebrae

Insertion: medial margin of the scapula between the superior angle and the root of the spine of the scapula

Innervation: branches of the cervical plexus (C3, C4) and the dorsal nerve of the scapula (C4, C5)

Action: at its origin the levator scapulae muscle elevates and helps to rotate the scapula so as to guide the movement of the glenoid cavity in a caudal direction. At its insertion the muscle acts unilaterally to flex laterally and rotate the cervical vertebrae on the same side. Acting bilaterally, it can contribute to extension of the cervical spine.

CLINICAL APPLICATIONS

- Disorders of the capsule-ligament apparatus
- Post-traumatic and post-surgical shoulder rehabilitation
- Stiffness and limited rotation of the cervical spine
- Winged scapulae
- Shoulder impingement syndromes

Combined Applications

- Deltoid ➡ page 161
- Splenius cervicis ➡ page 129
- Sternocleidomastoid ➡ page 131

MUSCLE TEST

Patient: seated

Test: adduction and elevation of the scapula on one side (medial rotation of the inferior angle) against resistance and with the head turned to the same side (useful for location and good visualization of the levator scapulae)

Pressure: using one hand, the examiner applies pressure on the shoulder of the patient in the direction of lowering (depression) of the scapula.

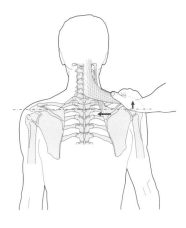

Levator Scapulae - Tape Application

TAPE SPECIFICATIONS

- 2 tapes
- Width 2.5 cm (1")
- Length 25 cm (10")
- Anchor 2 cm (0.75")
- Y-shaped

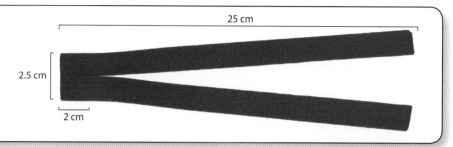

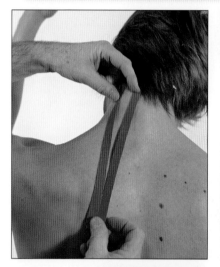
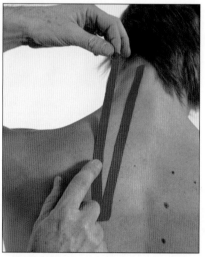
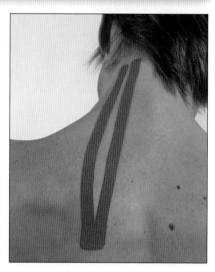

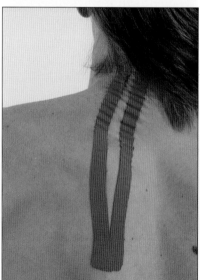

From 5 cm below the superomedial angle of the scapula to the hairline in the occipital region, plus 2 cm

Anterior flexion of the head and neck and their rotation away from the side of the muscle being treated

1. Anchor the tape just below the superomedial angle of the scapula, bilaterally.

2. For ease of application, remove the backing paper from the ends of the two strips of tape and lay them forward medially towards the descending part of the trapezius on both the left and the right.

3. Apply the internal strip, without tension, following the levator scapulae obliquely and medially as far as the transverse processes from C4 to C1, from which point it rises more vertically.

4. Then apply the external strip.

5. Repeat the operation on the opposite side. The head and neck are still flexed forward, but this time rotated in the other direction.

NOTE: As the levator scapulae influences body posture, being connected with the spinal column, the application of the tape must always be bilateral and symmetrical.

SERRATUS ANTERIOR

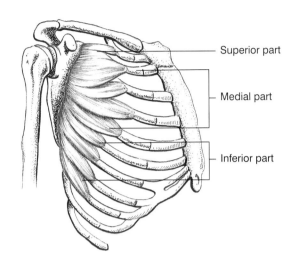

Superior part

Medial part

Inferior part

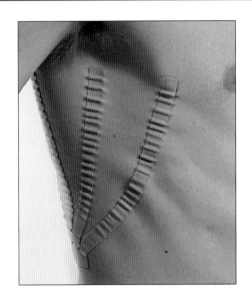

M. serratus anterior (Latin)

Origin: external surface and upper margin of the first eight or nine ribs

Insertion: medial margin and inferior angle of the scapula

Innervation: long thoracic nerve (C5, C6, C7, C8)

Action: rotation of the scapula with abduction and flexion of the arm, protraction of the scapula (forward thrust of the scapula that makes it adhere closely to the chest wall), which facilitates thrusting movements, such as push-ups

CLINICAL APPLICATIONS
- Panic attacks
- Dyspnea
- Painful contracture
- Chest pain not relieved by rest
- Rib injuries
- Winged scapulae
- Breast pain and sensitivity

Combined Applications

- Pectoralis major ➡ page 152
- Rectus abdominis ➡ page 200
- Rhomboid major ➡ page 148
- Rhomboid minor ➡ page 146
- Scalenus anterior ➡ page 118
- Scalenus posterior ➡ page 120
- Trapezius ➡ page 136

MUSCLE TEST

Patient: supine, shoulder flexed to 90°, slightly abducted, elbow extended

Test: the scapula is abducted (with protraction).

Pressure: on the distal end of the arm

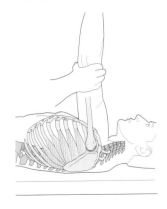

Serratus Anterior - Tape Application

TAPE SPECIFICATIONS

- 1 tape
- Width 5 cm (2")
- Length 30 cm (12")
- Anchor 2 cm (0.75")
- Fan-shaped with four strips

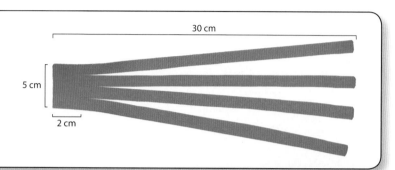

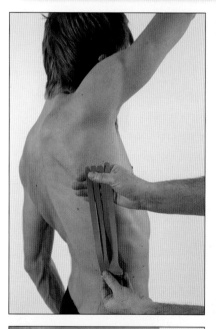

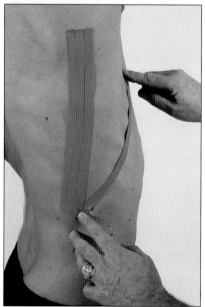

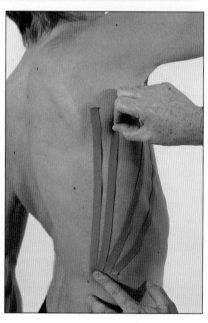

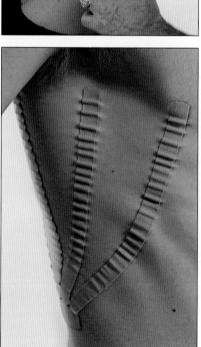

Application 1

 From the angle of the last rib to 2 cm beyond the inferior angle of the scapula

The patient inhales with the arm fully abducted

1. Apply the base to the floating rib for the tape to rise vertically.

2. Distribute the tape strips over the ribs, extending as far as the axillary fossa.

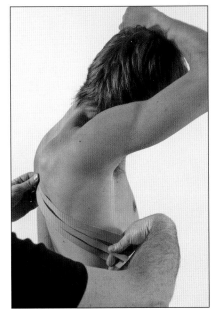
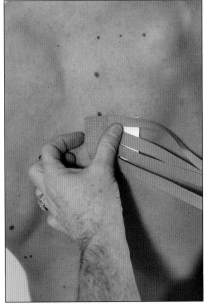
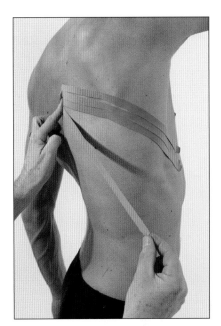

Application 2

🗒 From the transverse process of the eighth thoracic vertebra, following the curvature of the ribs as far as the costal arch

✝ The patient inhales with their arm fully abducted

1. Apply the tape anchor at the level of the eighth thoracic vertebra for the tape to extend horizontally.

2. Distribute the tape strips over the intercostal spaces as far as the sternum.

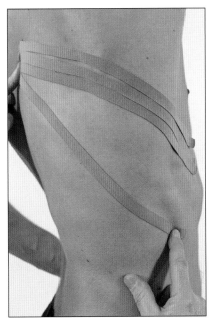
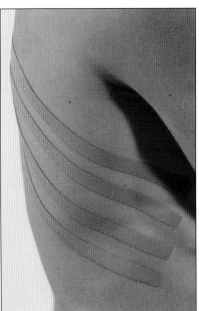

RHOMBOID MINOR

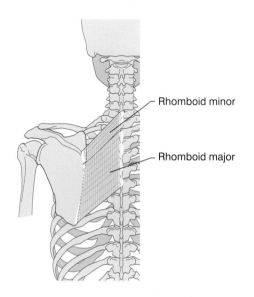

Rhomboid minor

Rhomboid major

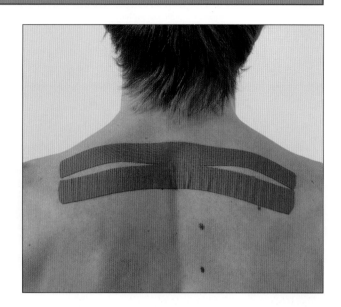

M. rhomboideus minor (Latin)

Origin
- Lower part of the nuchal ligament
- Spinous processes of the seventh cervical and first thoracic vertebrae

Insertion: medial margin of the scapula above the spine of the scapula

Innervation: dorsal nerve of the scapula (C5)

Action: the rhomboid muscle assists with downward, medial and lateral rotation of the scapula. Also, together with the latissimus dorsi, it contributes to maintaining correct posture. When good posture is not maintained, this influences the pectoralis minor and serratus anterior, causing the scapula to tilt to one side.

CLINICAL APPLICATIONS

- Pain at the base of the scapula (C7-T5)
- Neurological and motor rehabilitation of the shoulder
- Post-traumatic and post-surgical shoulder rehabilitation
- Shoulder stiffness
- Snapping scapula
- Rib subluxation

Combined Applications

- Infraspinatus ➥ page 172
- Latissimus dorsi ➥ page 158
- Scalenus anterior ➥ pagine 118
- Scalenus posterior ➥ pagine 120
- Descending part of the trapezius ➥ page 136

TAPE SPECIFICATIONS

- 1 tape
- Width 5 cm (2")
- Length 30 cm (12")
- Center anchor 2 cm (0.75")
- X-shaped

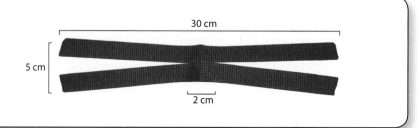

30 cm

5 cm

2 cm

Rhomboid Minor - Tape Application

🎗 From 2 cm before the supero-medial corner of the scapula to 2 cm beyond the superomedial corner of the scapula on the other side

🧍 Arms crossed with hands on shoulders and accentuated dorsal kyphosis

1. Cut the tape in an X-shape by folding it in half and then in half again for a further 5 cm, and cutting longitudinally as far as the first fold. The center of the X should be positioned over the spinous process of C7.

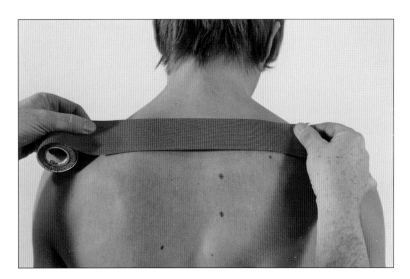

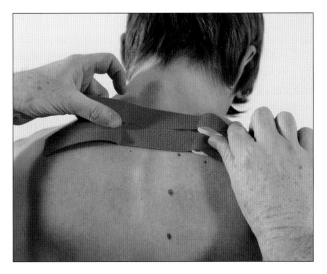

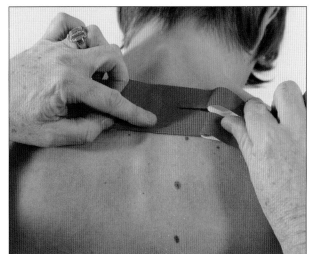

2. Remove the paper by tearing it at the center. The paper is then folded back. Holding the paper, apply the tape gently to the skin over the spinous process of C7.

3. Apply the four strips of tape forming the X, still without adding any tension, so that they end beyond the upper angle of the medial margin of the scapula.

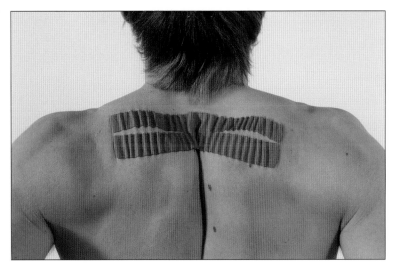

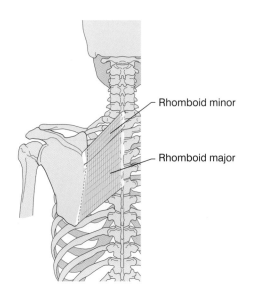

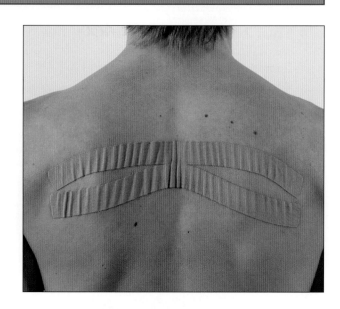

M. rhomboideus major (Latin)

Origin: spinous processes and corresponding supraspinous ligament of the first four thoracic vertebrae

Insertion: medial margin of the scapula between the spinal root and inferior angle of the scapula

Innervation: dorsal nerve of the scapula (C4-C6)

Action: the rhomboid major muscle aids the downward, medial and lateral rotation of the scapula. Also, together with the latissimus dorsi, it contributes to maintaining correct posture. When good posture is not maintained, this influences the pectoralis minor and serratus anterior, causing the scapula to tilt to one side.

the lever action that generates the pressure required for this test, the arm must be positioned as shown here. With the elbow flexed, the humerus is adducted toward the side of the body in slight extension and slight lateral rotation. This test determines the ability of the rhomboid major and rhomboid minor to hold the scapula in the test position during application of pressure against the arm.

Pressure: with one hand, the examiner applies pressure against the patient's arm in the direction of the abduction of the scapula and the lateral rotation of the inferior angle, and (using the other hand) against the patient's shoulder in the direction of its depression.

MUSCLE TEST

Patient: prone

Stabilization: not necessary on the part of the examiner. It is assumed that the adductor muscles of the shoulder have been found to be strong enough to support the arm which is used as a lever in this test.

Test: adduction and elevation of the scapula with medial rotation of its inferior angle. In order to obtain this position of the scapula and

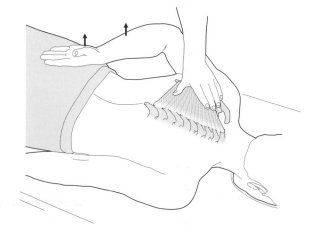

Rhomboid Major

CLINICAL APPLICATIONS

- Pain at the base of the scapula (C7-T5)
- Neurological and motor rehabilitation of the shoulder
- Post-traumatic and post-surgical shoulder rehabilitation
- Shoulder stiffness
- Snapping scapula
- Rib subluxation

Combined Applications

- Deltoid ➡ page 161
- Pectoralis major ➡ page 152
- Scalenus anterior ➡ page 118
- Scalenus posterior ➡ page 120
- Sternocleidomastoid ➡ page 131
- Trapezius ➡ page 136

TAPE SPECIFICATIONS

- 1 tape
- Width 5 cm (2")
- Length 35 cm (14")
- Center anchor 2 cm (0.75")
- X-shaped

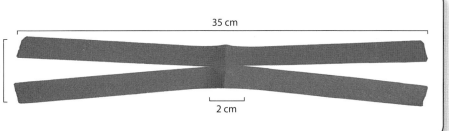

Rhomboid Major - Tape Application

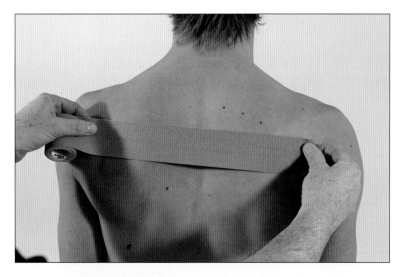

From 2 cm before the medial margin of the scapula to 2 cm beyond the medial margin of the scapula on the other side

Arms crossed with hands on shoulders and accentuated dorsal kyphosis

1. Cut the tape in an X-shape by folding it in half and then in half again for a further 5 cm, and cutting longitudinally as far as the first fold.

2. Position the center of the X midway between the spinous processes of T2 and T4.

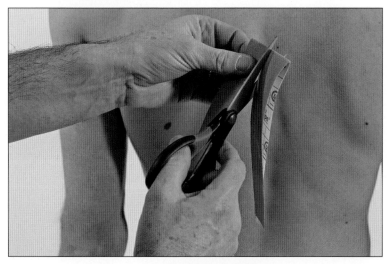

3. Remove the paper by tearing at the center. Fold the paper back on itself and apply the tape gently between the spinous processes of T2 and T4.

4. Apply the four tails of the X, still without adding tension, to beyond the medial margin of the scapula, ensuring that the ends of the upper and lower strips converge.

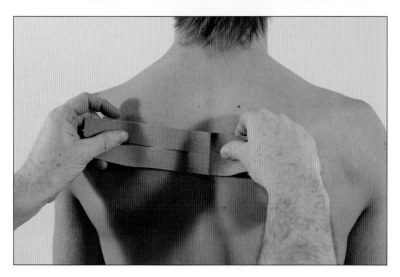

Rhomboid Major - Tape Application

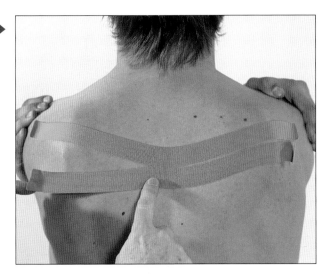
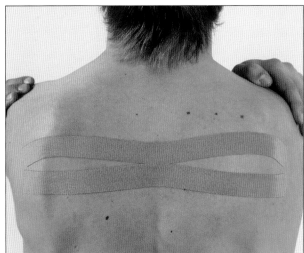

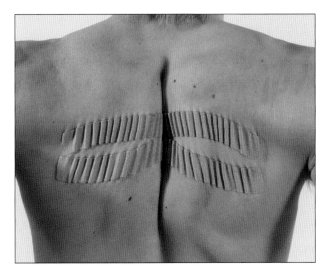
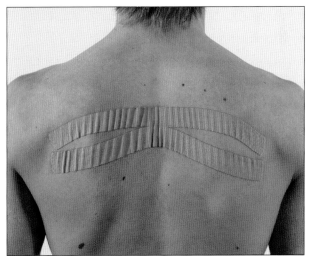

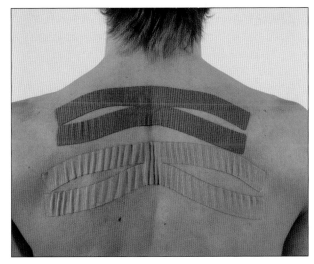

NOTE: A combined application can also be used to treat the rhomboid major and rhomboid minor muscles.

PECTORALIS MAJOR

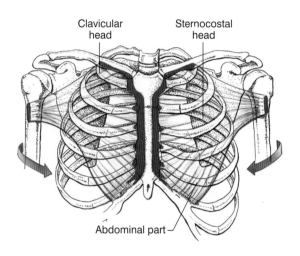

Clavicular head — Sternocostal head

Abdominal part

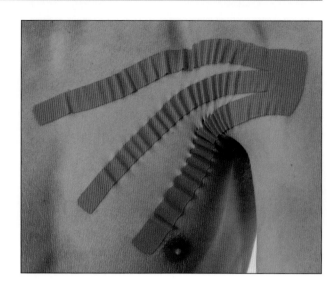

M. pectoralis major (Latin)

Origin
- *Clavicular part*: medial half of the anterior margin of the clavicle
- *Sternocostal part*: anterior surface of the sternum and costal cartilage of the second to sixth ribs
- *Abdominal part*: upper part of the rectus abdominis sheath

Insertion: crest of the greater tubercle of the humerus

Innervation: medial and lateral pectoral nerves (C5-C8 and T1)

Action: adducts and rotates the arm medially. From the point attached to the humerus, it raises the trunk. The clavicular part of the pectoralis major, together with the clavicular part of the deltoid, assists in flexion and adduction of the humerus. The sternocostal part enables upward and downward movements of the arm.

MUSCLE TEST

Clavicular and sternocostal parts

Patient: supine

Stabilization: the examiner holds the opposite shoulder firmly on the table; the triceps brachii keeps the elbow extended.

Test: with the elbow extended and the shoulder flexed to 90° and slightly rotated medially, the humerus is adducted toward the sternal end of the clavicle.

Pressure: against the distal end of the arm in the direction of horizontal abduction

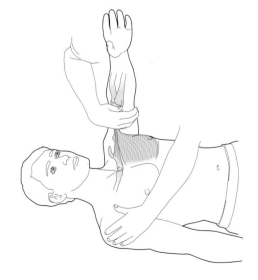

Abdominal part

Patient: supine

Stabilization: the examiner places one hand on the contralateral iliac crest to hold the pelvis firmly on the table. The anterior parts of the external and internal oblique muscles stabilize the thorax on the pelvis. In the presence of abdominal weakness, the thorax must be stabilized instead of the pelvis. The triceps brachii keeps the elbow extended.

Test: with the elbow extended and the shoulder flexed and slightly rotated medially, the arm is adducted obliquely toward the contralateral iliac crest.

Pressure: on the anterior surface of the arm, just above the elbow joint

CLINICAL APPLICATIONS

- Bronchitis and asthma
- Midscapular back pain
- Chest pains
- Anterior shoulder pain
- Pain in hands and paresthesia (numbness)
- Facilitation of chest cavity enlargement prior to breast implant surgery
- Shoulder girdle disorders
- Post-surgical or post oncological rehabilitation of the breast
- Post-surgical cardiac rehabilitation
- Post-myocardial infarction rehabilitation

Combined Applications

- Coracobrachialis ➡ page 210
- Latissimus dorsi ➡ page 158
- Rhomboid major ➡ page 148
- Rhomboid minor ➡ page 146
- Supraspinatus ➡ page 165
- Teres minor ➡ page 170
- Descending and transverse parts of the trapezius ➡ page 136

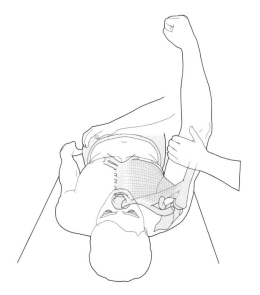

TAPE SPECIFICATIONS

- 1 tape
- Width 5 cm (2")
- Length 25 cm (10")
- Anchor 2 cm (0.75")
- W-shaped or Y-shaped

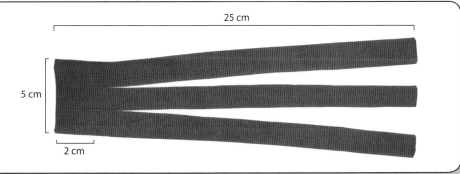

25 cm

5 cm

2 cm

Pectoralis Major - Tape Application

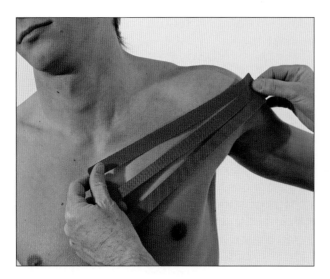 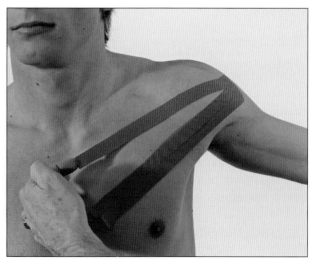

🎞️ From 5 cm beyond the intertubercular (or bicipital) groove of the humerus

🤸 Arm abducted to 90° and slightly extended, head turned in the opposite direction

1. Cut the tape in a Y-shape or W-shape. Position the tape base 5 cm beyond the intertubercular groove of the humerus.

2. At this point, remove the backing paper from the tape, except for the last 2.5 cm, and position the two or three strip ends momentarily at the center of the sternum.

3. Take the uppermost strip end beyond the front surface of the sternal end of the clavicle; apply it without tension. Then take the central strip and position it beyond the insertion of the sixth costal cartilage into the sternum.

4. Finally, take the lower strip beyond the abdominal part of the anterior layer of the rectus abdominis muscle sheath and apply it without tension. As the three strips are applied, the patient should progressively increase the abduction of the arm.

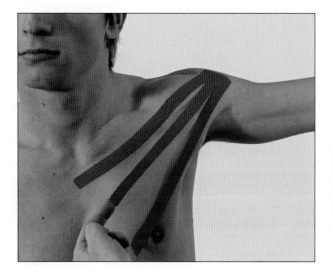 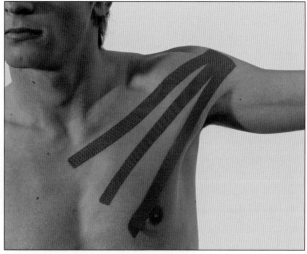

PECTORALIS MINOR

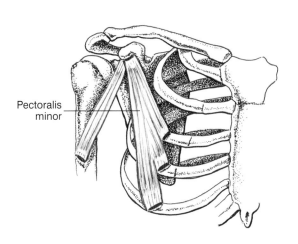

Pectoralis minor

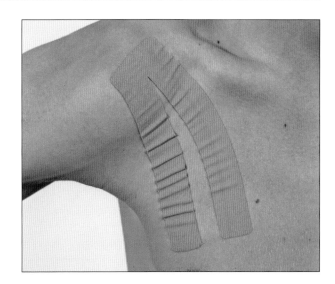

M. pectoralis minor (Latin)

Origin: upper surfaces of the second, third and fourth ribs

Insertion: coracoid process of the scapula

Innervation: medial and lateral pectoral nerves (C5-C8 and T1)

Action: adduction and internal rotation of the arm: with the end fixed on the humerus, it raises the trunk. It is divided into two parts: one is inserted in the coracoid process of the scapula and the other originates from the ribs. The first, together with the clavicular part of the deltoid, assists in horizontal flexion of the humerus, while the second allows upward and downward movements of the arm.

MUSCLE TEST

Patient: supine

Stabilization: not necessary on the part of the examiner, unless the abdominal muscles are weak, in which case the ipsilateral rib cage should be firmly held down.

Test: push the shoulder forward with the arm lying along the side. The patient should not exert any downward pressure with the hand to push the shoulder forward (if necessary, raise the patient's hand and elbow from the table).

Pressure: against the anterior surface of the shoulder, downwards in the direction of the table

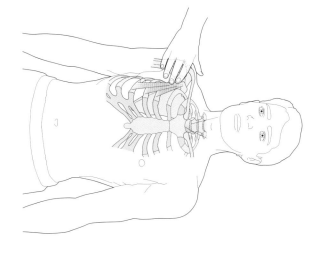

Pectoralis Minor

CLINICAL APPLICATIONS

- Bronchitis and asthma
- Anterior shoulder pain
- Midscapular back pain
- Chest pains
- Pain in hands and paresthesia (numbness)
- Facilitation of chest cavity enlargement prior to breast implant surgery
- Shoulder girdle disorders
- Post-surgical and post-oncological rehabilitation of the breast

- Post-surgical cardiac rehabilitation
- Post-myocardial infarction respiratory rehabilitation

Combined Applications

- Latissimus dorsi ➠ page 158
- Supraspinatus ➠ page 165
- Teres minor ➠ page 170
- Transverse part of the trapezius ➠ page 136

TAPE SPECIFICATIONS

- 1 tape
- Width 5 cm (2")
- Length 20 cm (8")
- Anchor 2 cm (0.75")
- Y-shaped

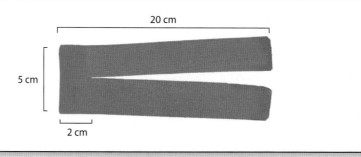

Pectoralis Minor - Tape Application

From 2 cm above the coracoid process of the scapula to the fifth rib

Arm abducted to 90° and slightly extended, head turned away from the side of the application

1. Position the tape anchor 2 cm beyond the coracoid process of the scapula.

2. In this position, apply the medial strip, without tension, directing it downward towards the second rib. Then apply the lateral strip towards the fifth rib.

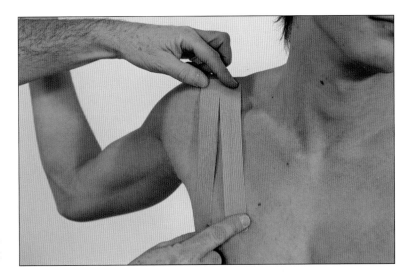

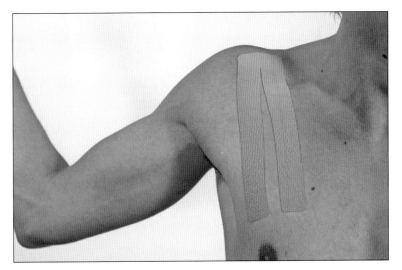

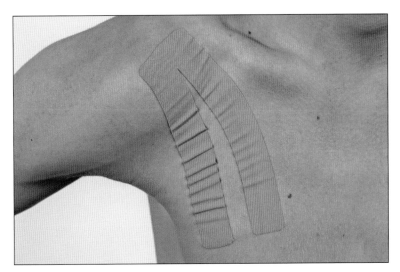

LATISSIMUS DORSI

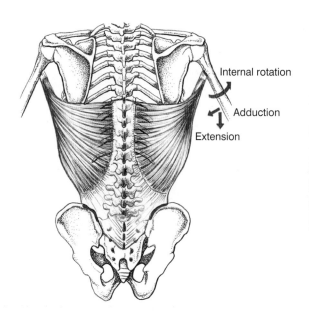

Internal rotation

Adduction

Extension

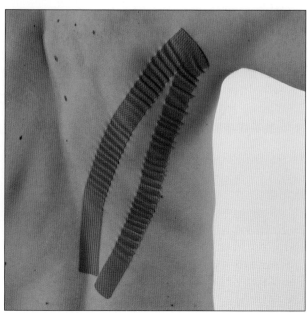

M. latissimus dorsi (Latin)

Origin
- Posterior lamina of the thoracolumbar fascia which originates from the spinous processes of the last six thoracic vertebrae and the lumbar vertebrae; median sacral crest; posterior surface of the iliac crest
- Last three or four ribs: inferior angle of the scapula

Insertion: intertubercular groove of the humerus

Innervation: thoracodorsal nerve (C6, C7, C8)

Action: the latissimus dorsi is a wide, thin, triangu-

lar muscle. From the last six thoracic vertebrae and the lumbar vertebrae the muscle belly gradually becomes thinner; its bands are oriented in an upward and lateral direction, passing the last three or four ribs dorsally, before insertion into the crest of the lesser tubercle of the humerus.

In adduction and medial rotation of the shoulder or glenohumeral joint, and especially in adduction of the arm, the latissimus dorsi exerts its main force on the pectoralis major. At the same time this muscle pushes back the humerus and the scapula. If this action is missing, the weight of the body cannot be sustained.

MUSCLE TEST

Patient: prone

Test: extension of the shoulder held in adduction with the arm lying along the side of the body, rotated medially, and the palm of the hand turned upward.

Pressure: the examiner applies pressure to the posteromedial aspect of the arm.

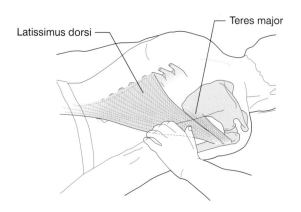

Latissimus dorsi — Teres major

Latissimus Dorsi - Tape Application

CLINICAL APPLICATIONS

- Chest pain
- Idiopathic scoliosis
- Frozen shoulder (adhesive capsulitis)

Combined Applications

- Biceps brachii ➡ page 177

- Pectoralis major ➡ page 152
- Rhomboid major ➡ page 148
- Rhomboid minor ➡ page 146
- Scalenus anterior ➡ page 118
- Scalenus posterior ➡ page 120
- Subscapularis ➡ page 174
- Transverse part of the trapezius ➡ page 136

TAPE SPECIFICATIONS

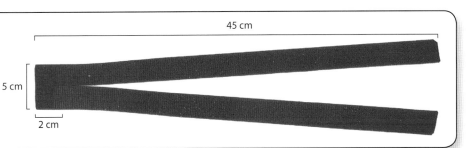

- 2 tapes
- Width 5 cm (2")
- Length 45 cm (18")
- Anchor 2 cm (0.75")
- Y-shaped

45 cm

5 cm

2 cm

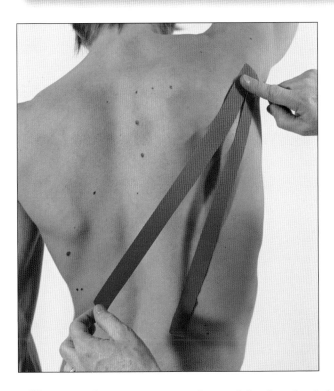
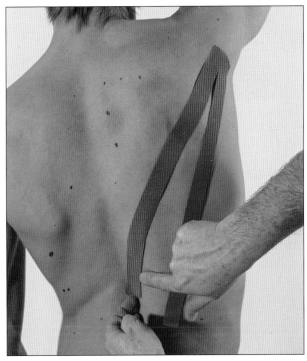

From the posterior surface of the head of the humerus to the spinous processes of the third and fourth lumbar vertebrae

Slight forward flexion of the trunk, which is bent to the side opposite to that of the muscle to be treated; the ipsilateral arm is raised

1. Apply the tape anchor below the posterior surface of the head of the humerus.

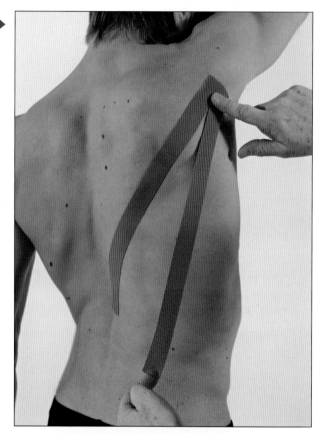

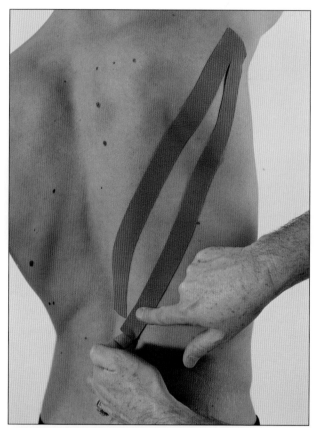

2. Apply the medial strip without tension in the direction of the last costovertebral joints then vertically down as far as the transverse process of the third lumbar vertebra.

3. Apply the lateral strip without tension in the direction of the transverse process of the fourth lumbar vertebra.

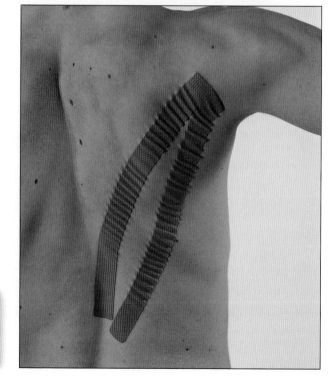

NOTE: As the latissimus dorsi influences body posture, being connected with the spinal column, the application of the tape must always be bilateral and symmetrical.

DELTOID

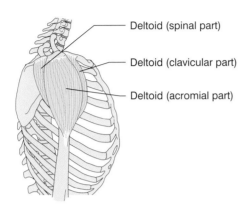

- Deltoid (spinal part)
- Deltoid (clavicular part)
- Deltoid (acromial part)

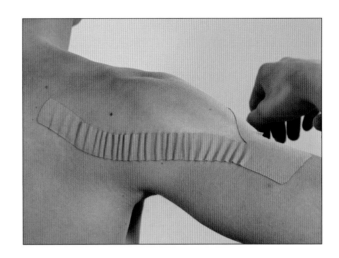

M. deltoideus (Latin)

Origin
- *Clavicular part*: anterior margin and upper surface of the lateral third of the clavicle
- *Acromial part*: lateral margin and upper surface of the acromion
- *Spinal part*: posterior margin of the spine of the scapula

Insertion: deltoid tuberosity, located in the middle third of the anterolateral surface of the humeral diaphysis; the rough surface of the humerus is also known as the "deltoid V".

Innervation: axillary nerve (C5-C6)

Action
- *Clavicular part*: flexes and medially rotates the humerus.
- *Acromial part*: abducts the humerus at the shoulder joint after activation of the supraspinatus.
- *Spinal part*: extends and laterally rotates the humerus.

The clavicular part enables the arm to move forward and rotate medially; the acromial part enhances abduction while the spinal part is responsible for backward movement and external rotation, thereby checking the strong pressure applied among the muscles.

MUSCLE TEST

Clavicular part

Patient: seated

Stabilization: if the scapular stabilizing muscles are weak, the examiner should stabilize the scapula. When pressure is applied on the arm (distal third), counter pressure should be applied posteriorly on the shoulder girdle.

Test: abduction and slight flexion of the shoulder with the humerus slightly rotated externally. With the patient sitting upright, position the humerus in slight external rotation so as to increase the effect of gravity on the clavicular part of the deltoid. (The natural action of this part of the muscle, which involves slight medial rotation, is part of the test performed in the supine position.)

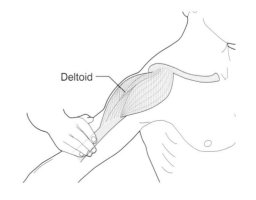

Deltoid

Deltoid

Pressure: against the ventral medial surface of the arm in the direction of adduction and slight extension

Spinal part

Patient: seated

Stabilization: if the scapular stabilizing muscles are weak, the examiner should stabilize the scapula. When pressure is applied on the arm, counter pressure should be applied anteriorly on the shoulder girdle.

Test: abduction and slight extension of the shoulder with the humerus in slight medial rotation; with the patient sitting upright, position the humerus in slight medial rotation in order to make the spinal part of the deltoid work against gravity. (The natural action of this part of the muscle, which involves slight external rotation, is part of the test performed in the prone position.)

Pressure: against the posterolateral surface of the arm, above the elbow, in the direction of adduction and slight flexion

CLINICAL APPLICATIONS

- Subacromial bursitis
- Acromioclavicular dislocation
- Chronic instability of the shoulder
- Neurological and motor rehabilitation of the shoulder
- Post-traumatic and post-surgical shoulder rehabilitation
- Reduced movement and range of motion particularly in abduction
- Impingement syndrome
- Tendonitis of the rotator cuff and osteoarthritis of the acromioclavicular joint

Combined applications

- Infraspinatus ➥ page 172
- Rhomboid major ➥ page 148
- Rhomboid minor ➥ page 146
- Supraspinatus ➥ page 165
- Teres minor ➥ page 170
- Descending part of the trapezius ➥ page 136

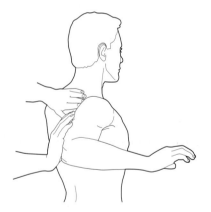

TAPE SPECIFICATIONS

- 1 tape
- Width 5 cm (2")
- Length 25 cm (10")
- Anchor 5 cm (2")
- Y-shaped

25 cm

5 cm

5 cm

Deltoid - Tape Application

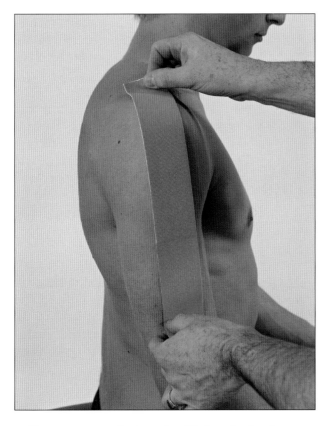 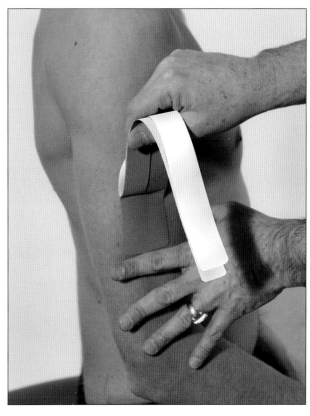

📏 From 5 cm below the "deltoid V" tuberosity of the humerus to 2.5 cm beyond the acromioclavicular joint

🧍 Arm hanging down the side

1. The patient is in a natural position with the arm hanging down the side. The therapist should remove the backing paper only from the tape anchor and position it below and slightly in front of the "deltoid V", leaving the two tape strips free with their backing on.

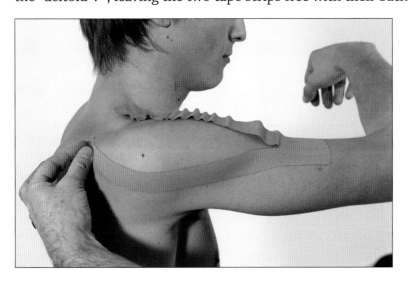

2. For ease of application, remove the backing paper from the two tails, except for the last 2.5 cm. Lay the strips on the center of the acromioclavicular joint.

▶

Deltoid - Tape Application

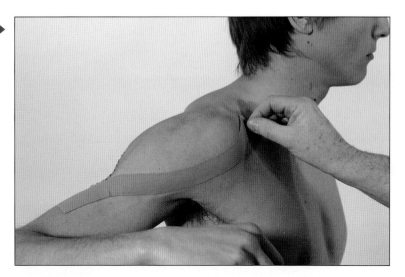

3. At this point, the patient should flex the elbow to 90°, and then abduct their arm to shoulder level, at 90°.

4. With the patient extending the arm, apply the tape to the clavicular part of the deltoid without any tension, outlining the edges of the muscle without applying the tape over the muscle belly. To avoid irritation, the tape end should not be applied in the area of the upper opening of the thorax.

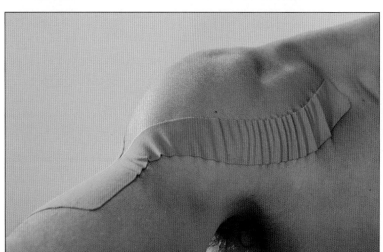

5. With the patient flexing the arm forward 90°, apply the tape to the spinal part of the deltoid, with no tension. Take care that the posterior strip does not overlap the anterior one.

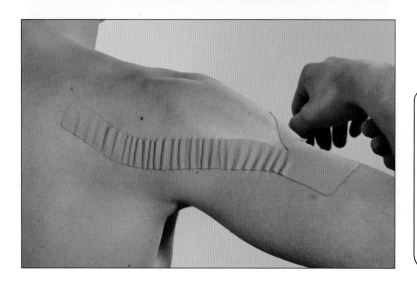

NOTE: With this application the deltoid will receive a continuous anteroposterior eccentric stimulus during normal daily movements. The final effect is a decoaptation action on the glenohumeral joint. Since this is a muscle that is not connected with the spine, application on one side only is appropriate.

SUPRASPINATUS

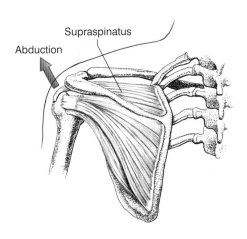

Abduction

Supraspinatus

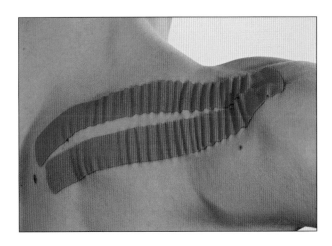

M. sopraspinatus (Latin)

Origin: medial two thirds of the supraspinatus fossa of the scapula

Insertion: upper facet of the greater tubercle of the humerus and glenohumeral joint capsule

Innervation: suprascapular nerve (C4, C5, C6)

Action: abducts the shoulder joint and stabilizes the head of the humerus in the glenoid cavity during movement of this joint.

CLINICAL APPLICATIONS

- Subacromial bursitis
- Idiopathic capsulitis
- Loss of strength in abduction
- Neurological and motor rehabilitation of the shoulder
- Post-traumatic and post-surgical shoulder rehabilitation
- Impingement syndrome of the rotator cuff
- Calcific tendonitis
- Rotator cuff tendonitis

Combined applications

- Biceps brachii ➥ page 177
- Deltoid ➥ page 161
- Latissimus dorsi ➥ page 158
- Pectoralis major ➥ page 152
- Teres minor ➥ page 170

MUSCLE TEST

Patient: sitting or standing with the arm hanging at the side, head and neck extended and bent laterally to the same side: face turned toward the opposite side

Stabilization: not necessary, since the test does not require great pressure

Test: initiation of abduction of the humerus

Pressure: against the forearm in the direction of adduction

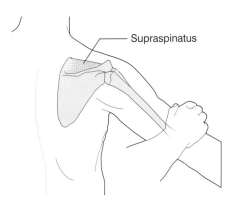

Supraspinatus

Supraspinatus - Tape Application

TAPE SPECIFICATIONS

- 1 tape
- Width 5 cm (2")
- Length 25 cm (10")
- Anchor 2 cm (0.75")
- Y-shaped

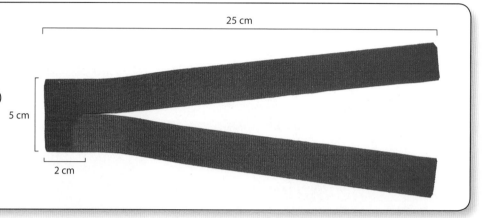

25 cm

5 cm

2 cm

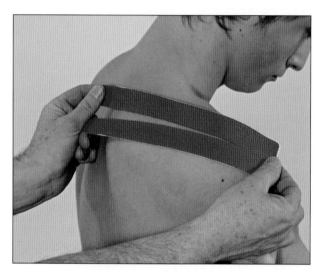

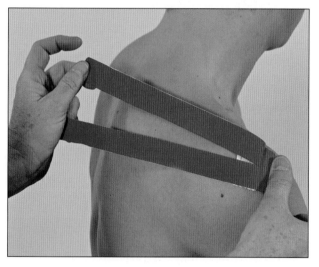

From the greater tubercle of the humerus to 2 cm beyond the superior angle of the scapula

Arm naturally adducted down the patient's side and rotated medially, with elbow flexed and forearm resting on the abdomen

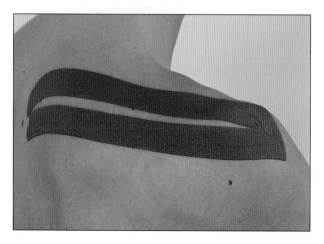

1. Place the tape anchor over the greater tubercle of the humerus.

2. Remove the backing paper from the two strips of tape, leaving the final 2.5 cm and then, for ease of application, lay these momentarily below the spine of the scapula.

3. Apply the upper strip just above the supraspinatus fossa of the scapula, outlining the superior angle of the scapula. Apply the lower strip parallel to the first, just below the spine of the scapula.

TERES MAJOR

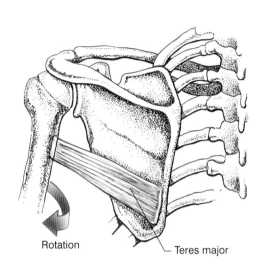

Rotation — Teres major

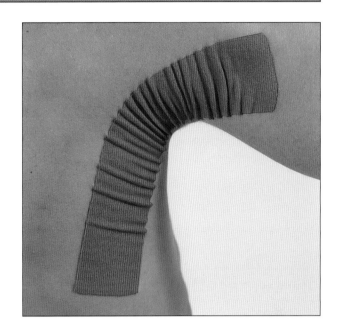

M. teres major (Latin)

Origin: posterior surface of the inferior angle of the scapula

Insertion: crest of the lesser tubercle or medial lip of the intertubercular groove of the humerus

Innervation: lower subscapular nerve (C5-C7)

Action: the teres major is in relation with the latissimus dorsi, the long head of the triceps brachii, and with the subscapularis and coracobrachialis muscles. Its lower margin, together with the latissimus dorsi and teres minor, forms the posterior wall of the axillary fossa. Its main actions are adduction, extension and internal rotation of the humerus. It works in synergy with the latissimus dorsi. It also plays an important role in arm retroversion. It stabilizes the glenohumeral joint. When the teres major contributes to the medial rotation of the humerus, it succeeds in raising the humerus to about 90°.

MUSCLE TEST

Patient: prone

Stabilization: not usually required, since the weight of the trunk provides sufficient stabilization. If necessary, the contralateral shoulder can be held down on the table.

Test: extension and adduction of the humerus in the medially rotated position with the hand resting on the posterior part of the iliac crest

Pressure: against the arm, above the elbow, in the direction of adduction and flexion

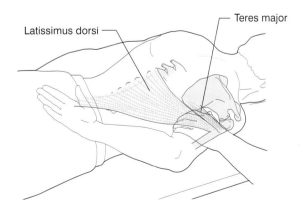

Latissimus dorsi — — Teres major

Teres Major

CLINICAL APPLICATIONS

- Calcific tendonitis of the supraspinatus
- Frozen shoulder (adhesive capsulitis)
- Shoulder pain caused by playing golf or baseball
- Cervical pain syndrome
- Shoulder impingement syndrome
- Rotator cuff tendonitis

Combined Applications

- Biceps brachii ➡ page 177
- Pectoralis major ➡ page 152
- Rhomboid major ➡ page 148
- Rhomboid minor ➡ page 146
- Supraspinatus ➡ page 165
- Descending part of the trapezius ➡ page 136

TAPE SPECIFICATIONS

- 1 tape
- Width 5 cm (2")
- Length 25 cm (10")
- I-shaped

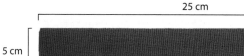

25 cm

5 cm

Teres Major - Tape Application

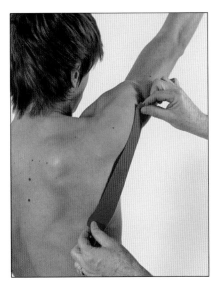 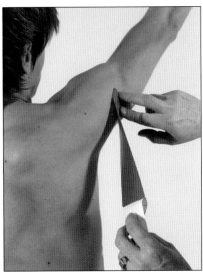 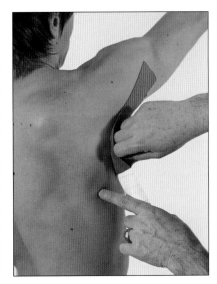

From 5 cm below the lower angle of the scapula to 5 cm beyond the intertubercular groove of the humerus

Arm flexed to 120°, slightly abducted and externally rotated

1. In neutral position, secure the tape anchor 5 cm before the origin on the scapula while the patient performs an external rotation and abduction of the arm with elbow extended.

2. Remove the backing paper from the tape except for the last 5 cm. Fold the paper back and take the free end of the tape in one hand; apply it with no tension along the belly of the teres major, ending 5 cm beyond its humeral insertion.

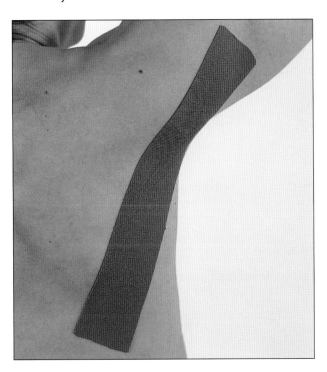 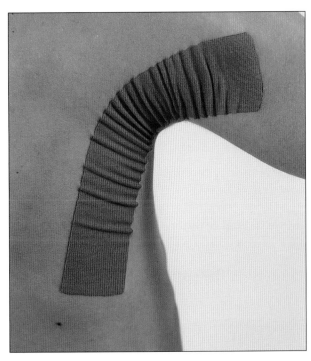

TERES MINOR

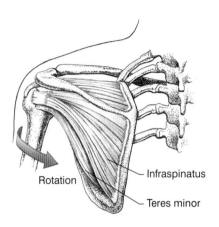

Rotation — Infraspinatus — Teres minor

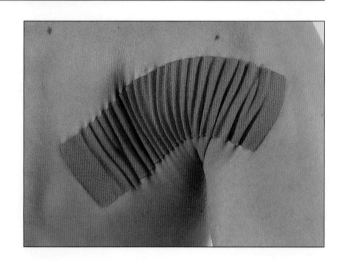

M. teres minor (Latin)

Origin: upper two thirds of the posterior surface of the scapula, near the lateral margin

Insertion: medial lip of the intertubercular groove of the humerus

Innervation: axillary nerve (C5, C6)

Action: the teres minor together with the infraspinatus aids in external rotation of the humerus. In addition, the supraspinatus and subscapularis muscles (external rotators) keep the head of the humerus in the glenoid cavity.

CLINICAL APPLICATIONS

- Subacromial bursitis
- Adhesive capsulitis
- Rotator cuff injuries
- Brachial neuralgia
- Tendinopathy of the biceps brachii

Combined applications

- Biceps brachii ➥ page 177
- Pectoralis major ➥ page 152
- Rhomboid major ➥ page 148
- Rhomboid minor ➥ page 146
- Supraspinatus ➥ page 165
- Descending part of the trapezius ➥ page 136

MUSCLE TEST

Patient: prone, shoulder abducted to 90° and elbow bent 90°

Test: external rotation of the shoulder with the back of the hand facing up

Pressure: on the posterior surface of the forearm just above the wrist

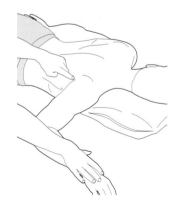

Teres Minor - Tape Application

TAPE SPECIFICATIONS
- 1 tape
- Width 5 cm (2")
- Length 20 cm (8")
- I-shaped

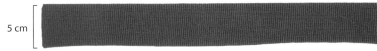

20 cm

5 cm

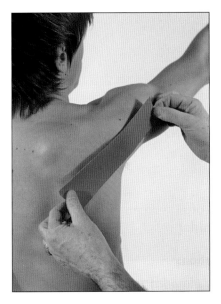 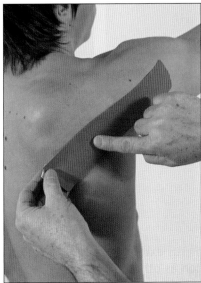 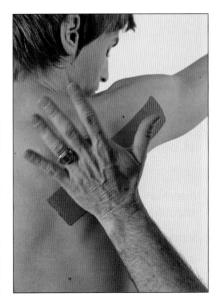

From 5 cm beyond the lateral margin of the scapula to the intertubercular groove of the humerus

Arm flexed and abducted about 120° forward, elbow extended

1. Secure the tape anchor 5 cm beyond the intertubercular groove of the humerus.

2. Remove the backing paper from the tape except for the last 5 cm and fold it back. Take the free end of the tape in one hand and apply it with no tension along the belly of the teres minor, ending 5 cm beyond the lateral margin of the scapula.

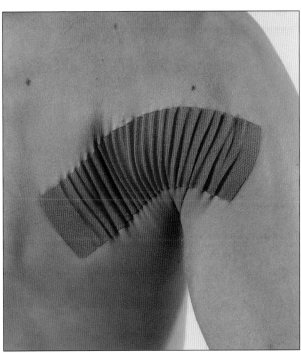

SUBSCAPULARIS

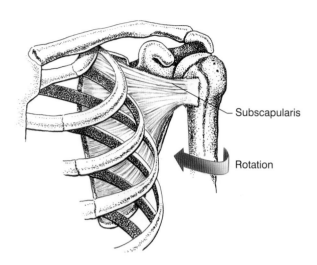

Subscapularis

Rotation

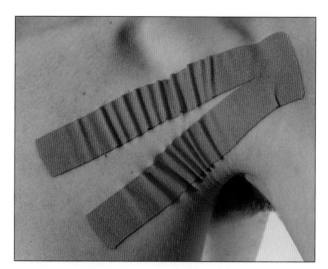

M. subscapularis (Latin)

Origin: subscapular fossa of the scapula

Insertion: lesser tubercle of the humerus, shoulder joint capsule

Innervation: upper and lower subscapular nerves (C5, C6, C7)

Action: like the other components of the rotator cuff, this muscle stabilizes the glenohumeral joint. It works mainly by preventing the head of the humerus from being pushed upward by the deltoid and biceps brachii muscles and by the long head of the triceps brachii. It rotates the humerus medially.

CLINICAL APPLICATIONS

- Adhesive capsulitis
- Limited abduction and external rotation movements
- Shoulder impingement syndrome
- Rotator cuff tendonitis

Combined applications

- Infraspinatus ➥ page 172
- Rhomboid major ➥ page 148
- Rhomboid minor ➥ page 146

MUSCLE TEST

Patient: prone, shoulder abducted 90° and elbow flexed 90°

Test: internal rotation of the shoulder with the palm of the hand facing up

Pressure: against the forearm just above the wrist with the elbow kept at a right angle

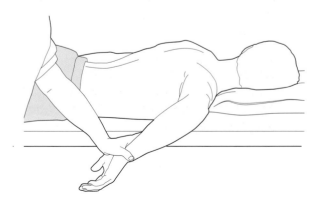

Teres Minor - Tape Application

TAPE SPECIFICATIONS
- 1 tape
- Width 5 cm (2")
- Length 20 cm (8")
- I-shaped

5 cm

20 cm

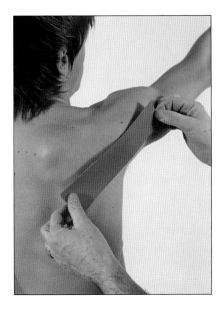
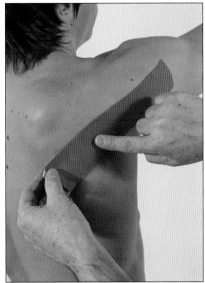
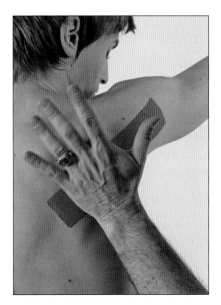

From 5 cm beyond the lateral margin of the scapula to the intertubercular groove of the humerus

Arm flexed and abducted about 120° forward, elbow extended

1. Secure the tape anchor 5 cm beyond the intertubercular groove of the humerus.

2. Remove the backing paper from the tape except for the last 5 cm and fold it back. Take the free end of the tape in one hand and apply it with no tension along the belly of the teres minor, ending 5 cm beyond the lateral margin of the scapula.

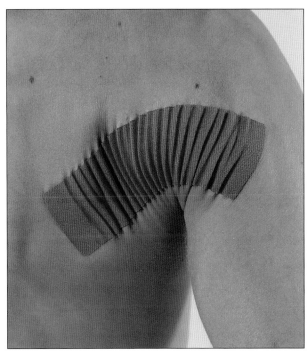

INFRASPINATUS

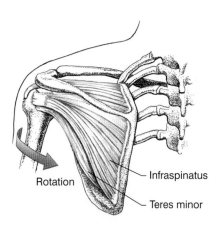

Rotation
— Infraspinatus
— Teres minor

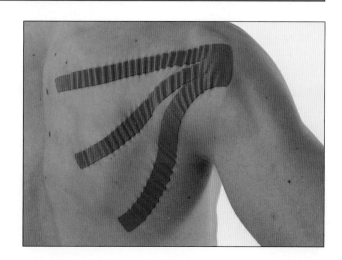

M. infraspinatus (Latin)

Origin: infraspinatus fossa of the scapula

Insertion: greater tubercle of the humerus and shoulder joint capsule

Innervation: suprascapular nerve (C4, C5, C6)

Action: this muscle rotates the humerus externally. It has exactly the same function as other components of the rotator cuff and helps prevent dislocation of the shoulder.

CLINICAL APPLICATIONS

- Adhesive capsulitis
- Hemiplegia
- Neuropathy
- Reduced range of movement
- Rotator cuff tendonitis

Combined Applications

- Biceps brachii ➥ page 177
- Levator scapulae ➥ page 141
- Pectoralis major ➥ page 152
- Subscapularis ➥ page 174
- Descending part of the trapezius ➥ page 136

MUSCLE TEST

Patient: prone, shoulder abducted 90° and elbow flexed 90°

Test: external rotation of the shoulder with the back of the hand facing up

Pressure: on the posterior surface of the forearm just above the wrist

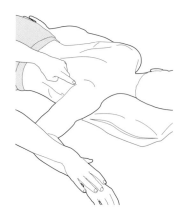

Infraspinatus - Tape Application

TAPE SPECIFICATIONS

- 1 tape
- Width 5 cm (2")
- Length 20 cm (8")
- Anchor 2 cm (0.75")
- W-shaped

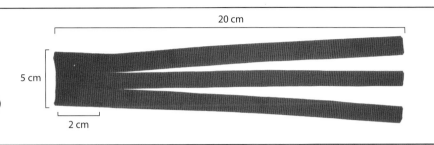

20 cm

5 cm

2 cm

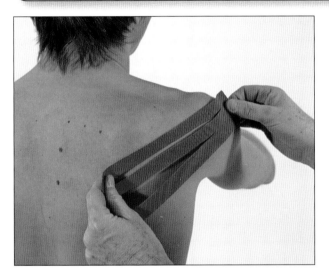

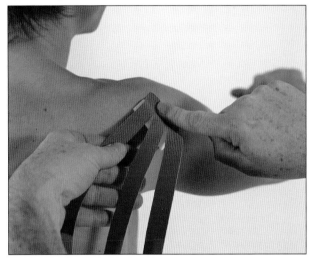

🔖 From the greater tubercle of the humerus to 2 cm beyond the medial margin of the scapula

👕 Arm flexed forward 90°, slightly internally rotated

1. Fix the tape anchor below the acromion, on the greater tubercle of the humerus.

2. With no tension, secure the ends of the W over the upper margin, at the center and toward the inferior angle of the scapula respectively.

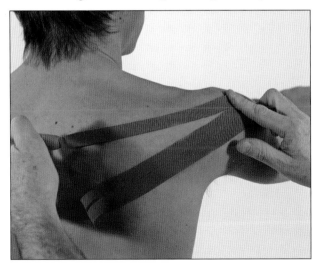

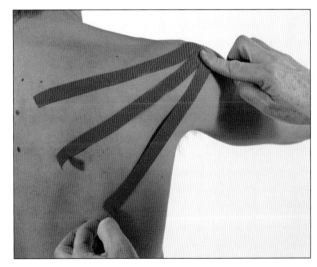

SUBSCAPULARIS

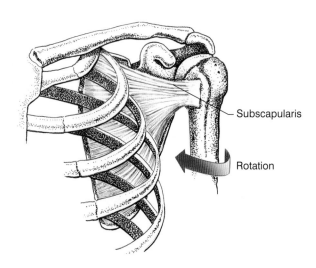

Subscapularis

Rotation

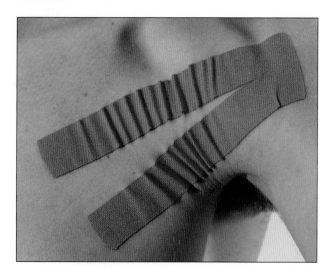

M. subscapularis (Latin)

Origin: subscapular fossa of the scapula

Insertion: lesser tubercle of the humerus, shoulder joint capsule

Innervation: upper and lower subscapular nerves (C5, C6, C7)

Action: like the other components of the rotator cuff, this muscle stabilizes the glenohumeral joint. It works mainly by preventing the head of the humerus from being pushed upward by the deltoid and biceps brachii muscles and by the long head of the triceps brachii. It rotates the humerus medially.

CLINICAL APPLICATIONS

- Adhesive capsulitis
- Limited abduction and external rotation movements
- Shoulder impingement syndrome
- Rotator cuff tendonitis

Combined applications

- Infraspinatus ➥ page 172
- Rhomboid major ➥ page 148
- Rhomboid minor ➥ page 146

MUSCLE TEST

Patient: prone, shoulder abducted 90° and elbow flexed 90°

Test: internal rotation of the shoulder with the palm of the hand facing up

Pressure: against the forearm just above the wrist with the elbow kept at a right angle

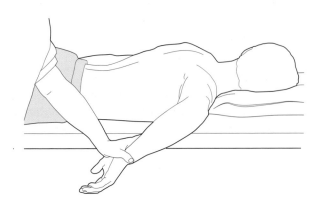

Subscapularis - Tape Application

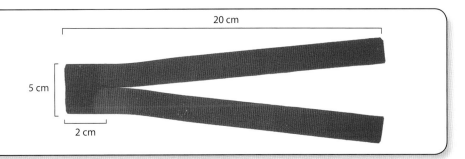

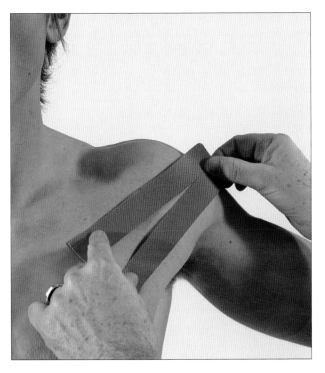
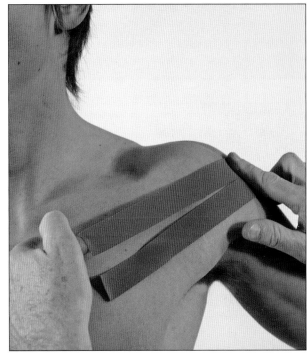

From 5 cm beyond the intertubercular groove of the humerus to the medial third of the clavicle

Upper limb abducted to about 45°, slightly extended and externally rotated

Y-shaped application

1. Position the tape anchor 5 cm beyond the intertubercular groove of the humerus.

2. For ease of application, remove the backing paper from the tape, except for the last 2.5 cm and place the two tape ends at the center of the sternum.

3. Apply the upper strip, without tension, in the direction of the third rib. Apply the lower strip, directing it toward the sixth rib.

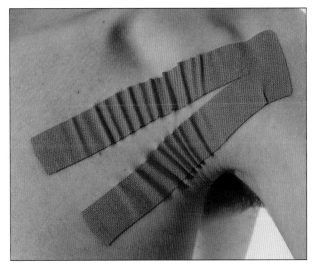

Subscapularis - Tape Application

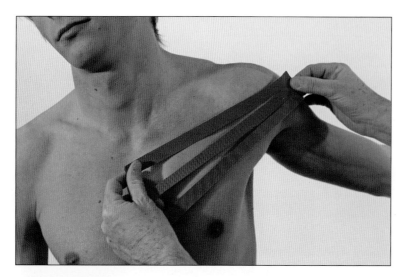

W-shaped application

1. Position the tape anchor 5 cm beyond the intertubercular groove of the humerus.

2. For ease of application, remove the backing paper from the tape, except for the last 2.5 cm, and place the three tape ends at the center of the sternum.

3. Apply the upper strip, without tension, in the direction of the third rib, the lower strip, toward the sixth rib and apply the central strip between the first two.

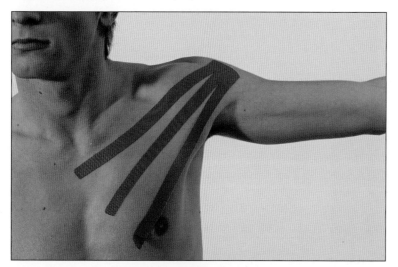

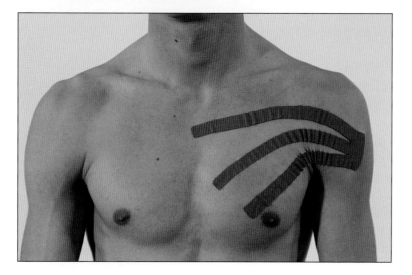

BICEPS BRACHII

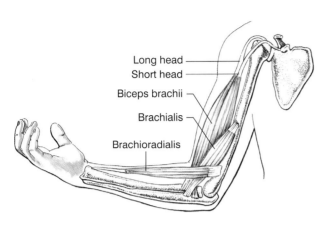

Long head
Short head
Biceps brachii
Brachialis
Brachioradialis

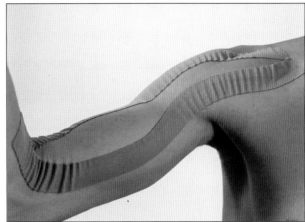

M. biceps brachii (Latin)

Origin
- *Short head*: apex of the coracoid process of the scapula
- *Long head*: supraglenoid tubercle of the scapula

Insertion: tuberosity of the radius

Innervation: musculocutaneous nerve (C5, C6)

Action: the two heads of the biceps brachii unite in a strong tendon that connects to the tuberosity of the radius at the elbow. Its function is to both flex and medially rotate the humerus as well as to aid the triceps brachii in stabilizing the shoulder joint.

CLINICAL APPLICATIONS

- Subacromial bursitis
- Adhesive capsulitis
- Reduced elbow extension
- Pain on arm extension
- Tennis elbow
- Neurological and motor rehabilitation of the shoulder
- Post-traumatic and post-surgical shoulder rehabilitation
- Tendinopathy of the biceps brachii

Combined Applications

- Coracobrachialis ➡ page 210
- Subscapularis ➡ page 174
- Supinator ➡ page 241
- Supraspinatus ➡ page 165
- Teres major ➡ page 167
- Descending part of the trapezius ➡ page 136
- Triceps brachii ➡ page 180

MUSCLE TEST

Patient: seated or supine

Stabilization: the examiner places one hand under the patient's elbow to protect it from pressure from the table.

Test: flexion of the elbow slightly less than or to a right angle, with the forearm in supination

Pressure: against the distal forearm in the direction of extension

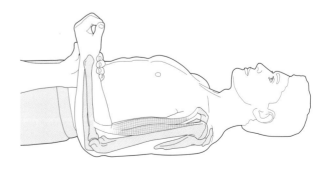

Biceps Brachii - Tape Application

TAPE SPECIFICATIONS

- 1 tape
- Width 5 cm (2")
- Length 35 cm (14")
- Anchor 2 cm (0.75")
- Y-shaped

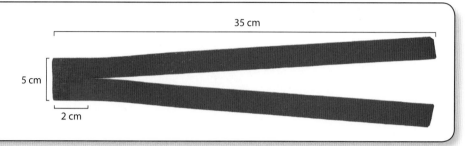

35 cm

5 cm

2 cm

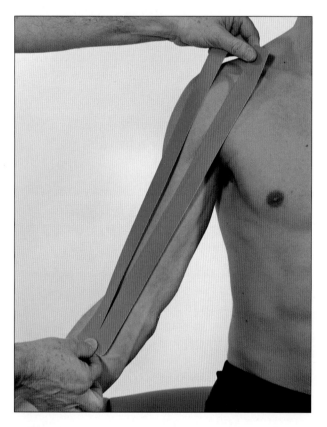
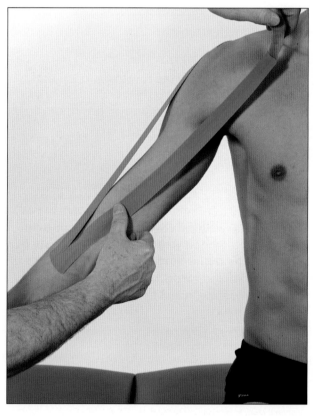

From 2 cm before the tuberosity of the radius to 2 cm past the lateral third of the clavicle

Arm adducted 45° down the patient's side and forearm in supination

1. Apply the tape anchor just below the tuberosity of the radius, so that it coincides with the center of the bifurcation of the Y.

2. The patient extends the elbow and abducts the shoulder moving their arm backward and outward. Remove the backing paper from the tape, except for the last 2.5 cm, and, for ease of application, lay the strips momentarily externally to the points of origin of the muscle on the shoulder.

Biceps Brachii - Tape Application

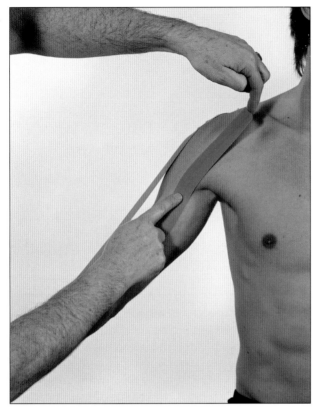

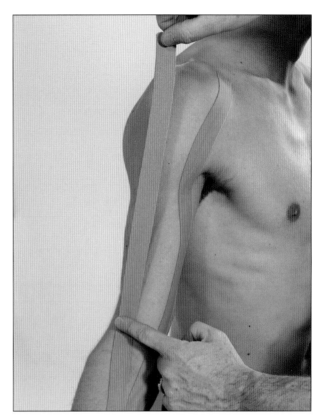

3. Apply the internal strip without tension. Holding it in one hand, direct the tape first towards the midline of the body before returning laterally to apply the tape just outside of the axillary fold and beyond the coracoid process of the scapula. The purpose of all this is to outline the most medial part of the muscle.

4. The patient slightly reduces the abduction of the shoulder. Outline the external margin using the same method used to apply the internal strip. Apply the end of the external tape beyond the supraglenoid tubercle of the scapula.

5. In order to outline the muscle margins correctly, separate the application immediately, directing the internal tape medially and the external tape laterally so that the distance between the two tapes is increased. Then bring them back together again centrally, ending on the scapular origins of the muscle.

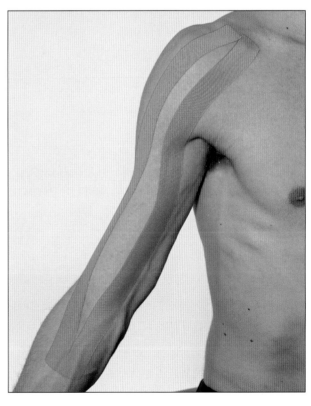

TRICEPS BRACHII

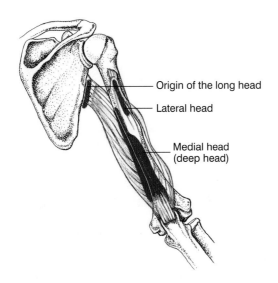

Origin of the long head
Lateral head
Medial head
(deep head)

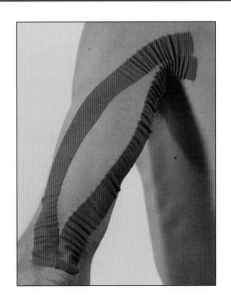

M. triceps brachii (Latin)

Origin
- *Long head*: infraglenoid tubercle of the scapula
- *Lateral head*: posterior surface of the humerus above the groove for the radial nerve
- *Medial head*: posterior surface of the humerus below the groove for the radial nerve

Insertion: olecranon of the ulna

Innervation: radial nerve (C6-C8, T1)

Action: as its name suggests, the triceps brachii has three heads: a long head, a lateral head and a medial head. It is the most important posterior muscle of the arm. Functioning as an antagonist of the biceps brachii, it is the most voluminous of the arm muscles and is the main extensor muscle of the forearm.

By means of its long head, which acts in synergy with the latissimus dorsi, it also contributes to adduction of the humerus.

MUSCLE TEST

Patient: supine

Stabilization: the shoulder is flexed about 90°, and the arm is supported in a position perpendicular to the table.

Test: elbow extension slightly less than full extension

Pressure: against the forearm in the direction of flexion

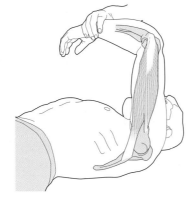

CLINICAL APPLICATIONS

- Arthritis of the elbow
- Deformation of the elbow joint
- Tennis elbow pain on flexion of the elbow
- Radial nerve injury and ulnar neuropathy
- Neurological and motor rehabilitation of the shoulder
- Post-traumatic and post-surgical shoulder rehabilitation

Combined Applications

- Biceps brachii ➥ page 177
- Brachioradialis ➥ page 230
- Latissimus dorsi ➥ page 158
- Pectoralis major ➥ page 152

Triceps Brachii - Tape Application

- Rhomboid major ➥ page 148
- Rhomboid minor ➥ page 146

- Subscapularis ➥ page 174
- Descending part of the trapezius ➥ page 136

TAPE SPECIFICATIONS

- 1 tape
- Width 5 cm (2")
- Length 35 cm (14")
- Anchor 2 cm (0.75")
- Y-shaped

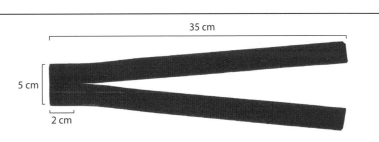

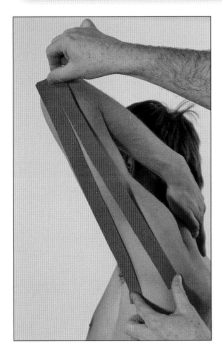 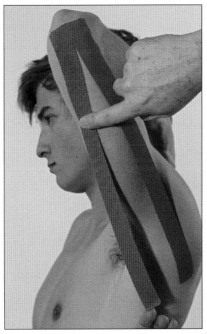 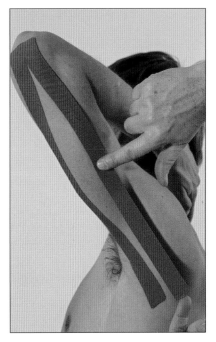

From the olecranon to 2 cm past the infraglenoid tubercle of the scapula

Forward flexion of the arm and flexion of the elbow, so as to place the palm of the hand on the back of the neck

1. The patient flexes the elbow to its maximum and flexes the arm forward, bringing the palm of the hand as close to the back of the neck as possible.

2. With the patient in this position, place the tape anchor just below the olecranon.

3. Apply the tape, without tension, up to 5 cm above the olecranon. For ease of application, remove the backing paper from the two strips of tape, leaving the last 2.5 cm, and lay them centrally towards the shoulder.

Triceps Brachii - Tape Application

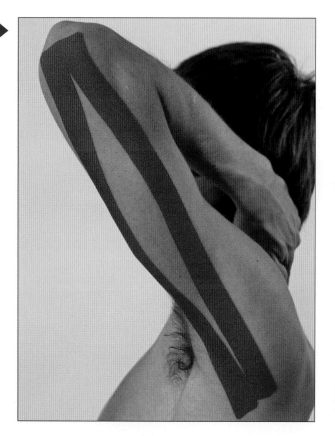 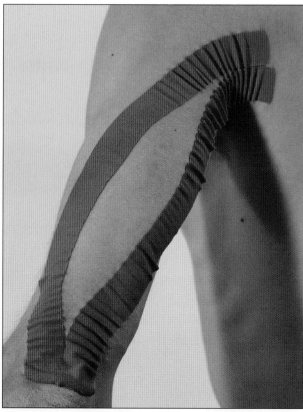

4. Apply the internal tape end, with no tension, opening outwards about 20°, carefully following the medial head edge of the muscle, then take the tape up laterally towards the point of origin on the shoulder. Apply the external strip, outlining the lateral edge of the muscle head before rising in a medial direction toward the infraglenoid tubercle of the scapula.

5. The two tape ends must be attached at least 2.5 cm beyond the points of origin of the muscle itself.

6

Trunk and Abdomen

- **Diaphragm**
- **Thoracic part
  of the iliocostalis lumborum**
- **Lumbar part
  of the iliocostalis lumborum**

- **Multifidus lumborum**
- **Semispinalis thoracis**
- **Rectus abdominis**
- **Internal oblique**
- **External oblique**

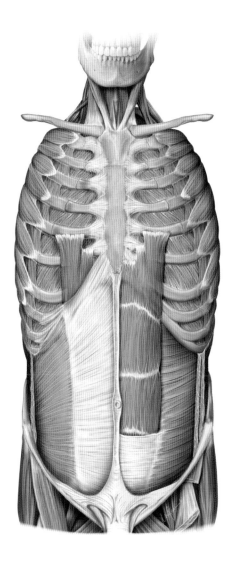
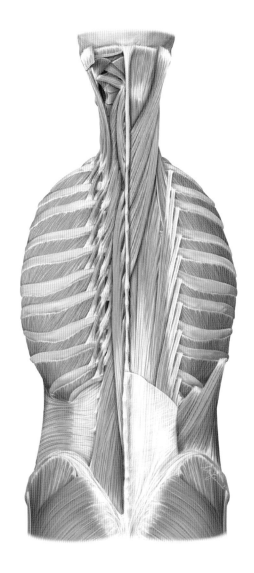

DIAPHRAGM

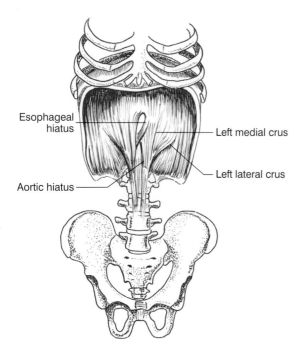

Esophageal hiatus

Left medial crus

Aortic hiatus

Left lateral crus

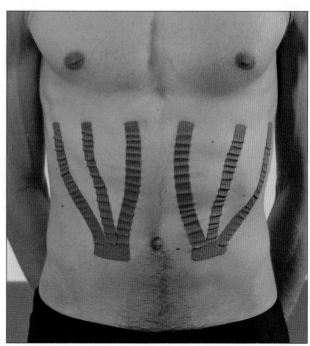

Diaphragma (Latin)

Origin
- *Sternal part*: posterior surface of the xiphoid process of the sternum
- *Costal part*: ribs (from the seventh to the twelfth)
- *Lumbar part*: lumbar vertebrae

Insertion: tendinous center of the diaphragm

Innervation: phrenic nerve (C3, C4, C5)

Action: the diaphragm is a thin, dome-shaped muscle that, through skeletal attachments to the sternum, ribs and lumbar vertebrae, separates the thoracic cavity from the abdominal cavity. In the center of the diaphragm there is the central tendon shaped like an inverted V. The diaphragm is the most important muscle for breathing. It works during inhalation by lowering in contraction and increasing the volume of the chest. Contraction of the diaphragm enables inhalation, exhalation and external expansion of the lower ribs.

Malfunction of this muscle can result in hiccups, breathing difficulties, digestive problems, angina pectoris, visceroptosis, etc.

CLINICAL APPLICATIONS

- Medial back pain
- Respiratory rehabilitation
- Raising of the diaphragm (chest pressure)

Combined APPLICATIONS

- Lumbar part of the iliocostalis lumborum ➡ page 192
- Rhomboid major ➡ page 148
- Rhomboid minor ➡ page 146

TAPE SPECIFICATIONS

Anterior part of the diaphragm

Application 1

- 2 tapes
- Width 5 cm (2")
- Length 25-30 cm (10-12")
- I-shaped

Application 2

- 2 tapes
- Width 5 cm (2")
- Length 20 cm (8")
- Anchor 2 cm (0.75")
- W-shaped

Posterior part of the diaphragm

- 2 tapes
- Width 5 cm (2")
- Length 20 cm (8")
- Anchor 2 cm (0.75")
- W-shaped

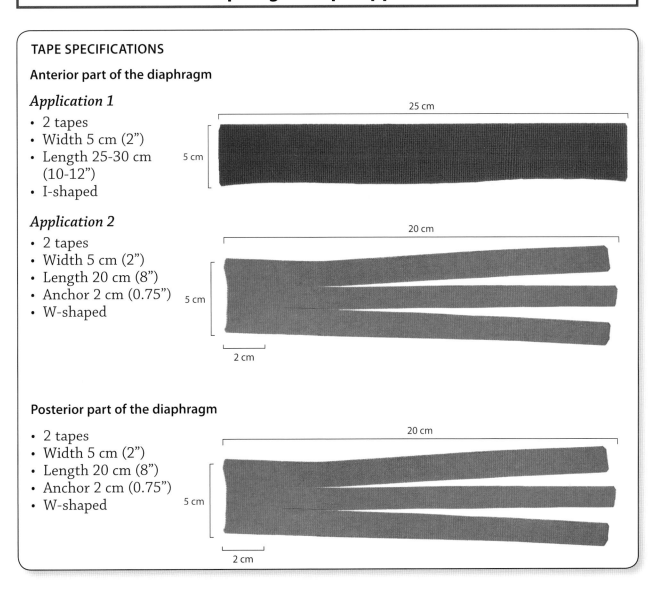

Diaphragm - Tape Application

Anterior part of the diaphragm - Application 1

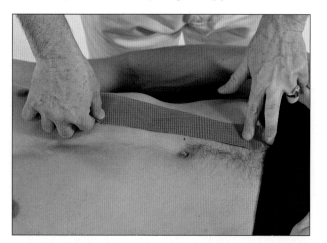 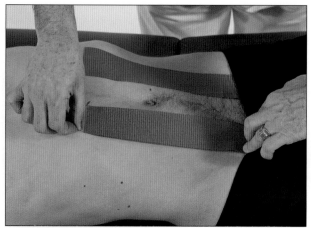

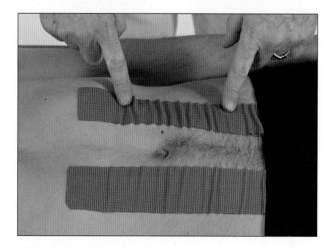

📏 From the pubis to 2 cm above the last rib

⚕ The patient is supine with arms abducted above their head to allow good expansion of the rib cage. The patient should inhale, drawing the air deep into the abdomen below the angle of the ribs. The lower limbs are relaxed.

1. Apply the tape anchor just above the pubis, 2 cm laterally to the midline.

2. Remove the backing paper from the tape, folding back the final 2 cm.

3. With one hand, at the level of the tape anchor, pull the patient's skin towards the pubis. With the other hand, apply the tape with no tension upwards towards the last rib, deviating slightly away from the midline.

> NOTE: Because the diaphragm is connected to the spinal column, it influences body posture; therefore tape application must always be bilateral and symmetrical.

Diaphragm - Tape Application

Anterior part of the diaphragm - Application 2

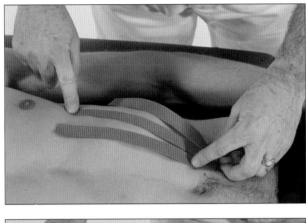
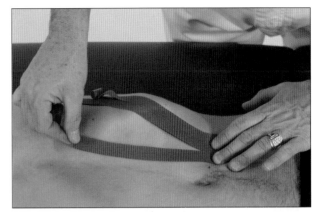
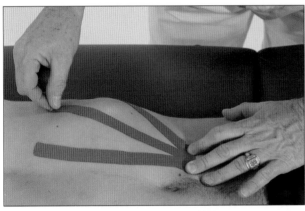
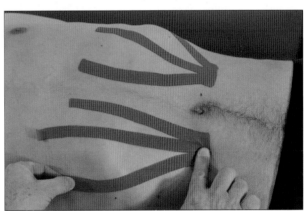
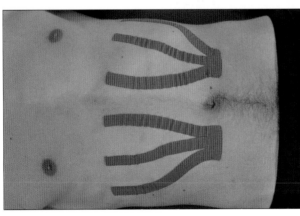
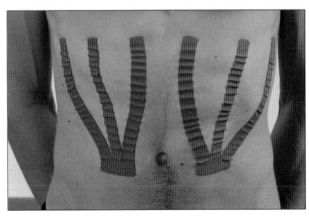

📏 From 2 cm to the side of the navel as far as the ribs, to the height of the xiphoid process

⊤ The patient is supine, lower limbs relaxed, arms raised as high as possible to stretch the abdominal muscles.

1. Apply the tape anchor to the side of the navel. Stretching the skin downward, apply the three tape strips to embrace the ribs.

2. Carry out two applications on the right and on the left of the linea alba.

Diaphragm - Tape Application

Posterior part of the diaphragm

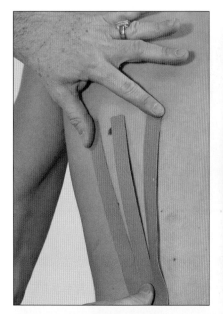 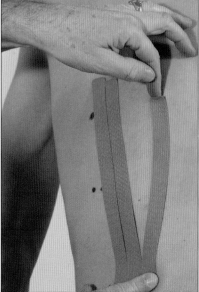 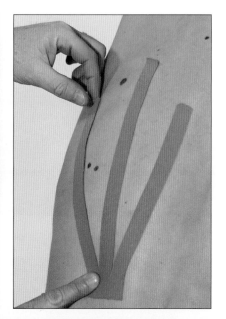

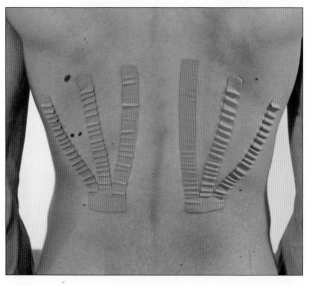 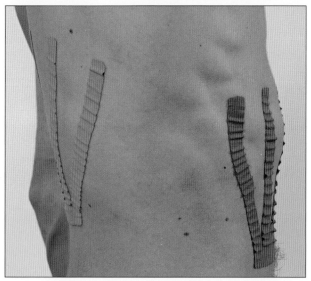

🧵 From the transverse process of the twelfth thoracic vertebra to 2 cm above the seventh thoracic vertebra

✂ The patient is forward flexed through 45° with their arms extended backward.

1. Apply the tape anchor at the level of the transverse process of the twelfth thoracic vertebra.

2. Ask the patient to inhale and, at the same time, to flex the trunk forward slightly, and bring the arms forward. This has the effect of enlarging the posterior section of the lower ribs. Apply the three tape tails without tension so that they embrace the ribs. As the external strips are applied, the patient should maintain the flexion and bend the trunk away from the side of the application.

THORACIC PART OF THE ILIOCOSTALIS LUMBORUM

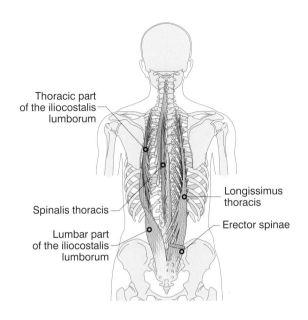

Thoracic part of the iliocostalis lumborum

Spinalis thoracis

Lumbar part of the iliocostalis lumborum

Longissimus thoracis

Erector spinae

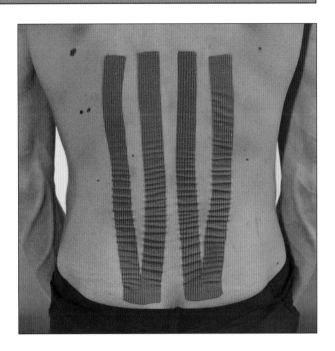

M. iliocostalis lumborum, pars thoracica (Latin)

Origin: costal angles from sixth to twelfth ribs

Insertion: costal angles from the first to the sixth ribs; transverse process of C7

Innervation: posterior branches of the spinal nerves (C4 to L3)

Action: extension and lateral bending of the trunk.

CLINICAL APPLICATIONS

- Lumbar deformation
- Symptomatic lumbar disc herniation
- Floating rib inflammation
- Low back pain symptoms (myofascial pain syndrome)

Combined Applications

- Piriformis ➠ page 276
- Rectus abdominis ➠ page 200
- Rhomboid major ➠ page 148
- Rhomboid minor ➠ page 146

NOTE: The erector spinae is a muscle group comprising the iliocostalis, longissimus and spinalis muscles, forming thick columns of muscle on both sides of the spinous processes of the vertebrae. These columns rise from the sacrum to the base of the cranium.

When standing, the center of gravity line is constantly tilted forward, so these muscles are well developed in order to oppose this force. Good elasticity of this muscle group is essential for maintaining proper curvature of the spine.

Thoracic Part of the Iliocostalis Lumborum - Tape Application

TAPE SPECIFICATIONS

- 2 tapes
- Width 5 cm (2")
- Length
  45 cm (18")
- Anchor
  2 cm (0.75")
- Y-shaped

45 cm

5 cm

2 cm

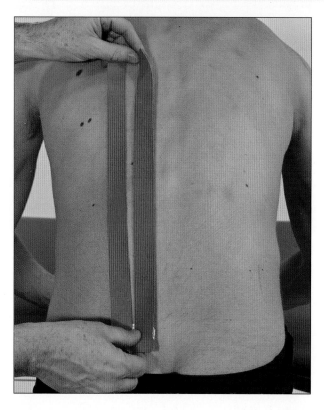 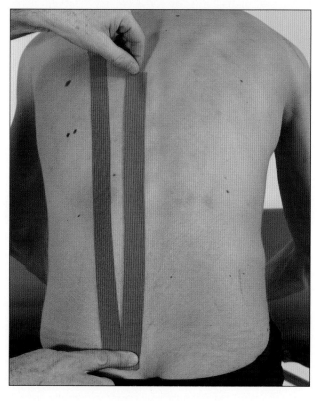

From 2 cm to the side of the gluteal cleft to the level of the sixth thoracic vertebra

The patient is standing or seated with the trunk slightly flexed forward.

1. Apply the tape anchor 5 cm below the supraspinous ligament and medial sacral crest, at the level of the gluteal cleft.

2. Position the internal strips of the two Ys, without tension, terminating over the costal processes of the thoracic vertebrae, as far as the sixth thoracic vertebra.

Thoracic Part of the Iliocostalis Lumborum - Tape Application

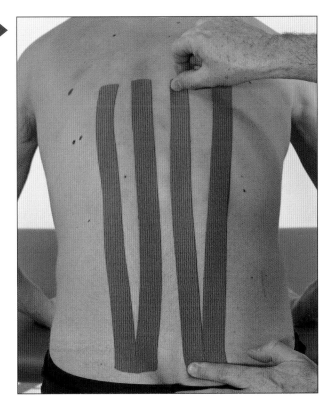 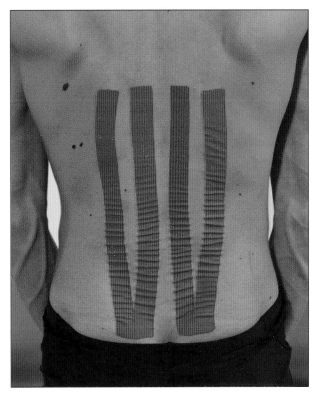

3. The patient should maintain forward flexion of 45°. Apply the external branch of the Y along the costal angle as far as the sixth rib, ending above it.

4. Repeat the procedure on the opposite side.

NOTE: The thoracic part of the iliocostalis lumborum is connected with the spinal column and influences body posture. Therefore this tape application must always be bilateral and symmetrical.

LUMBAR PART OF THE ILIOCOSTALIS LUMBORUM

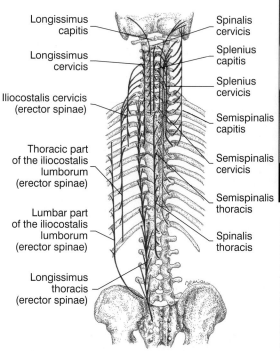

Longissimus capitis
Longissimus cervicis
Iliocostalis cervicis (erector spinae)
Thoracic part of the iliocostalis lumborum (erector spinae)
Lumbar part of the iliocostalis lumborum (erector spinae)
Longissimus thoracis (erector spinae)

Spinalis cervicis
Splenius capitis
Splenius cervicis
Semispinalis capitis
Semispinalis cervicis
Semispinalis thoracis
Spinalis thoracis

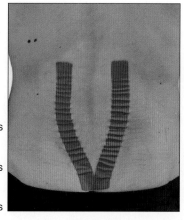

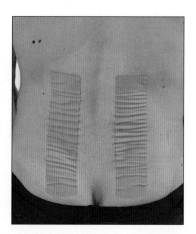

M. iliocostalis lumborum, pars lumbalis (Latin)

Origin: sacrum, iliac crest and posterior layer of the thoracolumbar fascia

Insertion: upper lumbar vertebrae and the last nine ribs

Innervation: posterior branches of the spinal nerves (C4-L3)

Action: extension and lateral bending of the trunk

CLINICAL APPLICATIONS

- Lumbar deformation
- Symptomatic lumbar disc herniation
- Floating rib inflammation
- Low back pain symptoms (myofascial pain syndrome)

Combined applications

- Piriformis ➡ page 276
- Rectus abdominis ➡ page 200
- Rhomboid major ➡ page 148
- Rhomboid minor ➡ page 146

TAPE SPECIFICATIONS

Application 1

- 1 tape
- Width 5 cm (2")
- Length 30 cm (12")
- Anchor 2 cm (0.75")
- Y-shaped

30 cm
5 cm
2 cm

Application 2

- 2 tapes
- Width 5 cm (2")
- Length 30 cm (12")
- *I*-shaped

30 cm
5 cm

Lumbar Part of the Iliocostalis Lumborum - Tape Application

Application of Y-shaped tape

> This application is indicated for low back pain or erector spinae muscle conditions at the level of the higher lumbar vertebrae from L1 to L4.

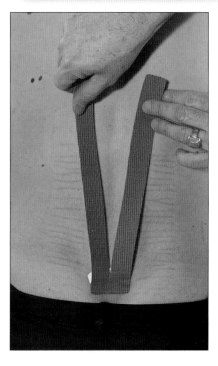 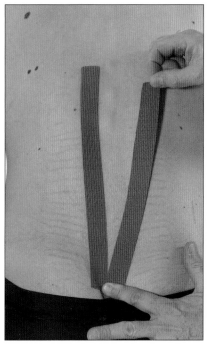 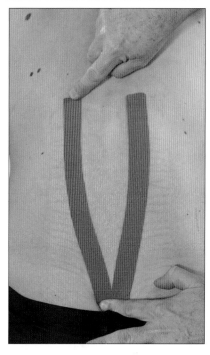

🎞 From the gluteal cleft to the tenth thoracic vertebra

🧍 The patient is standing, if possible near the treatment table, with feet apart at shoulder width.

1. The therapist applies the anchor of the Y at the level of the sacrum, between S2 and S4, at gluteal cleft height.

2. With hands on the treatment table, the patient progressively bends forward until the trunk is flexed forward at 45°. With the patient in this position, the therapist removes the backing paper from the tape and applies one tape strip along the lumbosacral muscles with no tension, immediately angling it outward by 5° so that a broadened "V" shape is formed when the strip is applied symmetrically on the other side.

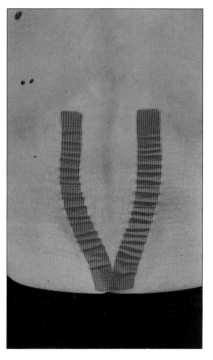

Lumbar Part of the Iliocostalis Lumborum - Tape Application

Application of I-shaped tape

> This application is indicated for low back pain or erector spinae muscle problems at the level of the lower lumbar and sacral vertebrae (L1 to S2-S3).

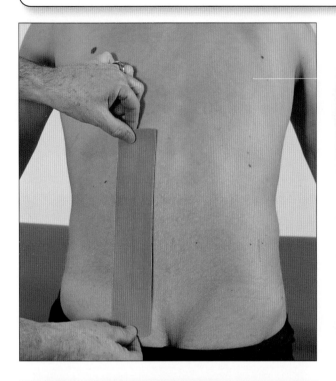

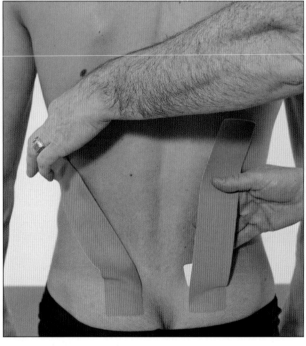

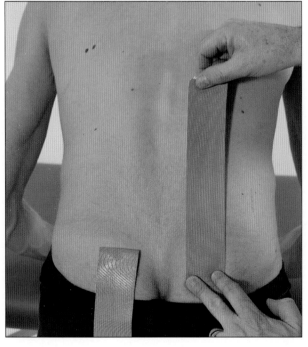

From the gluteal cleft to the twelfth thoracic vertebra

The patient is standing, if possible near the treatment table, with feet apart at shoulder width.

1. The therapist applies the anchor of each tape so that it is centred just below the two posterior superior iliac spines, level with the gluteal cleft and at about 2 cm from the midline.

2. With hands on the table, the patient bends progressively forward, until the trunk is forward flexed through 45°. With the patient in this position, the therapist removes the backing paper from the tape and applies one strip and then the other with no tension, making sure that both are parallel to the spine and end at the same height.

Lumbar Part of the Iliocostalis Lumborum - Tape Application

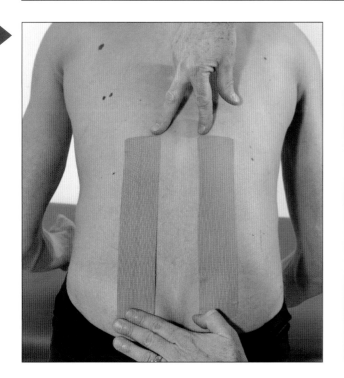 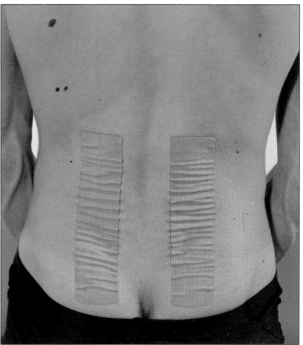

NOTE: The lumbar part of the iliocostalis lumborum is connected with the spinal column and influences body posture. Therefore tape application must always be bilateral and symmetrical.

MULTIFIDUS LUMBORUM

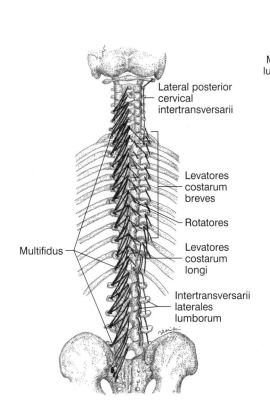

Lateral posterior cervical intertransversarii

Levatores costarum breves

Rotatores

Levatores costarum longi

Multifidus

Intertransversarii laterales lumborum

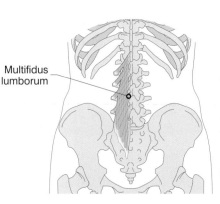

Multifidus lumborum

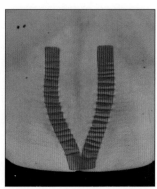

CLINICAL APPLICATIONS

- Kyphosis
- Coccydynia
- Lumbar deformation
- Symptomatic lumbar disc herniation
- Chronic low back pain
- Scoliosis
- Low back pain symptoms (myofascial pain syndrome)
- Mild spondylolisthesis

Mm. multifidi (Latin)

Origin
- *Sacral region*: posterior surface of the sacrum, erector spinae, posterior superior iliac spine and posterior sacroiliac ligament
- *Lumbar, thoracic and cervical regions*: transverse processes from C4 to L5

Insertion: spinous processes of the next four vertebrae above

Innervation: posterior branches of the spinal nerves (C3 - S4)

Action: extension and contralateral rotation of the trunk

Combined Applications

- Piriformis ➥ page 276
- Rectus abdominis ➥ page 200
- Rhomboid major ➥ page 148
- Rhomboid minor ➥ page 146

TAPE SPECIFICATIONS

- 1 tape
- Width 5 cm (2")
- Length 30 cm (12")
- Anchor 2 cm (0.75")
- Y-shaped

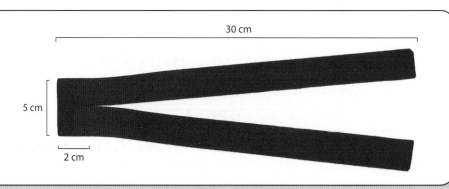

30 cm

5 cm

2 cm

Multifidus Lumborum - Tape Application

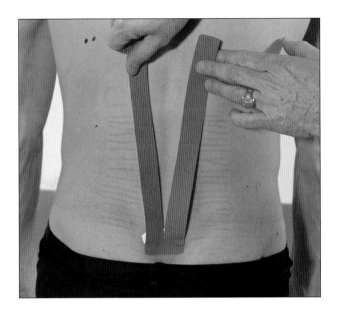

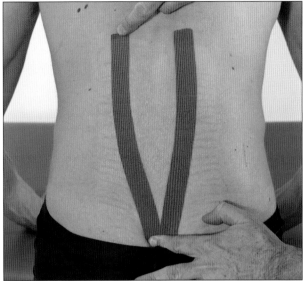

📏 From the gluteal cleft to the tenth thoracic vertebra

🪑 Seated

1. With the tape cut as a Y, fix the anchor below the posterior sacroiliac ligament and medial part of the posterior superior iliac spine, at the level of the gluteal cleft.

2. The patient flexes the neck and trunk forward, resting the elbows on the knees. To enable tape application over the right multifidus lumborum, the patient must twist the trunk to the left, placing the right elbow on the left forearm.

3. Repeat the application on the other side.

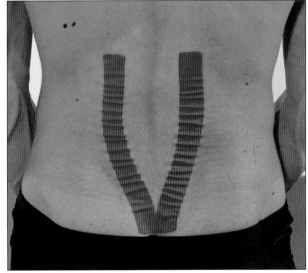

NOTE: The multifidus lumborum influences body posture as it is connected to the spinal column; tape application must therefore always be bilateral and symmetrical. The tape can be applied to the entire length of the spine or just to the affected section.

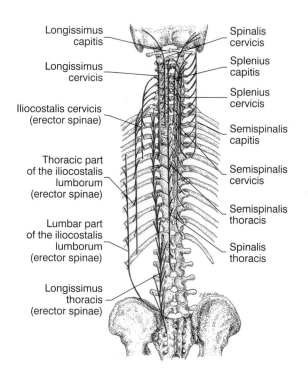

Longissimus capitis
Longissimus cervicis
Iliocostalis cervicis (erector spinae)
Thoracic part of the iliocostalis lumborum (erector spinae)
Lumbar part of the iliocostalis lumborum (erector spinae)
Longissimus thoracis (erector spinae)

Spinalis cervicis
Splenius capitis
Splenius cervicis
Semispinalis capitis
Semispinalis cervicis
Semispinalis thoracis
Spinalis thoracis

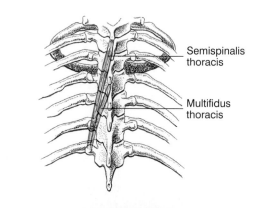

Semispinalis thoracis
Multifidus thoracis

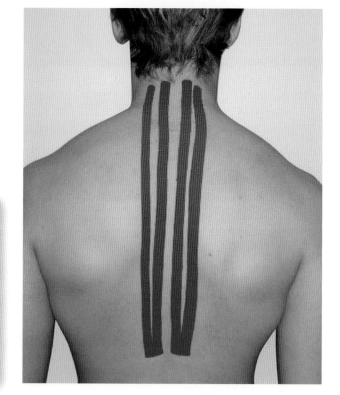

M. semispinalis thoracis (Latin)

Origin: transverse processes of the thoracic vertebrae from T6 to T10

Insertion: spinous processes of the thoracic vertebrae and cervical vertebrae

Innervation: posterior branches of the spinal nerves (C3-S4)

Action: extension and contralateral rotation of the trunk

CLINICAL APPLICATIONS

- Kyphosis
- Whiplash
- Discopathy
- Cervical hernia
- Reduced neck rotation
- Neck stiffness

- Scoliosis
- Spondyloarthropathy of the neck
- Torticollis

Combined Applications

- Sternocleidomastoid ➡ page 131

Semispinalis Thoracis - Tape Application

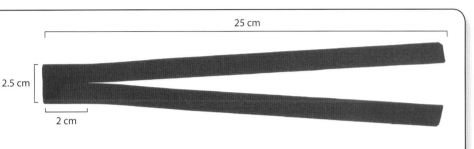

TAPE SPECIFICATIONS

- 2 tapes
- Width 2.5 cm (1")
- Length 25 cm (10")
- Anchor 2 cm (0.75")
- Y-shaped

25 cm

2.5 cm

2 cm

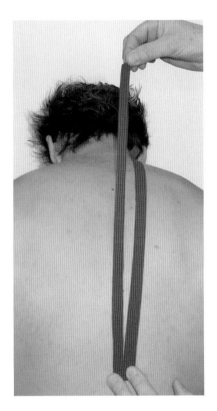
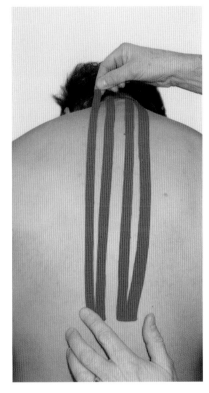
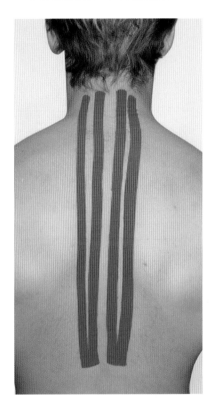

From the transverse process of the tenth thoracic vertebra to the hairline at the level of the occipital bone

The neck and trunk are flexed forward.

1. Apply the tape anchor on the transverse process of the tenth thoracic vertebra. With the patient's trunk flexed forward, apply the internal strip along the transverse processes of the vertebrae as far as the occipital bone with no tension and the external strip 0.5 cm distant to the inner strip.

2. Repeat the application on the other side.

NOTE: The semispinalis thoracis is connected with the spinal column and influences body posture; therefore tape application must always be bilateral and symmetrical.

RECTUS ABDOMINIS

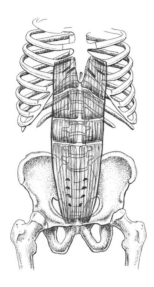

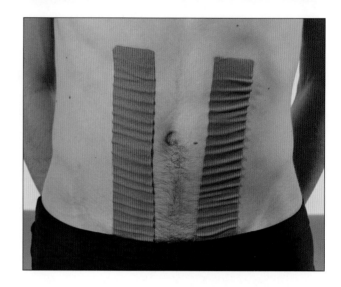

M. rectus abdominis (Latin)

Origin: costal cartilage from the fifth to the seventh ribs

Insertion: superior pubic ramus between the tubercle and the pubic symphysis

Innervation: last intercostal nerves and iliohypogastric nerve (T7-T12/L1)

Action: forward flexion of the trunk; when only one side of the muscle contracts, it assists in lateral flexion of the spine. In particular, it is involved in raising the head and when standing, it aids in bending the spine backward. When the rectus abdominis is weak, the lower back becomes fatigued and often painful. If only one side of the muscle is weakened, there will be a slowing of shoulder movement on the opposite side. The muscle often loses flexibility, agility and tone during pregnancy, possibly causing difficulties during delivery. The transversus abdominis muscle works with the rectus abdominis in flexion, abdominal contraction and exhalation.

CLINICAL APPLICATIONS

- Back pain
- Symptomatic lumbar disc herniation
- Parkinson's disease
- Pubic pain
- Spondylolysis
- Mild spondylolisthesis
- Symptomatic spinal canal stenosis

Combined applications

- Adductor muscles ➡ page 270
- Lumbar part of the iliocostalis lumborum ➡ page 192
- Rhomboid major ➡ page 148
- Rhomboid minor ➡ page 146

TAPE SPECIFICATIONS

- 2 tapes
- Width 5 cm (2")
- Length 35 cm (14")
- I-shaped

35 cm

5 cm

Rectus Abdominis - Tape Application

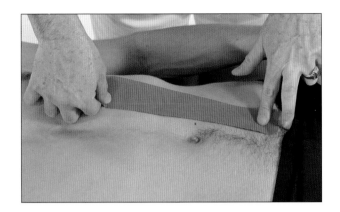
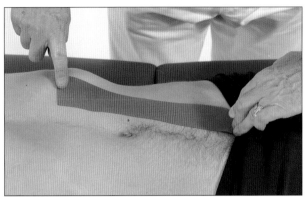
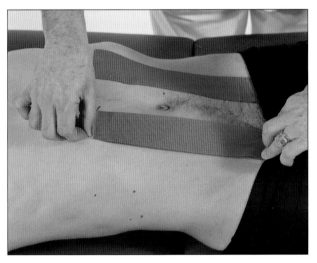
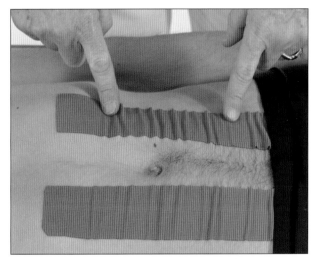

From the pubis to the costal arch

The patient is supine, arms along the sides, legs extended.

1. Apply the tape anchor over the pubis, 2.5 cm to the side of the linea alba.

2. The patient should bring both arms up and backward. With the patient in this position, remove the backing paper from the upper part of the tape and lay it in place. With no tension and stretching the skin downward apply the tape along a line parallel to the linea alba which corresponds to the rectus abdominis.

3. Apply the other tape in the same way.

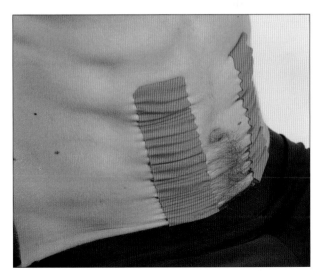

NOTE: the rectus abdominis influences body posture and is symmetrical with respect to the midline of the trunk; tape application must therefore always be bilateral and symmetrical.

INTERNAL OBLIQUE

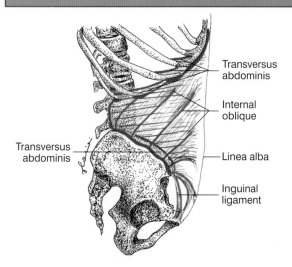

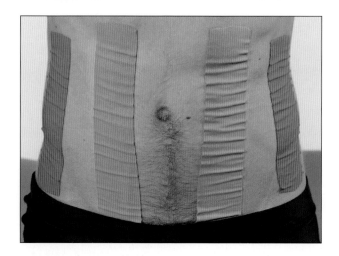

M. obliquus internus abdominis (Latin)

Origin: inguinal ligament; iliac crest; thoracolumbar fascia

Insertion: lower margin of the cartilage of the last three or four costal cartilages; upper margin of the pubis through an aponeurosis that helps to form the sheath of the rectus abdominis and the linea alba

Innervation: last intercostal nerves and iliohypogastric and ilioinguinal nerves (T6-L1)

Action: ipsilateral and contralateral rotation of the trunk and forward flexion of the chest. This muscle is mainly involved in active rotation of the spine. When it contracts bilaterally, it flexes the spine, lowers the ribs (exhalation function) and compresses the abdominal viscera.

CLINICAL APPLICATIONS

- Back pain
- Symptomatic lumbar disc herniation
- Inguinal hernia
- Low back pain
- Parkinson's disease
- Costal cartilage ossification
- Pubic pain
- Spondylolysis
- Mild spondylolisthesis
- Symptomatic spinal canal stenosis

Combined applications

- Adductor muscles ➥ page 270
- Lumbar part of the iliocostalis lumborum ➥ page 192
- Rhomboid major ➥ page 148
- Rhomboid minor ➥ page 146

TAPE SPECIFICATIONS

Anterior application

- 2 tapes
- Width 5 cm (2")
- Length 30 cm (12")
- I-shaped

Lateral application

- 2 tapes
- Width 5 cm (2")
- Length 20 cm (8")
- I-shaped

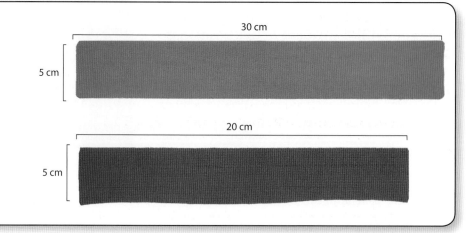

30 cm

5 cm

20 cm

5 cm

Internal Oblique – Tape Application

Anterior application

📏 From the pubis to the costal arch

🧍 The patient is supine, arms lying along the sides, legs extended.

1. Apply the tape anchor 5 cm below the anterior half of the iliac crest.

2. At this point, the patient should raise their arms and bend away from the side of the muscle to be treated. With the patient in this position, remove the backing paper from the tape and apply it, without tension, in an upward oblique direction, following the course of the muscle. The tape ends beyond, and medially to, the costal cartilage of the last three ribs.

3. Repeat the application on the other side.

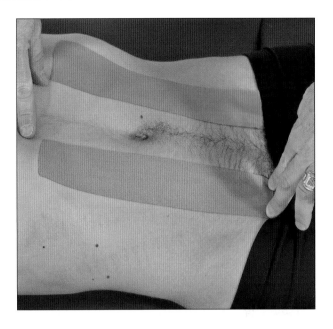

Lateral application

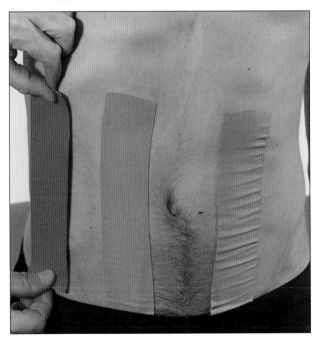
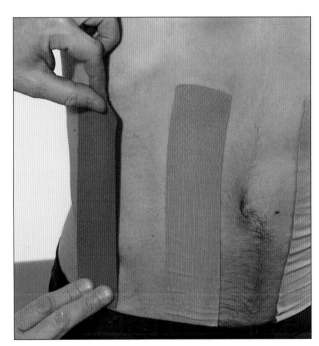

📏 From the iliac crest to 2 cm above the floating ribs

🧍 The patient is standing with the arm ipsilateral to the treated muscle raised and trunk slightly bent in the opposite direction.

1. Apply the tape at the iliac crest. The arm ipsilateral to the tape is raised and the trunk is slightly bent to the opposite side. ▶

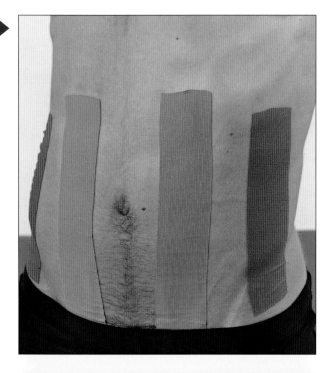

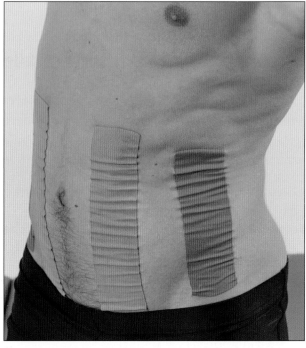

2. Apply the tape vertically over the abdomen, without imparting tension, as far as the level of the floating ribs.

3. Repeat the application on the other side.

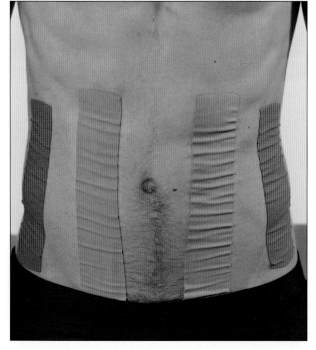

NOTE: The internal oblique is connected with the linea alba and influences body posture. Therefore tape application must always be bilateral and symmetrical.

EXTERNAL OBLIQUE

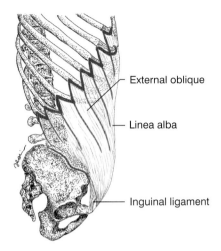

External oblique

Linea alba

Inguinal ligament

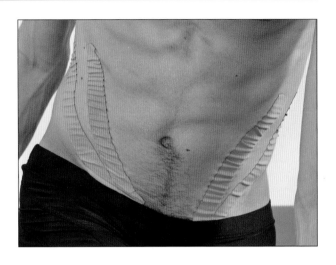

M. obliquus externus abdominis (Latin)

Origin: outer lip of the iliac crest, aponeurosis of the internal oblique which forms the linea alba from the xiphoid process to pubic symphysis and the inguinal ligament

Insertion: external and lower surfaces of the last eight ribs

Innervation: intercostal, iliohypogastric and ilio-inguinal nerves (T5 - T12)

Action: contralateral rotation of the trunk and forward flexion of the chest: when it contracts bilaterally, it flexes the vertebral column, lowers the ribs (exhalation function) and compresses the abdominal viscera.

CLINICAL APPLICATIONS

- Colitis
- Back pain
- Lumbar disc herniation
- Low back pain
- Parkinson's disease
- Costal cartilage ossification
- Pubic pain
- Spondylolysis
- Spondylolisthesis
- Symptomatic spinal canal stenosis

Combined Applications

- Adductor muscles ➡ page 270
- Lumbar part of the iliocostalis lumborum ➡ page 192
- Rhomboid major ➡ page 148
- Rhomboid minor ➡ page 146

TAPE SPECIFICATIONS

- 2 tapes
- Width 5 cm (2")
- Length 30 cm (12")
- Anchor 2 cm (0.75")
- Y-shaped

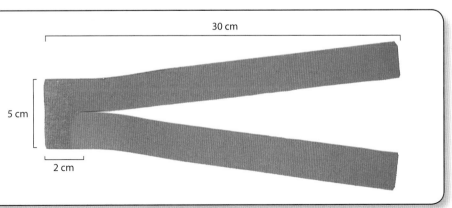

30 cm

5 cm

2 cm

External Oblique - Tape Application

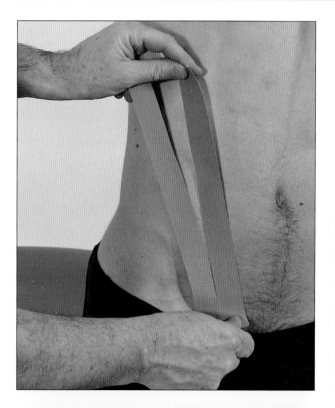

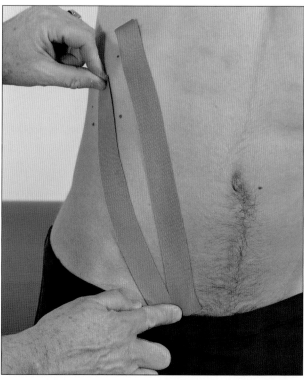

From the upper margin of the pubic symphysis to the lateral surface of the eighth and ninth ribs

The patient is standing with the trunk slightly bent away from the muscle being treated and the arms raised.

1. Apply the tape anchor just proximally and laterally to the pubic symphysis, remaining internal to the anterior superior iliac spine, and angled toward the lateral surface of the eighth and ninth ribs.

2. Remove the backing paper from the tape and apply the two tape strips, with no tension, following the course of the muscle in the direction of the lateral surfaces of the eighth and ninth ribs respectively.

3. Repeat the application on the opposite side.

External Oblique - Tape Application

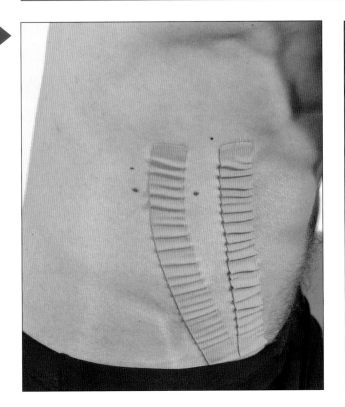

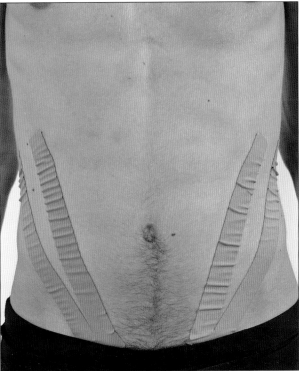

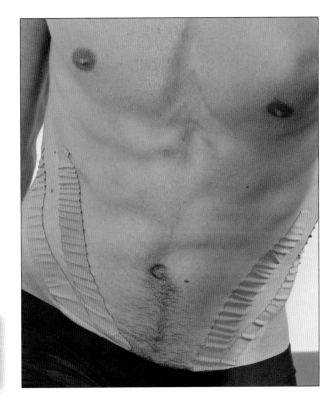

NOTE: The external oblique is connected with the linea alba and influences body posture. Therefore, tape application must always be bilateral and symmetrical.

7

Upper Limb

- Coracobrachialis
- Brachialis
- Pronator teres
- Flexor carpi radialis
- Palmaris longus
- Flexor carpi ulnaris
- Flexor digitorum profundus
- Pronator quadratus
- Brachioradialis
- Extensor carpi radialis longus

- Extensor carpi radialis brevis
- Extensor digitorum
- Extensor carpi ulnaris
- Supinator
- Extensor pollicis longus
- Abductor pollicis brevis
- Adductor pollicis
- Dorsal interossei, lumbricals, abductor digiti minimi

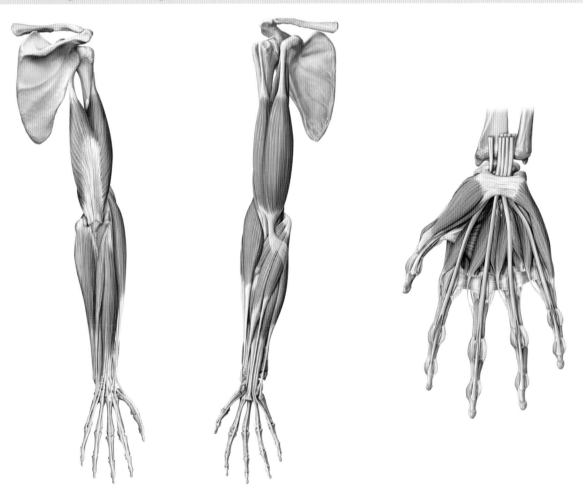

CORACOBRACHIALIS

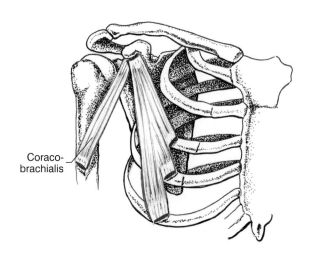

Coraco-
brachialis

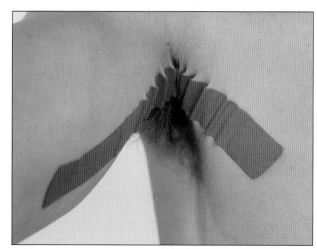

M. coracobrachialis (Latin)

Origin: coracoid process of the scapula

Insertion: anteromedial surface of the humerus

Innervation: musculocutaneous nerve

Action: shoulder flexion and adduction

CLINICAL APPLICATIONS

• Post breast implant surgery rehabilitation and treatment of scar tissue and adhesions
• Post breast cancer treatment rehabilitation

Combined Applications

• Deltoid ➥ page 161
• Latissimus dorsi ➥ page 158
• Triceps brachii ➥ page 180
• Descending part of the trapezius ➥ page 136

MUSCLE TEST

Patient: seated or supine

Stabilization: if the trunk is stable, there is no need for stabilization by the examiner.

Test: flexion in external rotation of the shoulder with the elbow fully flexed and the forearm in supination. In this position, the action of the coracobrachialis muscle during flexion of the shoulder is reduced, as the complete flexion of the elbow and supination of the forearm shorten this muscle to such a degree that it becomes ineffective in shoulder flexion.

Pressure: against the anteromedial surface of the lower third of the humerus in the direction of extension and slight abduction

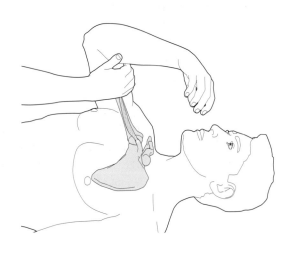

Coracobrachialis - Tape Application

TAPE SPECIFICATIONS

- 1 tape
- Width 2.5 cm (1")
- Length 35 cm (14")
- I-shaped

2.5 cm

35 cm

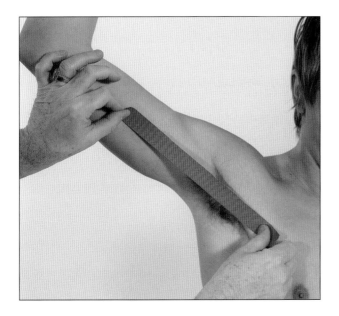

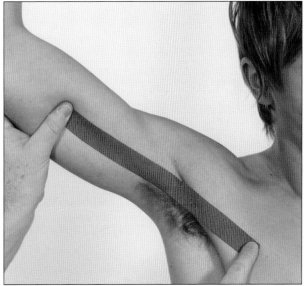

From the coracoid process of the scapula to mid humerus

Arm abducted to 120° and slightly extended, externally rotated

1. Fix the tape anchor below the coracoid process of the scapula.

2. Apply the tape, without tension, to beyond the muscle's insertion on the anteromedial surface of the humerus. Outline the upper margin of the axillary cavity, always remaining below the belly of the short head of the biceps brachii.

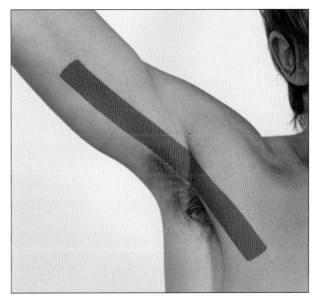

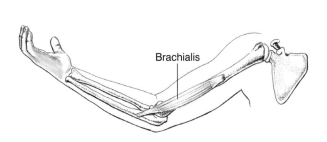

Brachialis

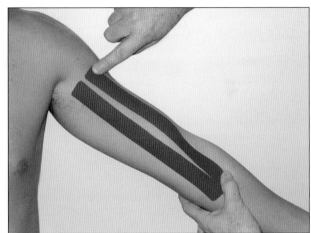

M. brachialis (Latin)

Origin: anteromedial and anterolateral surfaces of the humerus

Insertion: tuberosity of the ulna

Innervation: musculocutaneous and radial nerves (C5-C6)

Action: elbow flexion

CLINICAL APPLICATIONS

- Acute pain in the elbow joint
- Epicondylitis
- Rehabilitation after elbow fracture and surgery
- Rehabilitation after elbow replacement

Combined applications

- Brachioradialis ➥ page 230
- Extensor pollicis longus ➥ page 243
- Pronator quadratus ➥ page 228
- Triceps brachii ➥ page 180

TAPE SPECIFICATIONS

- 1 tape
- Width 5 cm (2")
- Length 25 cm (10")
- Anchor 2 cm (0.75")
- Y-shaped

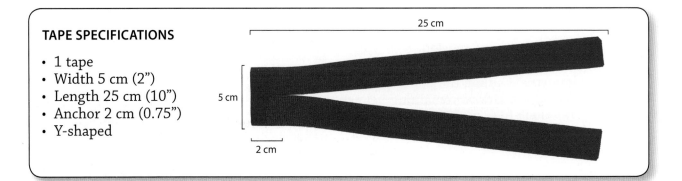

25 cm

5 cm

2 cm

Brachialis - Tape Application

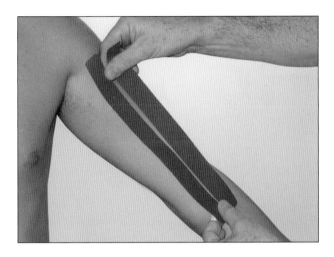 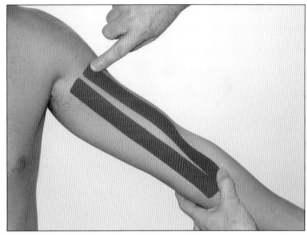

From 2 cm distal to the tuberosity of the ulna to the middle of the anterolateral surface of the humerus

Elbow extended, forearm supinated

1. Fix the tape anchor 2 cm distally to the tuberosity of the ulna.

2. Remove the backing paper and for ease of application lay the tape strips vertically on the humerus. With no tension, apply the lateral strip, taking it over the anterolateral portion of the bend of the elbow and then around the lateral margin of the brachialis, to end half way along the anterolateral surface of the humerus.

3. Apply the medial strip, again without tension, over the anteromedial portion of the bend of the elbow. It then passes around the medial margin of the brachialis before finally converging with the first tape tail toward the middle of the anterolateral surface of the humerus.

PRONATOR TERES

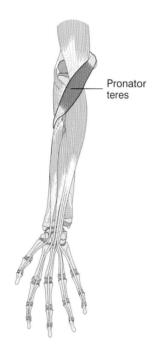

Pronator
teres

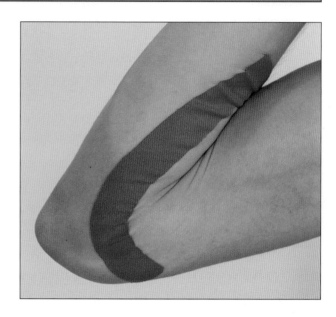

M. pronator teres (Latin)

Origin
- *Humeral head*: anterior surface of the medial epicondyle of the humerus, medial margin of the humerus, brachial fascia
- *Ulnar head*: medial surface of the coronoid process of the ulna

Insertion: lateral surface of the radius

Innervation: median nerve (C6-C7)

Action: elbow pronation. The pronator teres assists in internal rotation of the forearm. It is also a supporting muscle in flexion movements against resistance.

The pronator teres assists in external and internal rotation of the proximal radioulnar joint and in flexion and extension of the humeroradial joint.

MUSCLE TEST

Patient: seated or supine

Stabilization: the patient's elbow should be against their side, or held there by the examiner to prevent any abduction movement of the shoulder.

Test: pronation of the forearm with the elbow partially flexed

Pressure: against the lower part of the forearm above the wrist (to prevent twisting of the wrist) in the direction of forearm supination

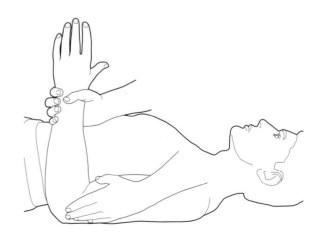

Pronator Teres - Tape Application

CLINICAL APPLICATIONS

- Acute pain in the elbow joint
- Acute pain on internal rotation of the forearm
- Wrist pain
- Pain in the carpometacarpal joint of the thumb
- Pain during supination
- Epicondylitis

- Functional impairment of the arm
- Radial head instability
- De Quervain's tenosynovitis

Combined Applications

- Brachioradialis ➥ page 230
- Extensor digitorum ➥ page 236
- Extensor carpi radialis longus ➥ page 232
- Palmaris longus ➥ page 219

TAPE SPECIFICATIONS

- 1 tape
- Width 2.5 cm (1")
- Length 20 cm (8")
- I-shaped

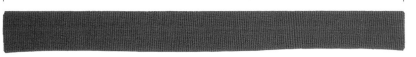

20 cm

2.5 cm

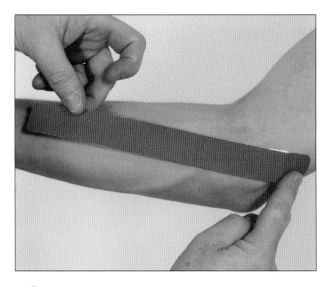
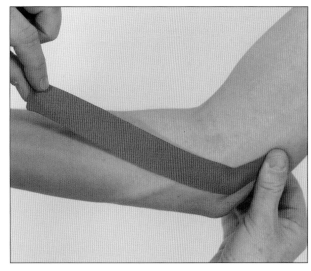

🎞 From 5 cm proximal to the medial epicondyle of the humerus to the middle of the anterolateral surface of the radius

⚕ Elbow slightly flexed, forearm supinated

1. Position the tape anchor 5 cm proximally to the medial epicondyle of the humerus.

2. Remove the backing paper from 10 cm of tape, folding it back. Apply the tape, with no tension, over the medial epicondyle of the humerus.

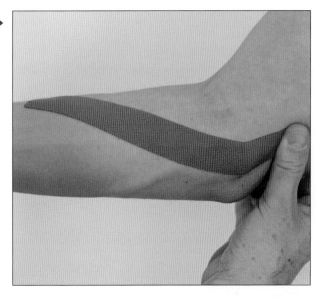 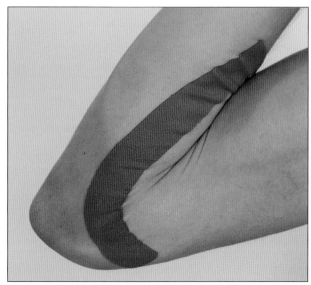

3. Remove the remaining backing paper, except for the last 2 cm, which is folded back. Apply the tape, with no tension, following the path of the muscle, and taking it beyond the radial insertion. The tape should end half way along the radius.

FLEXOR CARPI RADIALIS

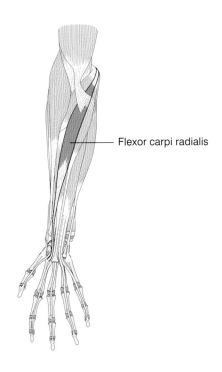

Flexor carpi radialis

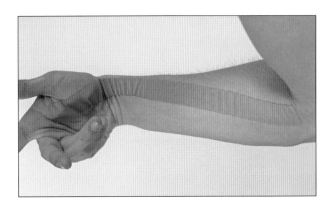

M. flexor carpi radialis (Latin)

Origin: medial epicondyle of the humerus

Insertion: base of the second and third metacarpals

Innervation: median nerve (C6-C7)

Action: flexion and radial abduction of the wrist and pronation of the elbow

---

CLINICAL APPLICATIONS

- Wrist joint dysfunction
- Elbow pain
- Pain in the fingers, hand and wrist
- Epicondylitis
- Hemiplegic hand patients (neurological and motor rehabilitation)
- Loss of hand and finger function
- Rehabilitation after wrist or finger fractures
- Carpal tunnel syndrome
- De Quervain's tenosynovitis

Combined Applications

- Brachioradialis ➡ page 230
- Extensor carpi radialis longus ➡ page 232
- Extensor digitorum ➡ page 236
- Palmaris longus ➡ page 219
- Supinator ➡ page 241

MUSCLE TEST

Patient: seated or supine

Stabilization: the forearm, in almost full supination, rests on the table or is supported by the examiner.

Test: flexion of wrist toward the radial side

Pressure: against the thenar eminence in the direction of extension toward the ulnar side

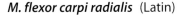

Flexor Carpi Radialis - Tape Application

TAPE SPECIFICATIONS

35 cm

- 1 tape
- Width 2.5 cm (1")   2.5 cm
- Length 35 cm (14")
- I-shaped

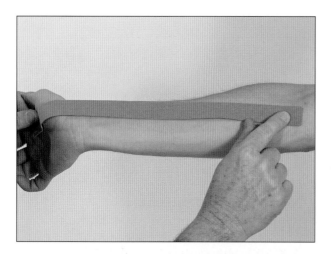
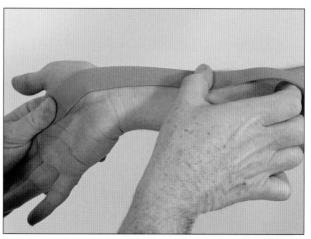
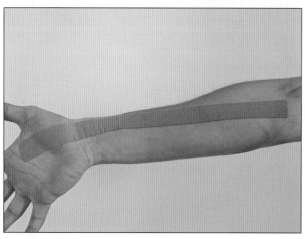
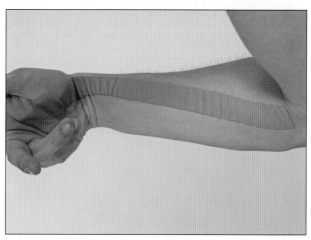

From the middle of the second metacarpal to 5 cm proximal to the medial epicondyle of the humerus

Elbow extended, forearm slightly supinated, wrist extended and in ulnar flexed position

1. Fix the tape anchor on the patient's palm, mid-way along the second metacarpal.

2. Remove the backing paper from the tape, except for the last 2 cm, which is folded back. Apply the tape, with no tension, passing over the trapezoid and then toward the medial epicondyle of the humerus.

3. The tape ends on the anterior surface of the medial epicondyle of the humerus.

PALMARIS LONGUS

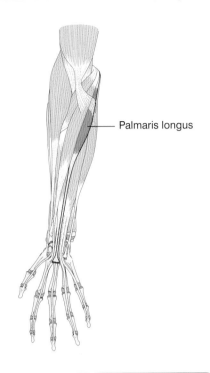

Palmaris longus

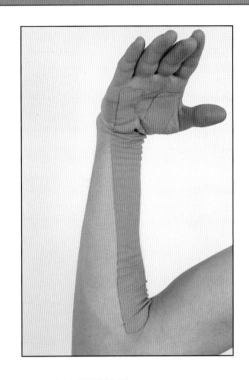

M. palmaris longus (Latin)

Origin: medial epicondyle of the humerus

Insertion: flexor retinaculum, palmar aponeurosis

Innervation: median nerve (C7-T1)

Action: hand flexion. The palmaris longus is the largest of the wrist flexor muscles.

CLINICAL APPLICATIONS

- Pain and tension in the hand or palm
- Epicondylitis
- Functional impairment of the hand
- Carpal tunnel syndrome
- De Quervain's tenosynovitis

Combined Applications

- Brachialis ➥ page 212
- Triceps brachii ➥ page 180

MUSCLE TEST

Patient: seated

Stabilization: the forearm, in supination, rests on the table for support.

Test: tensing of the palmar aponeurosis by cupping the hand firmly and flexing the wrist

Pressure: against the thenar and hypothenar eminences in the direction of the flattened part of the palm and against the hand in the direction of extension of the wrist

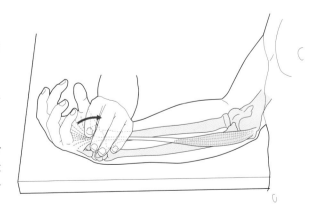

Palmaris Longus - Tape Application

TAPE SPECIFICATIONS

- 1 tape
- Width 5 cm (2")
- Length 35 cm (14")
- Y-shaped, with 10 cm strips

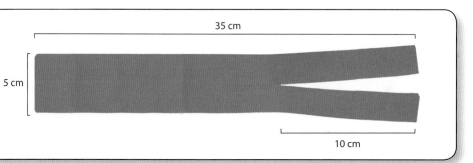

35 cm

5 cm

10 cm

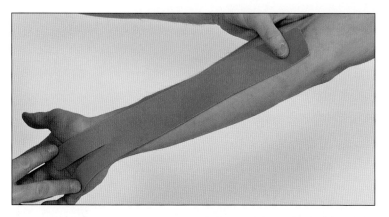

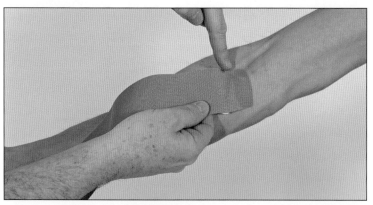

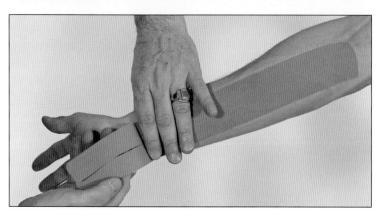

From the metacarpophalangeal joints to the anterior region of the elbow; the two tails of the Y are to be measured from the metacarpophalangeal joints to 2 cm beyond the wrist

The arm is slightly abducted, with the elbow and wrist fully extended.

1. Apply the tape anchor, which is 5 cm wide, just below the bend of the elbow.

2. Remove the backing paper as far as the bifurcation of the Y and fold it back. Apply the tape, with no tension, along the anterior surface of the forearm.

Palmaris Longus - Tape Application

▶ **3.** Remove the backing paper from the strips of tape and apply them with no tension along the fifth and second metacarpal bones.

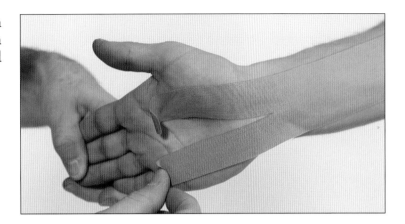

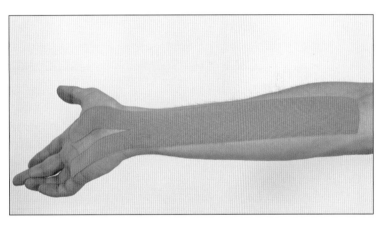

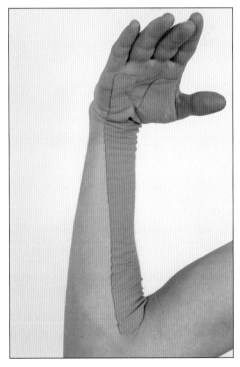

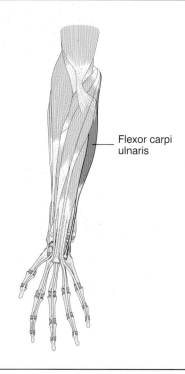

Flexor carpi ulnaris

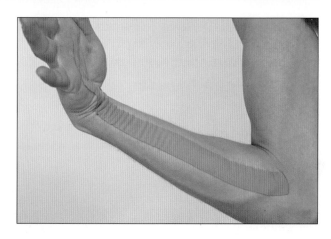

M. flexor carpi ulnaris (Latin)

Origin

- *Humeral head:* medial epicondyle of the humerus
- *Ulnar head:* medial margin of the olecranon and posterior margin of the ulna

Insertion: pisiform bone; hamate bone, base of the fifth metacarpal and flexor retinaculum

Innervation: ulnar nerve (C7-C8)

Action: flexion and ulnar abduction of the hand and wrist

CLINICAL APPLICATIONS

- Wrist joint dysfunction
- Elbow pain
- Pain in the fingers, hand and wrist
- Epicondylitis
- Hemiplegic hand patients (neurological and motor deficit rehabilitation)
- Loss of hand and finger function
- Rehabilitation after wrist and finger fractures
- Carpal tunnel syndrome
- De Quervain's tenosynovitis

Combined Applications

- Brachioradialis ➥ page 230
- Extensor digitorum ➥ page 236
- Extensor carpi radialis longus ➥ page 232
- Supinator ➥ page 241

MUSCLE TEST

Patient: seated or supine

Stabilization: the forearm, which is fully supinated, rests on the table or is supported by the examiner.

Test: flexion of the wrist toward the ulnar side

Pressure: against the hypothenar eminence in the direction of extension toward the radial side

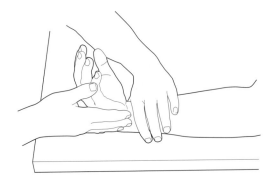

Flexor Carpi Ulnaris - Tape Application

TAPE SPECIFICATIONS

Application 1

- 1 tape
- Width 2.5 cm (1")
- Length 35 cm (14")
- I-shaped

Application 2

- 1 tape
- Width 5 cm (2")
- Length 35 cm (14")
- Y-shaped,
  with 10 cm strips

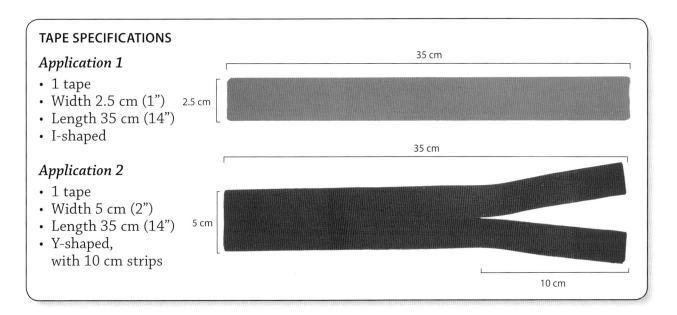

35 cm

2.5 cm

35 cm

5 cm

10 cm

Application 1

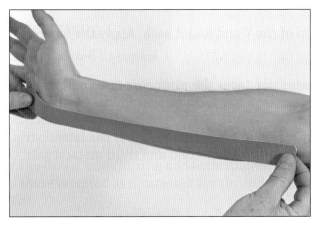

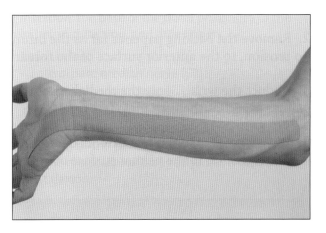

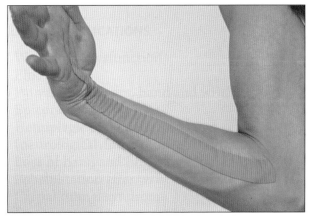

From the medial epicondyle of the humerus to the head of the fifth metacarpal bone

Elbow extended, wrist extended and in radial deviation

1. Fix the tape anchor proximally to the medial epicondyle of the humerus.

2. Extend the patient's elbow and extend and abduct the wrist and then apply the tape with no tension, taking it beyond the pisiform bone and the base of the fifth metacarpal.

Flexor Digitorum Profundus - Tape Application

Combined Applications
- Brachioradialis ➡ page 230
- Extensor carpi radialis longus ➡ page 232
- Extensor digitorum ➡ page 236
- Supinator ➡ page 241

TAPE SPECIFICATIONS

- 1 tape
- Width 5 cm (2")
- Length 45 cm (18")
- Fan-shaped, with four strips, each 20 cm long

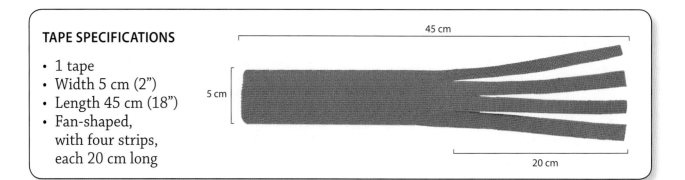

45 cm

5 cm

20 cm

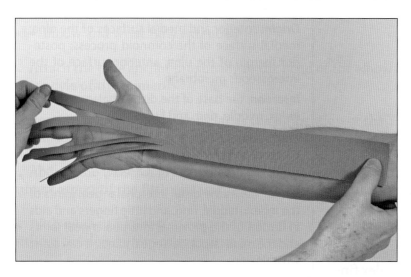

From the bend of the elbow to the tip of the middle finger: the strips of the fan are to be measured from the tip of the middle finger to 2 cm beyond the wrist. Each tape strip is then cut to the length of each finger so that it ends on each fingertip.

Elbow, wrist and fingers extended

1. Apply the end of the first strip to the tip of the index finger.

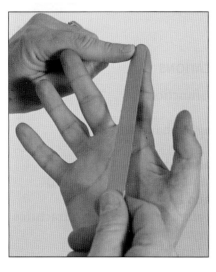

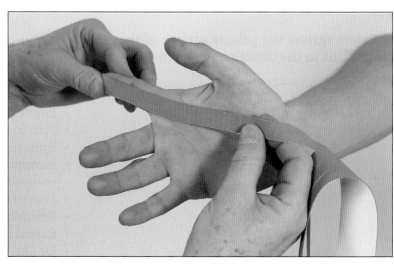

Flexor Digitorum Profundus - Tape Application

2. Remove the backing paper as far as wrist level and fold it back. With the patient's index finger held in the fully extended position, apply the strip without tension along the palmar surface of the finger and second metacarpal bone. Repeat the procedure for the middle, ring and little fingers.

3. Remove the backing paper, except for the last 2 cm, which is folded back. With the patient's wrist held in the fully extended position, apply the tape without tension along the anterior surface of the forearm.

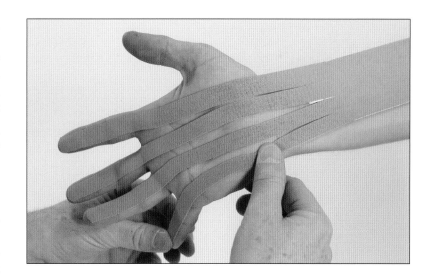

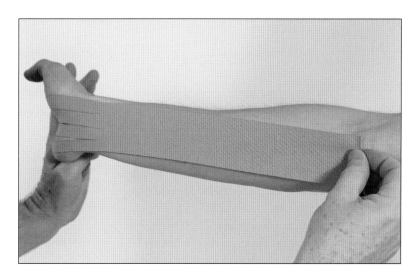

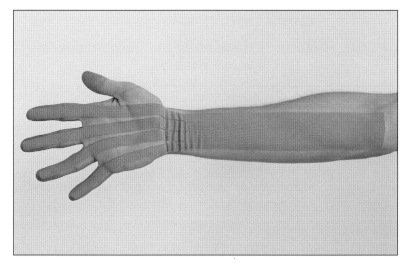

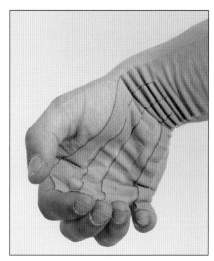

PRONATOR QUADRATUS

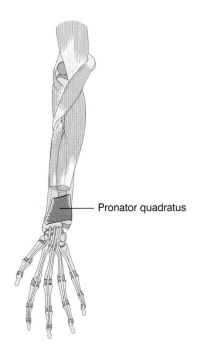

Pronator quadratus

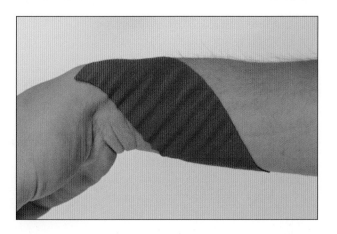

MUSCLE TEST

Patient: seated or supine

Stabilization: the elbow should be against the patient's side, or if necessary held by the examiner to prevent abduction of the shoulder.

Test: pronation of the forearm with the elbow fully flexed so as to shorten the humeral head of the pronator teres, thereby reducing its efficacy

Pressure: against the lower part of the forearm above the wrist (to prevent twisting of the wrist) in the direction of forearm supination

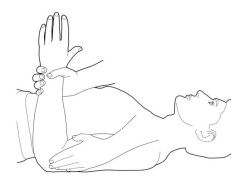

M. pronator quadratus (Latin)

Origin: anterior surface and anterior margin of the ulna

Insertion: anterior surface and anterior margin of the radius

Innervation: median nerve (C6-T1)

Action: pronation of the elbow: the pronator quadratus, together with the pronator teres, rotates the forearm medially. The considerable effect this muscle has on this movement compared with the pronator teres is clearly observable on an electromyogram.

CLINICAL APPLICATIONS

- Pain in the anterior forearm and/or wrist
- Carpal tunnel syndrome
- De Quervain's tenosynovitis

Combined Applications

- Brachialis ➥ page 212
- Brachioradialis ➥ page 230
- Extensor carpi radialis longus ➥ page 232
- Extensor digitorum ➥ page 236
- Pronator teres ➥ page 214

Pronator Quadratus - Tape Application

TAPE SPECIFICATIONS

- 1 tape
- Width 5 cm (2")
- Length 15 cm (6")
- I-shaped

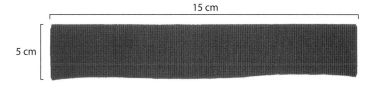

15 cm

5 cm

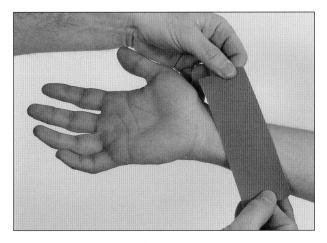
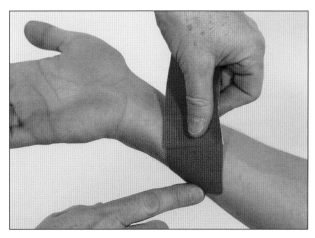
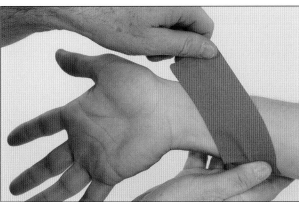
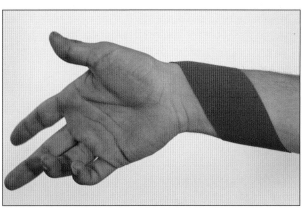

From the proximal part of the distal fourth of the ulna's medial aspect to the lateral surface of the radius, just proximal to the trapezoid

Arm in full external rotation, forearm supinated

1. Fix the tape anchor over the medial aspect of the ulna, on the proximal part of its distal quarter.

2. Apply the tape, without tension, wrapping it over the anterior surface of the forearm in a lateral-distal direction, ending on the lateral surface of the distal quarter of the radius, just proximal to the base of the first metacarpal bone.

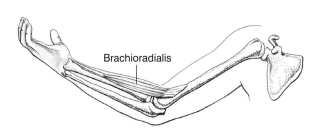

Brachioradialis

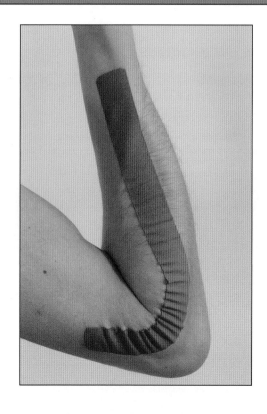

M. brachioradialis (Latin)

Origin: lateral supracondylar ridge and lateral epicondyle of the humerus

Insertion: styloid process of the radius

Innervation: radial nerve (C5-C6)

Action: elbow flexion, being a powerful flexor of the elbow joint, the brachioradialis is the initial motor in rapid movements. It supinates and pronates the forearm against resistance, and assists in prolonged flexion of the elbow against resistance.

MUSCLE TEST

Patient: seated or supine

Stabilization: the examiner places one hand under the patient's elbow to protect it against pressure from the table.

Test: elbow flexion with the forearm in a neutral position between pronation and supination; as the movement in question could be produced by other elbow flexors, the belly of the brachioradialis must be both observed and 'felt' during the test.

Pressure: against the most distal portion of the forearm in the direction of extension

CLINICAL APPLICATIONS

- Writer's cramp
- Elbow pain
- Pain along the brachioradialis
- Injuries due to overloading
- Rhizarthrosis
- De Quervain's tenosynovitis

Combined Applications

- Biceps brachii ➡ page 177
- Brachialis ➡ page 212

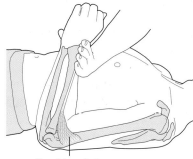

Brachioradialis

Brachioradialis - Tape Application

TAPE SPECIFICATIONS

- 1 tape
- Width 2.5 cm (1")
- Length 35 cm (14")
- I-shaped

35 cm

2.5 cm

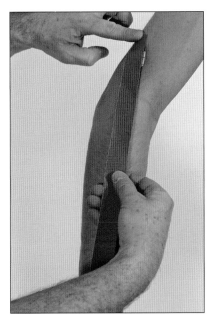 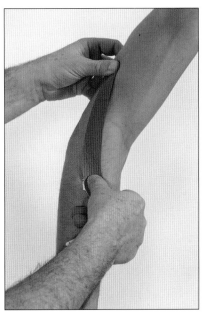 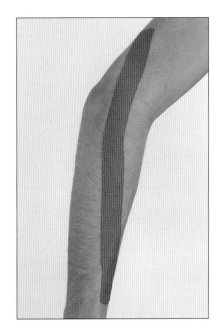

From 10 cm above the lateral epicondyle to the styloid process of the radius

The arm is forward flexed, elbow slightly flexed, forearm pronated and wrist flexed.

1. Fix the tape anchor 10 cm above the lateral epicondyle, over the lateral aspect of the humerus.

2. Remove 20 cm of backing paper and fold it back. Apply the tape, with no tension, passing medially to the lateral epicondyle.

3. Remove the remaining backing paper, except for the last 2 cm, and apply the tape, with no tension, as far as the styloid process of the radius.

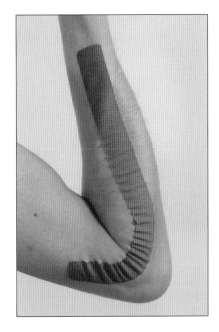

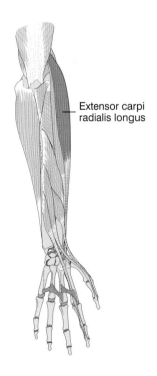

Extensor carpi
radialis longus

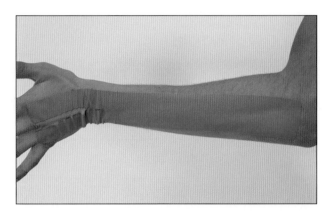

M. *extensor carpi radialis longus* (Latin)

Origin
• Lateral supracondylar ridge of the humerus
• Lateral epicondyle of the humerus

Insertion: dorsal surface of the base of the second metacarpal

Innervation: radial nerve (C6-C7)

Action: extension and radial abduction of the hand; assists in flexion of the elbow.

MUSCLE TEST

Patient: seated with the elbow bent about 30° short of 0° (full extension)

Stabilization: the forearm, which is almost fully pronated, rests on the table for support.

Test: extension of the wrist toward the radial side: the fingers should be allowed to flex when the wrist is extended.

Pressure: against the back of the hand along the second and third metacarpals in the direction of flexion toward the ulnar side

CLINICAL APPLICATIONS

• Wrist joint dysfunction
• Elbow pain
• Pain in the fingers, hand and wrist
• Epicondylitis
• Hemiplegic hand patients (neurological and motor rehabilitation)
• Loss of hand and finger function
• Rehabilitation after wrist and finger fractures
• Carpal tunnel syndrome
• De Quervain's tenosynovitis

Combined Applications

• Palmaris longus ➡ page 219
• Pronator teres ➡ page 214

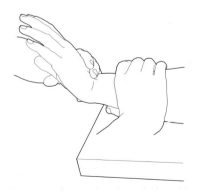

Extensor Carpi Radialis Longus - Tape Application

TAPE SPECIFICATIONS

- 1 tape
- Width 5 cm (2")
- Length 35 cm (14")
- Y-shaped, with 10 cm strips

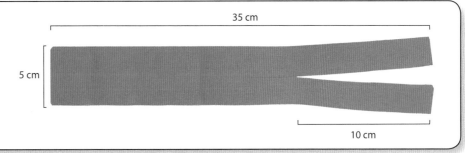

35 cm

5 cm

10 cm

From the elbow to the metacarpophalangeal joints, plus 2 cm: the two tails of the Y are to be measured from the metacarpophalangeal joints to 2 cm beyond the wrist.

Elbow and wrist are flexed, wrist in ulnar deviation, fingers flexed.

1. Fix the tape anchor just distal to the olecranon.

2. Remove the backing paper as far as the bifurcation of the Y and fold it back. Apply the tape, with no tension, on the posterior surface of the forearm.

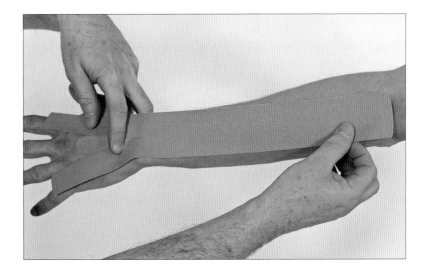

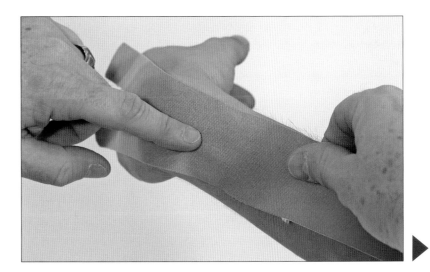

3. Remove the backing paper from the two tails of the Y. Apply the radial strip along the space between the second and third metacarpal bones and the ulnar strip along the fourth metacarpal to end beyond the metacarpophalangeal joints.

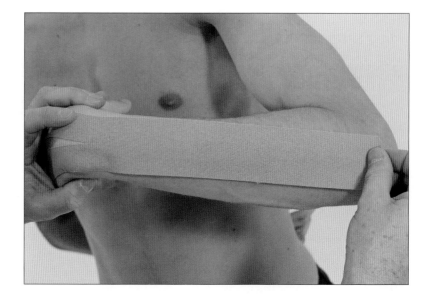

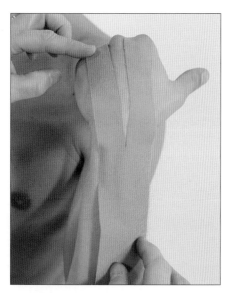

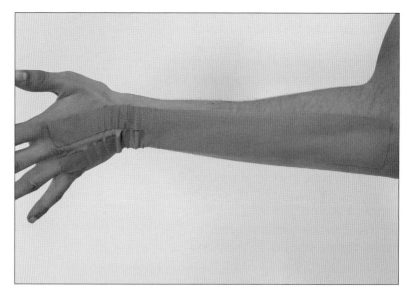

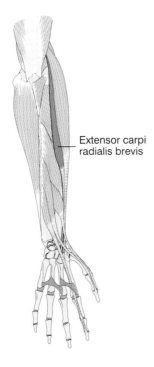

Extensor carpi
radialis brevis

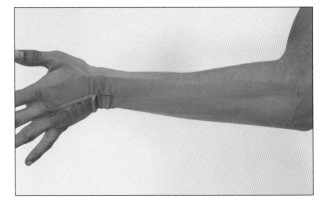

M. extensor carpi radialis brevis (Latin)

Origin: lateral epicondyle of the humerus, radial collateral ligament

Insertion: dorsal surface of the base of the third metacarpal bone

Innervation: radial nerve - posterior interosseous nerve (C7)

Action: extension and radial abduction of the hand

CLINICAL APPLICATIONS

- Wrist joint dysfunction
- Elbow pain
- Pain in the fingers, hand or wrist
- Epicondylitis
- Hemiplegic hand patients (neurological and motor rehabilitation)
- Loss of hand and finger function
- Rehabilitation after wrist and finger fractures
- Carpal tunnel syndrome
- De Quervain's tenosynovitis

Combined Applications

- Palmaris longus ➡ page 219
- Pronator teres ➡ page 214

NOTE: Use the same technique as for the extensor carpi radialis longus ➡ page 232.

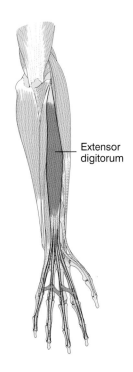

Extensor digitorum

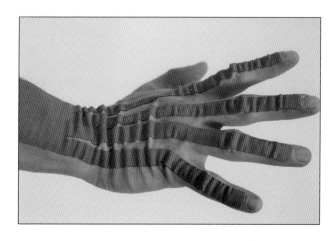

M. extensor digitorum (Latin)

Origin: lateral epicondyle of the humerus

Insertion: dorsal surfaces of the base of the middle and distal phalanges of the index, middle, ring and little fingers

Innervation: posterior interosseous nerve (C7-C8)

Action: extension and abduction of the fingers

CLINICAL APPLICATIONS

- Elbow pain
- Ulnar pain
- Pain in the fingers, hand and wrist
- Inflammation of the tendon sheath of the little finger
- Hemiplegic hand patients (neurological and motor rehabilitation)
- Rehabilitation after wrist and finger fractures

Combined Applications

- Palmaris longus ➡ page 219
- Pronator teres ➡ page 214
- Supinator ➡ page 241

TAPE SPECIFICATIONS

- 1 tape
- Width 5 cm (2")
- Length 50 cm (20")
- Fan-shaped, with four strips, each 20 cm long

50 cm

5 cm

20 cm

Extensor Digitorum - Tape Application

From the lateral epicondyle of the humerus to the tip of the middle finger; the tape strips are to be measured from the tip of the middle finger to 2 cm beyond the wrist. Each strip should then be cut according to the length of the finger concerned, so that it ends at the base of the nail.

Elbow is slightly flexed, forearm in the intermediate position between pronation and supination.

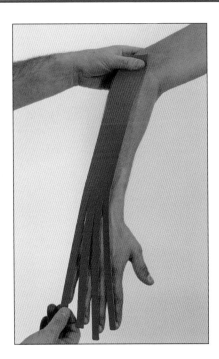
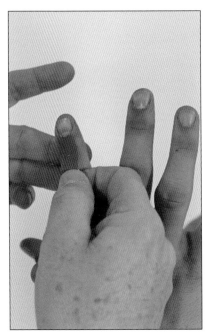

1. Apply the end of the first strip to the base of the index fingernail.

2. Remove the backing paper of the first strip to just beyond the level corresponding to the metacarpophalangeal joint and fold it back. With the patient forming a fist, apply the strip of tape, without tension, along the dorsum of the phalanges. Repeat the procedure for the middle, ring and little fingers.

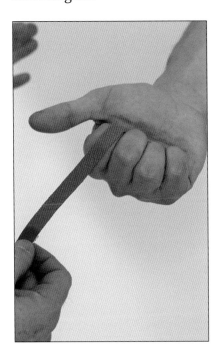
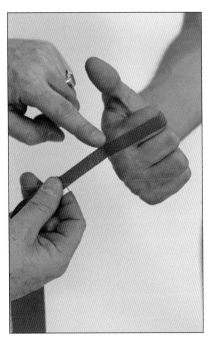
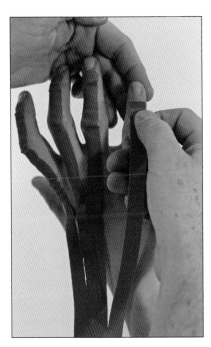

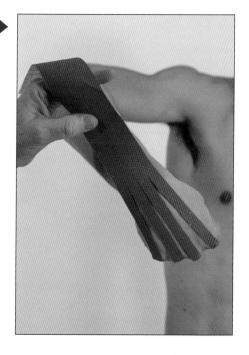

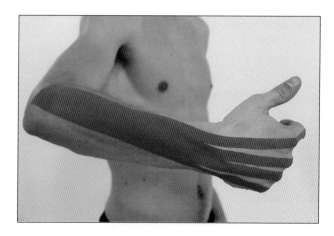

3. Remove the backing paper to just below the branching of the strips and fold it back. With the patient flexing the wrist, apply the strips of tape, which should be well spaced, without tension, to the back of the hand, each one over its respective metacarpal bone.

4. Once the remaining backing paper has been removed, apply the remaining tape, without tension, along the posterior surface of the forearm, in the direction of the lateral epicondyle of the humerus.

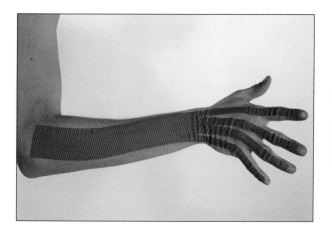

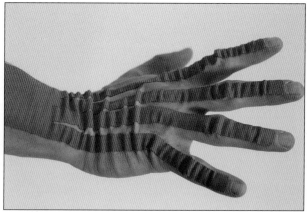

EXTENSOR CARPI ULNARIS

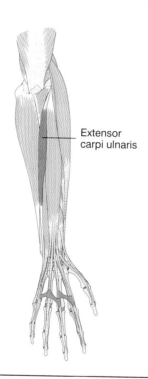

Extensor carpi ulnaris

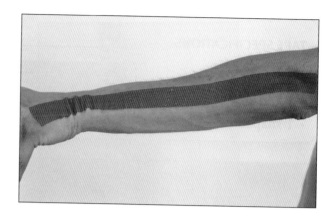

M. extensor carpi ulnaris (Latin)

Origin: lateral epicondyle of the humerus, posterior margin of the ulna

Insertion: ulnar surface of the base of the fifth metacarpal

Innervation: radial nerve (posterior interosseous nerve) (C7-C8)

Action: extension and ulnar abduction of the hand

CLINICAL APPLICATIONS

- Wrist joint dysfunction
- Elbow pain
- Pain in the fingers, hand and wrist
- Epicondylitis
- Hemiplegic hand patients (neurological and motor rehabilitation)
- Loss of hand and finger function
- Rehabilitation after wrist and finger fractures
- Carpal tunnel syndrome
- De Quervain's tenosynovitis

Combined Applications

- Palmaris longus ➡ page 219
- Pronator teres ➡ page 214

MUSCLE TEST

Patient: seated or supine

Stabilization: the forearm, which is fully pronated, rests on the table or is supported by the examiner.

Test: extension of the wrist toward the ulnar side

Pressure: against the back of the hand along the fifth metacarpal in the direction of flexion toward the radial side

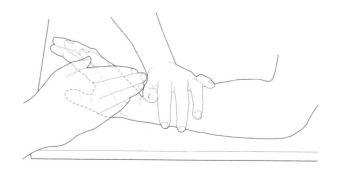

Extensor Pollicis Longus - Tape Application

CLINICAL APPLICATIONS

- Synovial (myxoid) cyst
- Hemiplegic hand patients (neurological and motor rehabilitation)
- Rehabilitation after wrist and finger fractures
- Extensor tendinitis

Combined applications

- Palmaris longus ➡ page 219
- Pronator teres ➡ page 214
- Supinator ➡ page 241

TAPE SPECIFICATIONS

- 1 tape
- Width 2.5 cm (1")
- Length 35 cm (14")
- I-shaped

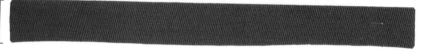

2.5 cm

35 cm

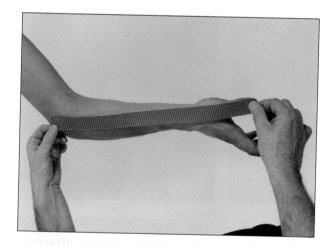

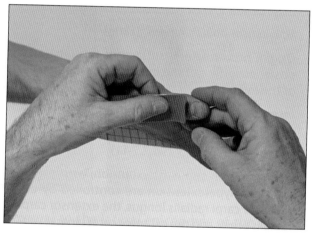

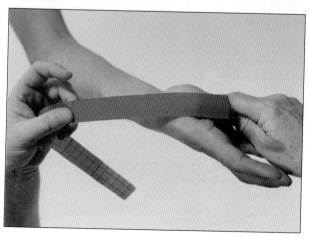

From 5 cm proximal to the lateral epicondyle of the humerus to the base of the thumbnail

Elbow is slightly flexed, forearm in the intermediate position between pronation and supination, wrist in ulnar deviation and thumb fully flexed.

1. Fix the tape anchor at the base of the thumbnail.

▶

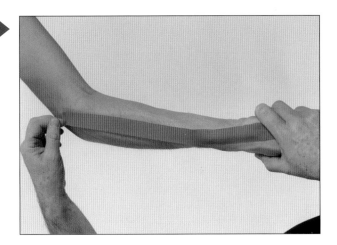

2. Remove the backing paper and apply the tape, without tension, along the dorsal surface of the thumb and then, once it is beyond the wrist, in the direction of the lateral epicondyle of the humerus. End 5 cm proximal to the lateral epicondyle of the humerus.

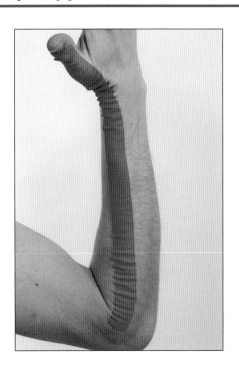

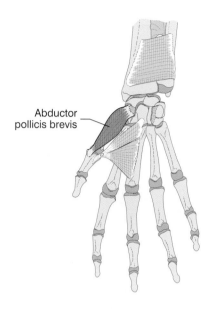

Abductor pollicis brevis

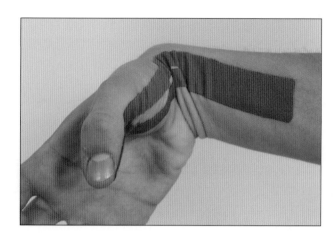

M. abductor pollicis brevis (Latin)

Origin: flexor retinaculum, tubercle of the scaphoid bone and tubercle of the trapezoid, abductor pollicis longus muscle

Insertion: radial surface of the base of the proximal phalanx of the thumb

Innervation: median nerve (C8-T1)

Action: abduction of the proximal phalanx of the thumb and of the first metacarpal

CLINICAL APPLICATIONS

- Wrist joint dysfunction
- Pain in the fingers, hand and wrist
- Hemiplegic hand patients (neurological and motor rehabilitation)
- Loss of hand and finger function
- Rehabilitation after wrist and finger fractures
- Carpal tunnel syndrome
- De Quervain's tenosynovitis

Combined Applications

- Brachioradialis ➡ page 230
- Extensor carpi radialis longus ➡ page 232
- Extensor digitorum ➡ page 236
- Pronator teres ➡ page 214
- Supinator ➡ page 241

Abductor Pollicis Brevis - Tape Application

TAPE SPECIFICATIONS

Application 1

- 1 tape
- Width 2.5 cm (1")
- Length 35 cm (14")
- I-shaped

Application 2

- 1 tape
- Width 2.5 cm (1")
- Length 25 cm (10")
- Y-shaped,
  with 10 cm strips

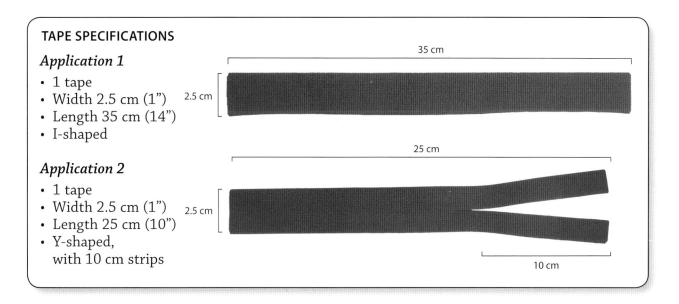

Application 1

From the tip of the thumb to mid forearm

Thumb extended toward the back of the hand

1. Position the tape anchor mid-way along the anterior surface of the radius.

2. Apply the tape, without tension, along the radius and thumb, to reach a point beyond and external to the base of the distal phalanx of the thumb.

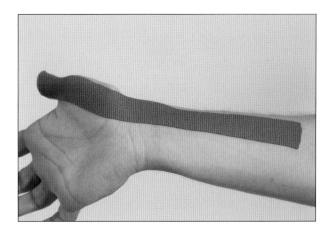

Abductor Pollicis Brevis - Tape Application

Application 2

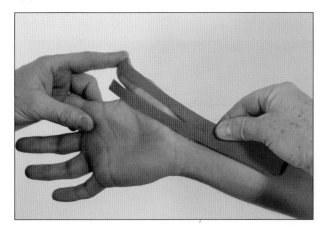
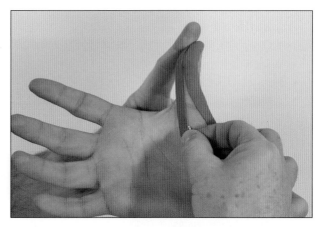
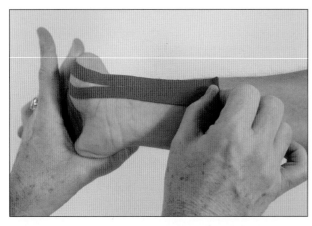
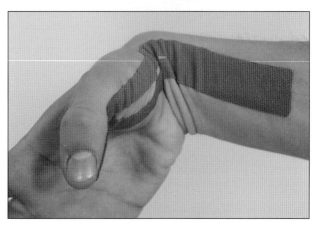

From the tip of the thumb to the distal third of the radius: the tails of the Y are to be measured from the tip of the thumb to the wrist.

Thumb extended

1. Position the end of the external strip of tape distal to the base of the distal phalanx of the thumb, on the radial side of the thumb-pad.

2. With the wrist in neutral position, extend the patient's thumb and apply the strip, without tension, in the direction of the trapezoid.

3. With the thumb fully abducted, position the internal end on the tip of the thumb, medially to the first, and apply the tape, without tension, along the thumb and thenar eminence, before finally converging with the first strip in a position proximal to the trapezoid.

4. Extend the wrist and apply the tape (2.5 cm wide), without tension, along the anterior aspect of the radius.

ADDUCTOR POLLICIS

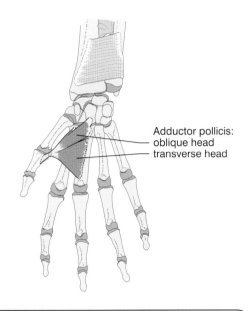

Adductor pollicis:
oblique head
transverse head

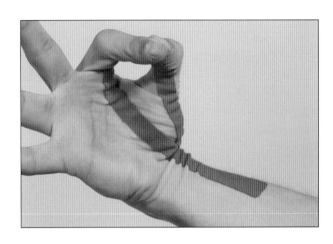

M. adductor pollicis (Latin)

Origin
- *Oblique head*: capitate bone and base of the second and third metacarpals
- *Transverse head*: shaft of the third metacarpal bone

Insertion: ulnar surface of the base of the proximal phalanx of the thumb

Innervation: ulnar nerve (C8-T1)

Action: adducts and flexes the proximal phalanx of the thumb and the first metacarpal. Assists in thumb-to-little finger opposition movement.

CLINICAL APPLICATIONS

- Wrist joint dysfunction
- Pain in the fingers, hand and wrist
- Hemiplegic hand patients (neurological and motor rehabilitation)
- Loss of hand and finger function
- Rehabilitation after wrist and finger fractures
- Carpal tunnel syndrome
- De Quervain's tenosynovitis

Combined Applications
- Brachioradialis ➡ page 230
- Extensor carpi radialis longus ➡ page 232
- Extensor digitorum ➡ page 236
- Pronator teres ➡ page 214
- Supinator ➡ page 241

MUSCLE TEST

Patient: seated or supine

Stabilization: the patient's hand may be held by the examiner or it may rest on the table for support.

Test: adduction of the thumb toward the palm

Pressure: against the medial surface of the thumb in the direction of abduction away from the palm

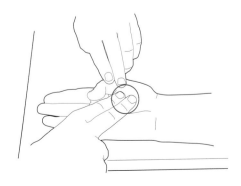

Adductor Pollicis - Tape Application

TAPE SPECIFICATIONS

- 1 tape
- Width 2.5 cm (1")
- Length 25 cm (10")
- Y-shaped,
  with 10 cm long strips

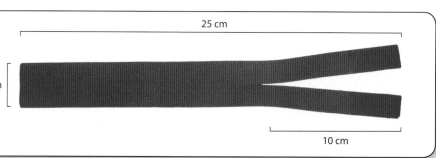

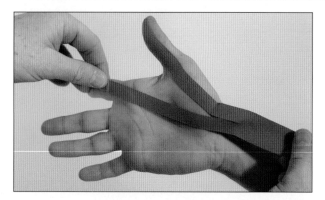
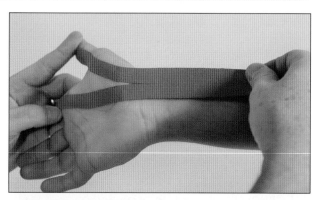
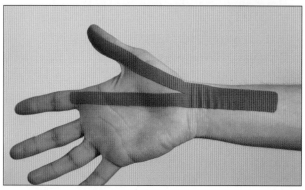
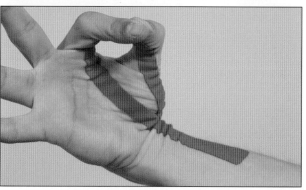

From the tip of the thumb to the distal third of the radius: the two tails of the Y are to be measured from the tip of the thumb to 2 cm beyond the trapezoid.

Thumb extended and abducted

1. Position the end of the external strip on the tip of the thumb distally to the base of the distal phalanx.

2. Extend and abduct the thumb and apply the strip as far as the bifurcation of the Y, with no tension, along the thumb and thenar eminence, in the direction of the carpometacarpal joint of the thumb.

3. Extend the patient's index finger and apply the end of the internal strip distally to the metacarpophalangeal joint. Then apply the tape, with no tension, along the second metacarpal, converging towards the first strip.

4. Extend the wrist and position the tape (2.5 cm wide), without tension, along the palmar surface of the radius.

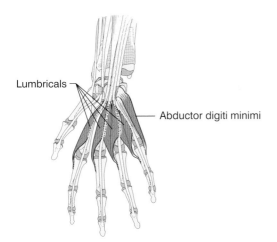

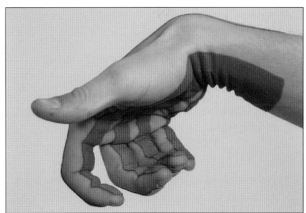

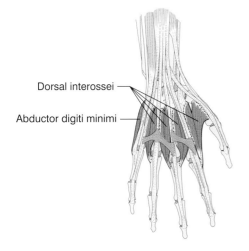

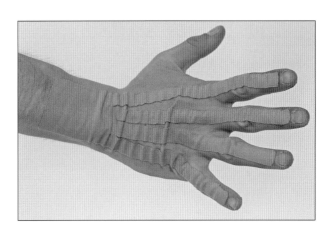

M. interossei dorsales, M. lumbricales, M. abductor digiti minimi (Latin)

Origin
- *Dorsal interossei*: each muscle arises from the adjacent sides of two metacarpals.
- *Lumbricals*: tendons of the flexor digitorum profundus
- *Abductor digiti minimi*: pisiform bone, pisohamate ligament and flexor carpi ulnaris tendon

Insertion
- *Dorsal interossei*: bases of the proximal phalanges of the index, middle and ring fingers
- *Lumbricals*: lateral margin of the tendons of the extensor digitorum
- *Abductor digiti minimi*: ulnar surface of the base of the proximal phalanx of little finger

Innervation
- *Dorsal interossei*: ulnar nerve (C8-T1)
- *Lumbricals*: first and second: median nerve (C8-T1); third and fourth: ulnar nerve
- *Abductor digiti minimi*: ulnar nerve (C8-T1)

Action
- *Dorsal interossei*: abduction of the fingers away from the middle finger and ulnar or radial abduction of the middle finger; these muscles assist in flexion and extension of the phalanges.
- *Lumbricals*: extension of the middle and distal phalanges and flexion of the proximal phalanges of the index, middle and ring fingers
- *Abductor digiti minimi*: abduction of the little finger

Small Muscles of the Hand - Tape Application

CLINICAL APPLICATIONS

- Arthritis of the fingers
- Pain on closing the hand or on grasping
- Inflammation and reduced mobility of the fingers
- Hemiplegic hand patients (neurological and motor rehabilitation)
- Paralysis of the hand
- Loss of hand or finger function
- Rehabilitation after wrist and finger fractures
- Stiffness and pain in the fingers

- Biceps brachii ➡ page 177
- Brachioradialis ➡ page 230
- Deltoid ➡ page 161
- Pronator teres ➡ page 214
- Supinator ➡ page 241
- Triceps brachii ➡ page 180

Combined Applications

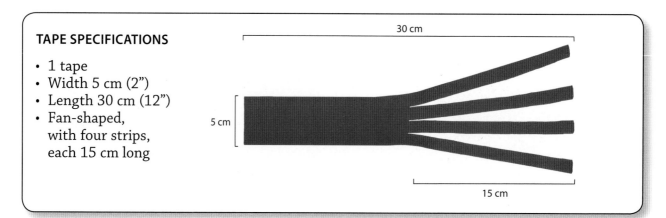

TAPE SPECIFICATIONS

- 1 tape
- Width 5 cm (2")
- Length 30 cm (12")
- Fan-shaped, with four strips, each 15 cm long

30 cm

5 cm

15 cm

Small Muscles of the Hand - Tape Application

Palmar application

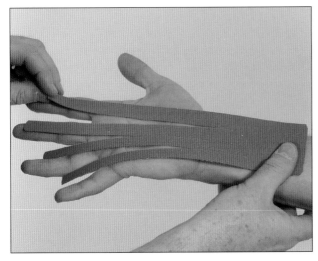
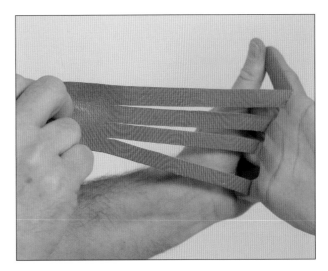
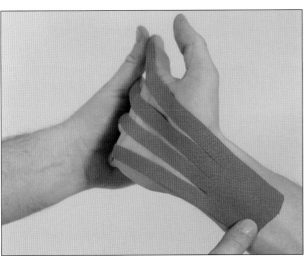
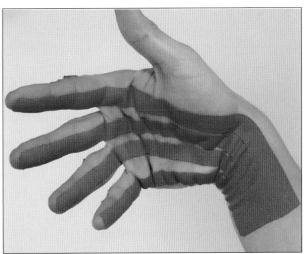

From the tip of the middle finger to the distal third of the forearm: the strips of the fan are to be measured from the tip of the middle finger to 2 cm beyond the wrist. Each strip is then cut according to the length of the finger concerned, so that it ends on the fingertip.

Fingers and wrist extended

1. Apply the anchor of the first strip to the index fingertip.

2. Remove the paper from the first strip up to the level corresponding to the metacarpophalangeal joint. Bring the patient's index finger to full extension and apply the strip, without tension, along the palmar surface of the finger. Repeat for the middle, ring and little fingers.

3. Remove the rest of the paper and apply the tape, with no tension and ensuring that the strips are well spaced. The tape ends on the distal third of the forearm.

Small Muscles of the Hand - Tape Application

Dorsal application

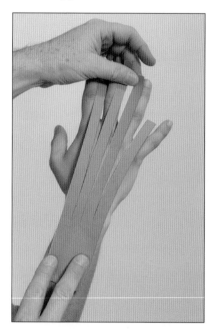 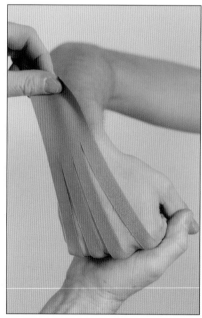 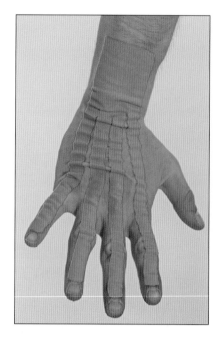

From the tip of the middle finger to the distal third of the forearm: the strips of the fan are to be measured from the tip of the middle finger to 2 cm beyond the wrist. Each strip is then shortened according to the length of the finger concerned, so that it ends at the base of the fingernail.

Fingers and wrist flexed

1. Apply the end of the first strip to the base of the index fingernail.

2. Remove the backing paper up to 2 cm beyond the metacarpophalangeal joints. Ask the patient to form a fist with the hand and apply the strip, without tension, along the dorsal surface of the index finger. Repeat the procedure for the middle, ring and little fingers.

3. Remove the rest of the backing paper. Ask the patient to flex the wrist and apply the remaining tape, still with no tension and ensuring that the tape tails are well spaced. The tape ends on the distal third of the forearm.

Combined application

Carry out the palmar and dorsal applications as previously described.

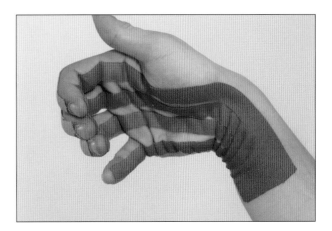

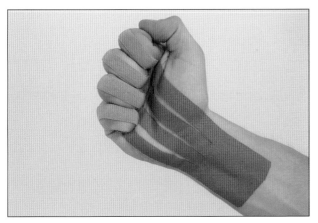

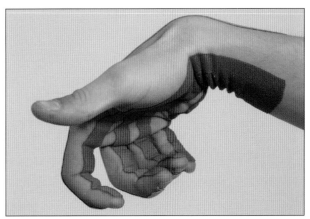

8

Hip and Lower Limb

- **Quadratus lumborum**
- **Iliopsoas**
- **Sartorius**
- **Pectineus**
- **Adductor muscles**
- **Piriformis**
- **Gluteus maximus**
- **Tensor fasciae latae**
- **Gluteus medius and gluteus minimus**
- **Hamstring muscles (biceps femoris, semimembranosus and semitendinosus)**
- **Quadriceps femoris**
- **Tibialis anterior**
- **Gastrocnemius**
- **Soleus**
- **Tibialis posterior**
- **Fibularis (peroneus) longus, brevis and tertius**
- **Flexor hallucis brevis**
- **Flexor digitorum brevis**
- **Flexor digitorum longus and hallucis longus**
- **Abductor hallucis**
- **Extensor digitorum brevis and hallucis brevis**
- **Extensor hallucis longus**
- **Extensor digitorum longus**
- **Plantaris**

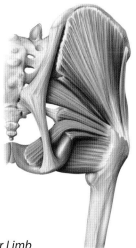

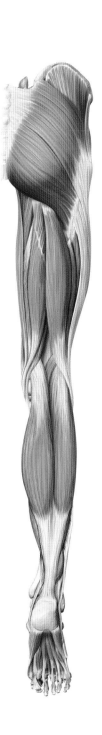

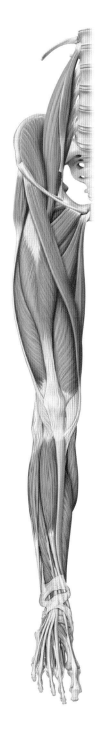

QUADRATUS LUMBORUM

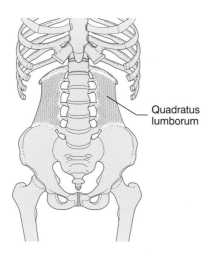

Quadratus
lumborum

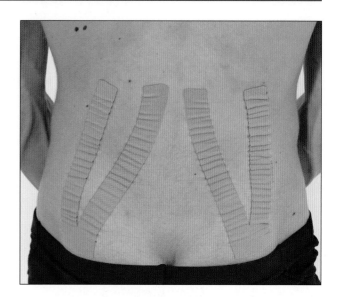

M. quadratus lumborum (Latin)

Origin: iliolumbar ligament, iliac crest

Insertion: inferior margin of the twelfth rib, transverse processes of the first four lumbar vertebrae

Innervation: last intercostal nerve, anterior branches of the first lumbar nerves (T12, L1, L2, L3)

Action: the quadratus lumborum assists in extension and lateral flexion of the spine and it depresses the last rib. Together with the diaphragm, it acts bilaterally to stabilize the last two ribs during breathing.

CLINICAL APPLICATIONS

- Hip bursitis
- Symptomatic lumbar disc herniation
- Scoliosis
- Low back pain symptoms (myofascial pain syndrome)
- Spondylosis
- Symptomatic spinal canal stenosis

Combined Applications

- Gluteus maximus ➡ page 278
- Gluteus medius and gluteus minimus ➡ page 284
- Iliopsoas ➡ page 261
- Piriformis ➡ page 276
- Rectus abdominis ➡ page 200
- Rhomboid major ➡ page 148
- Rhomboid minor ➡ page 146

TAPE SPECIFICATIONS

- 2 tapes
- Width 5 cm (2")
- Length 25 cm (10")
- Anchor 2 cm (0.75")
- Y-shaped

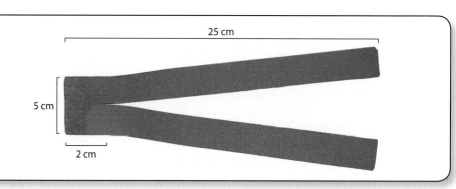

25 cm

5 cm

2 cm

Quadratus Lumborum - Tape Application

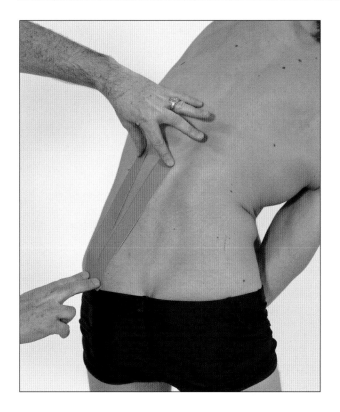

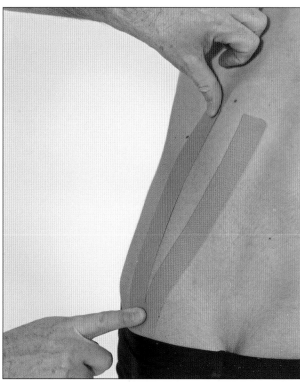

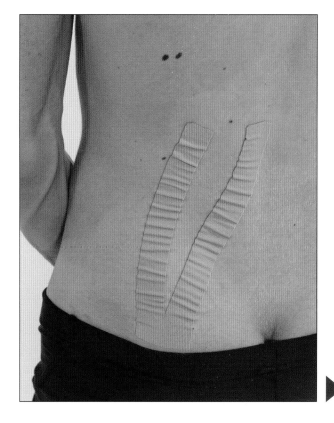

📏 From the posterior curve of the iliac crest to 2 cm beyond the transverse process of the first lumbar vertebra

🧍 Standing with feet together, trunk bent away from the side to be treated, and the arm on the side of the muscle to be treated, raised

1. Apply the anchors of the two tapes 5 cm below and laterally to the right and left iliolumbar ligaments, at the level of the top of the gluteal cleft.

2. Apply the medial strip of the Y, without tension, outlining the medial margin of the muscle towards the transverse process of the first lumbar vertebra. End just above this vertebra.

3. Apply the lateral strip of the Y without tension, ensuring that it is well spaced from the medial strip. End above the last rib.

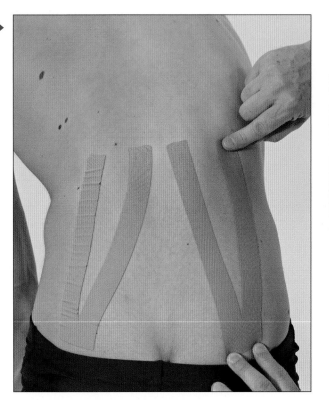
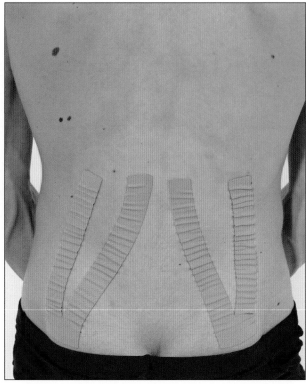

NOTE: The quadratus lumborum influences body posture due to its connection to the spinal column, so it must always receive bilateral and symmetrical tape applications.

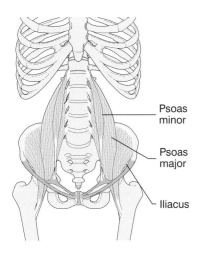

Psoas minor

Psoas major

Iliacus

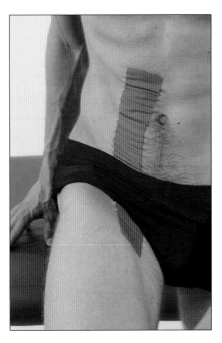

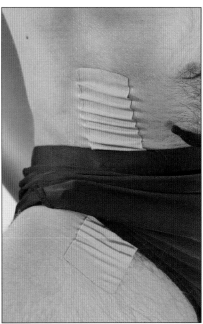

M. iliopsoas (Latin)

Origin

- *Psoas major*: anterior surfaces of the transverse processes of the lumbar vertebrae, lateral surfaces of the bodies and intervertebral discs of T12 and the lumbar vertebrae
- *Iliacus*: iliac fossa, inner lip of the iliac crest, anterior sacroiliac and iliolumbar ligaments, lateral part of the sacrum

Insertion

- *Psoas major*: lesser trochanter of the femur
- *Iliacus*: lesser trochanter of the femur, lateral surface of the tendon of the psoas major

Innervation

- *Psoas major*: anterior branches of the second and third lumbar nerves (L2, L3)
- *Iliacus*: anterior branches of the second and third lumbar nerves through the femoral nerve (L2, L3)

Action: forward flexion of the chest. The iliopsoas flexes the thigh on the trunk and can adduct and externally rotate the hip. With the insertion fixed, this muscle, contracting bilaterally, flexes the trunk on the thighs and increases lumbar lordosis. Contracting unilaterally, it contributes to lateral flexion of the trunk. Impairment of this muscle leads to difficulties in many activities of daily life, such as climbing stairs, standing up, sitting down, and walking uphill. If this muscle is severely impaired, during the gait there has to be a marked rotation of the pelvis toward the side of the weight-bearing limb so as to facilitate the advancement of the moving limb.

MUSCLE TEST

Patient: supine

Stabilization: the examiner holds the opposite iliac crest stabilized. The quadriceps femoris stabilizes the knee in extension.

Test: flexion of the hip in a slightly abducted and externally rotated position

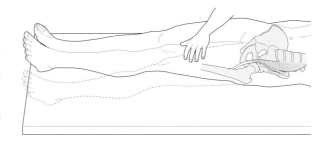

Pressure: against the anteromedial surface of the leg in the direction of extension and slight abduction and in a direction directly opposite to the orientation of the psoas major's line of pull, from its origin on the lumbar spine to its insertion on the lesser trochanter of the femur

CLINICAL APPLICATIONS

- Postural correction
- Coarthrosis
- Inguinal hernia
- Lumbar hernia
- Hyperlordosis
- Low back pain
- Pubic pain
- Rehabilitation after hip replacement
- Scoliosis

Combined Applications

- Lumbar part of the iliocostalis lumborum ➡ page 192
- Pectoralis major ➡ page 152
- Piriformis ➡ page 276
- Rhomboid major ➡ page 148
- Rhomboid minor ➡ page 146

TAPE SPECIFICATIONS

Psoas major
- 1 tape
- Width 5 cm (2")
- Length 40 cm (16")
- I-shaped

Iliacus
- 1 tape
- Width 5 cm (2")
- Length 20 cm (8")
- I-shaped

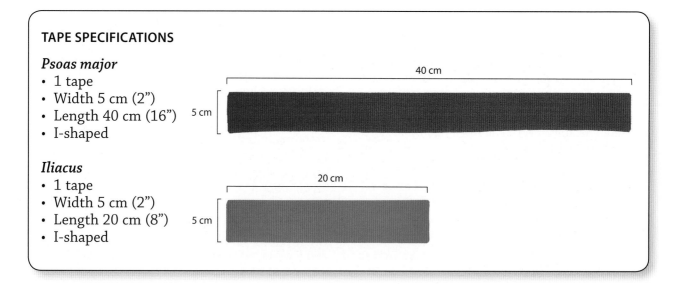

Iliopsoas - Tape Application

Psoas major

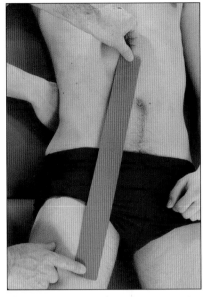
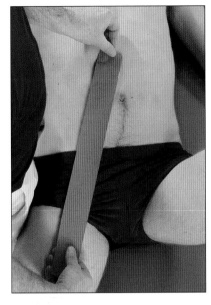
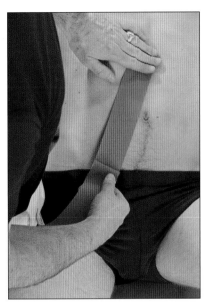
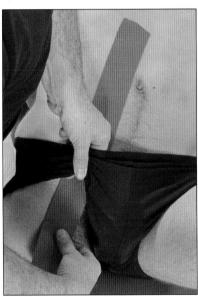
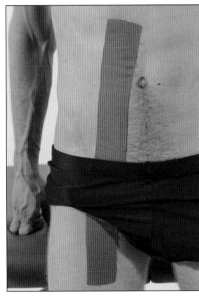
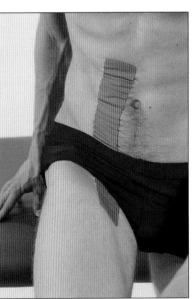

📏 From 10 cm above the navel to mid-thigh

⚕ Supine, with the leg on the side to be treated off the table and the other leg flexed on the table

1. Apply the tape anchor on the linea alba, 10 cm above the navel. The tape should be obliquely angled downward and outward so that it passes inside the anterior superior iliac spine.

2. Remove the backing paper from the tape, except for the last 5 cm. Then, following the muscle's line of projection, continue to apply the tape, without tension, in a downward direction, taking it inside the anterior superior iliac spine. End below the lesser trochanter of the femur.

Iliacus

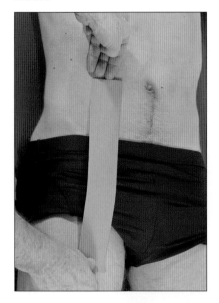
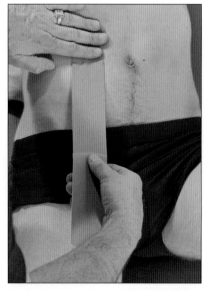
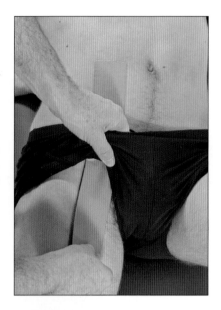

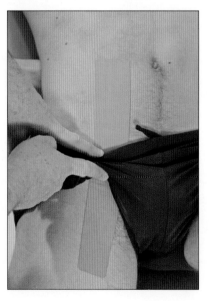
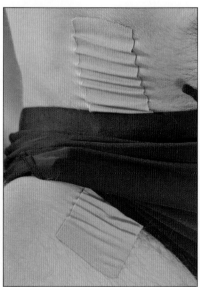

🗞 From the navel to the proximal third of the thigh

⚖ Supine, with the leg on the side to be treated off the table and the other leg flexed on the table

1. Apply the tape anchor around 5 cm laterally to the linea alba and navel. Applied vertically, the tape should follow the iliacus downward and externally, so that it passes inside the anterior superior iliac spine.

2. Remove the backing paper from the tape, except for the last 5 cm. Then, following the muscle's line of projection, continue to apply the tape, without tension, in a downward direction, taking it inside the anterior superior iliac spine. End below the lesser trochanter of the femur.

SARTORIUS

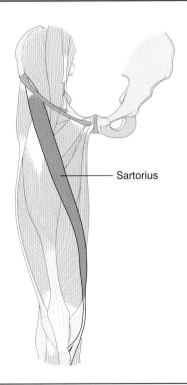

Sartorius

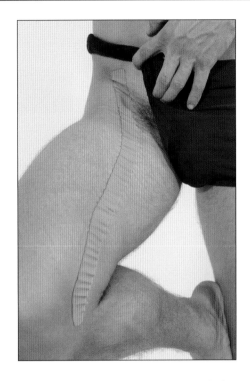

M. sartorius (Latin)

Origin: anterior superior iliac spine

Insertion: upper part of the medial surface of the tibia

Innervation: femoral nerve (L2-L3)

Action: flexion, external rotation, and abduction of the coxofemoral joint and internal rotation of the knee joint. Even though two-thirds of this muscle is located on the front of the thigh, it is not involved in knee extension, but contributes to internal flexion of the tibia during bending of the knee. Weakness of the sartorius causes pelvic pain, knee pain, and valgus knee.

MUSCLE TEST

Patient: supine

Stabilization: not necessary on the part of the examiner. The patient can use the table for support.

Test: external rotation, abduction and flexion of the thigh with flexion of the knee

Resistance: pressure is applied against the anterolateral and lateral surfaces of the lower thigh in the direction of the hip extension, adduction, and internal rotation, and against the leg in the direction of the knee extension. The examiner's hands are positioned in such a way as to oppose resistance to the external rotation of the hip through an action of pressure and counter-pressure. The examiner has to oppose the multiple actions involved in the test maneuvers through a combined movement of resistance.

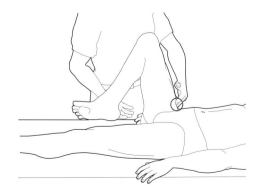

Sartorius - Tape Application

TAPE SPECIFICATIONS

- 1 tape
- Width 2.5 cm (1")
- Length 35-40 cm (14-16")
- I-shaped

35 cm

2.5 cm

CLINICAL APPLICATIONS

- Hip bursitis
- Coxarthrosis
- Coxitis
- Congenital dislocation of the hip
- Knee joint disorders
- Hip joint disorders
- Sciatica

Combined Applications

- Lumbar part of the iliocostalis lumborum ➡ page 192
- Piriformis ➡ page 276
- Quadratus lumborum ➡ page 258
- Rectus abdominis ➡ page 200

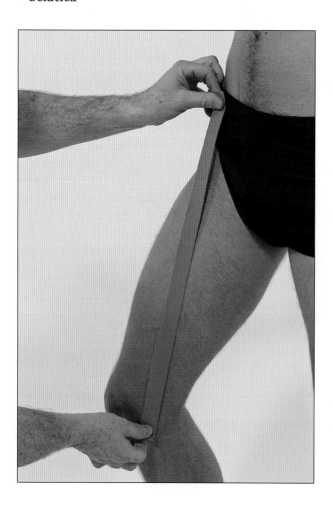
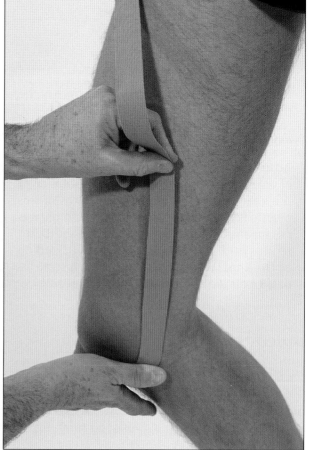

Sartorius - Tape Application

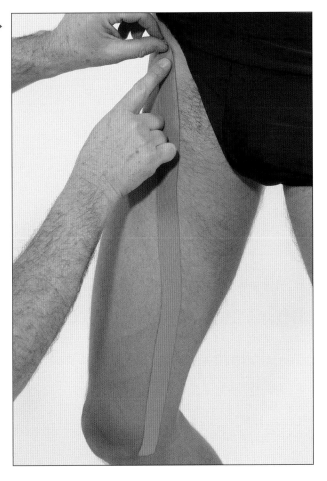 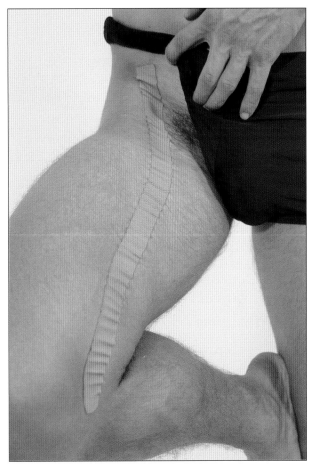

From 2 cm above the anterior superior iliac spine to 2 cm below the medial condyle of the tibia

Standing in front of the therapist, knee extended, and hip slightly extended, adducted, and externally rotated

1. Position the tape anchor below the medial condyle of the tibia.

2. Remove the backing paper and apply the tape, without tension, over the course of the muscle as far as a point just above the anterior superior iliac spine.

PECTINEUS

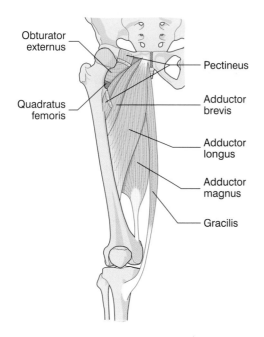

Obturator externus
Quadratus femoris
Pectineus
Adductor brevis
Adductor longus
Adductor magnus
Gracilis

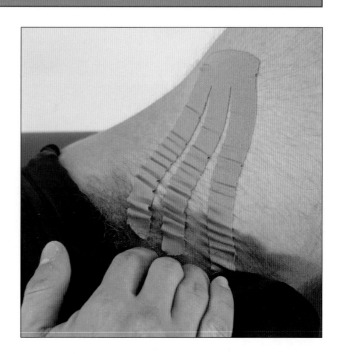

M. pectineus (Latin)

Origin: pectineal crest of the pubis and iliopubic eminence

Insertion: pectineal line of the femur

Innervation: femoral nerve (L2-L3)

Action: adduction and flexion of the coxofemoral joint.

CLINICAL APPLICATIONS

- Coxarthrosis
- Coxitis
- Congenital dislocation of the hip
- Inguinal hernia
- Hip joint disorders
- Pelvic disorders

Combined Applications

- Lumbar part of the iliocostalis lumborum ➥ page 192
- Piriformis ➥ page 276
- Quadratus lumborum ➥ page 258
- Rectus abdominis ➥ page 200
- Tensor fasciae latae ➥ page 281

TAPE SPECIFICATIONS

- 1 tape
- Width 5 cm (2")
- Length 15 cm (6")
- Anchor 2 cm (0.75")
- W-shaped

15 cm

5 cm

2 cm

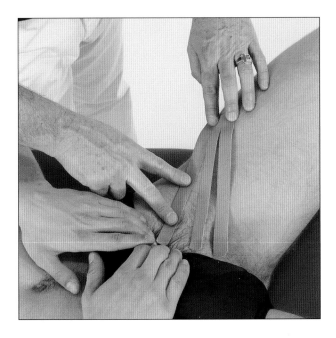
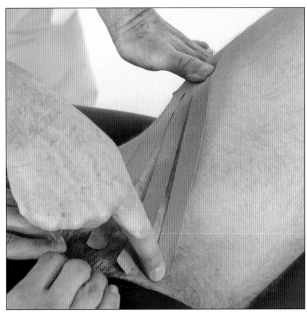
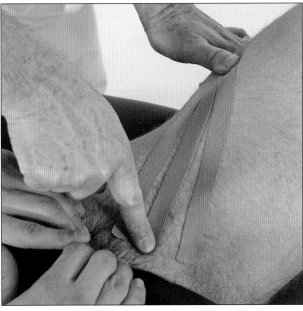
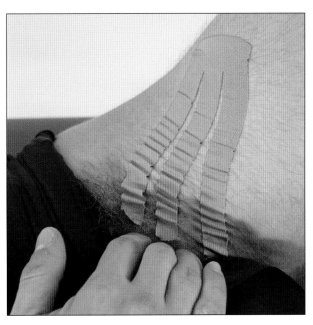

From the linea aspera of the femur (proximal third of the anteromedial thigh region) to the pectineal crest of the pubis at inguinal level

Supine, the hip flexed and externally rotated, knee flexed at 90°

1. The base of the tape is angled toward the groin and is applied on the proximal third of the anteromedial thigh region.

2. Apply the tape, with no tension. Distribute the three strips over the course of the muscle and have them diverge at the groin.

ADDUCTOR MUSCLES

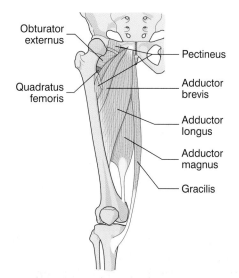

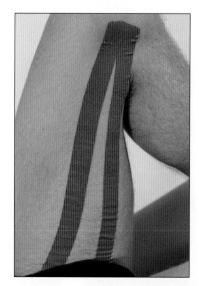

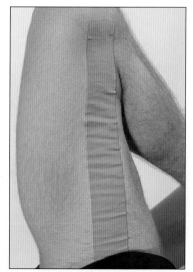

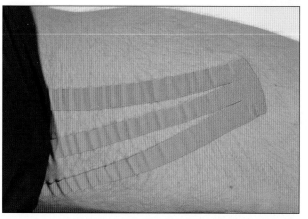

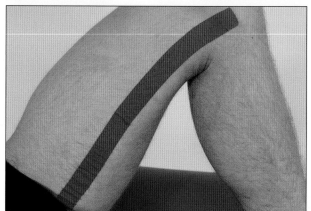

Obturator externus — **Pectineus** — **Quadratus femoris** — **Adductor brevis** — **Adductor longus** — **Adductor magnus** — **Gracilis**

M. adductor magnus, brevis, longus (Latin)

Origin
- *Adductor magnus*: external surface of the ramus of the ischium, ischial tuberosity
- *Adductor longus*: superior pubic ramus
- *Adductor brevis*: anterior surface of the inferior pubic ramus

Insertion
- *Adductor magnus*: medial lip of the linea aspera of the femur, medial supracondylar line of the femur, adductor tubercle
- *Adductor longus*: medial lip of the linea aspera of the femur
- *Adductor brevis*: medial lip of the linea aspera of the femur

Innervation
- *Adductor magnus*: obturator and tibial nerves (L3-L5)
- *Adductor longus*: obturator nerve (L1-L4)
- *Adductor brevis*: obturator nerve (L2-L4)

Action
- *Adductor magnus*: adduction, extension and external and internal rotation of the hip joint
- *Adductor longus and adductor brevis*: adduction and external rotation of the hip joint. These muscles participate, weakly, in hip flexion. If they are weak, the pelvis bends, which can cause knee pain. A hormonal effect may also occur, with frequent suspensions of the menstrual cycle.

Adductor Muscles - Tape Application

MUSCLE TEST

Patient: lying on the right side for testing of the right side, and vice-versa, with the body forming a straight line with the legs and the lumbar spine straight

Stabilization: the examiner supports the upper leg in abduction. The patient should hold onto the edge of the table for support.

Test: adduction of the underlying leg, which must be raised from the surface of the table without flexion, rotation, or extension and without tilting the pelvis

Pressure: against the medial surface of the distal end of the thigh in the direction of the abduction

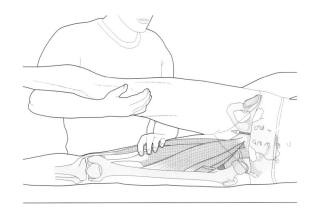

(downward, toward the table): pressure should be applied at a point above the knee in order to avoid stretching the tibial collateral ligament.

TAPE SPECIFICATIONS

Application 1
- 1 tape
- Width 5 cm (2")
- Length 50 cm (20")
- Anchor 2 cm (0.75")
- Y-shaped

Application 2
- 1 tape
- Width 5 cm (2")
- Length 50 cm (20")
- I-shaped

Application 3
- 1 tape
- Width 5 cm (2")
- Length 20 cm (8")
- Anchor 2 cm (0.75")
- W-shaped

Application 4
- 1 tape
- Width 2.5 cm (1")
- Length 50 cm (20")
- I-shaped

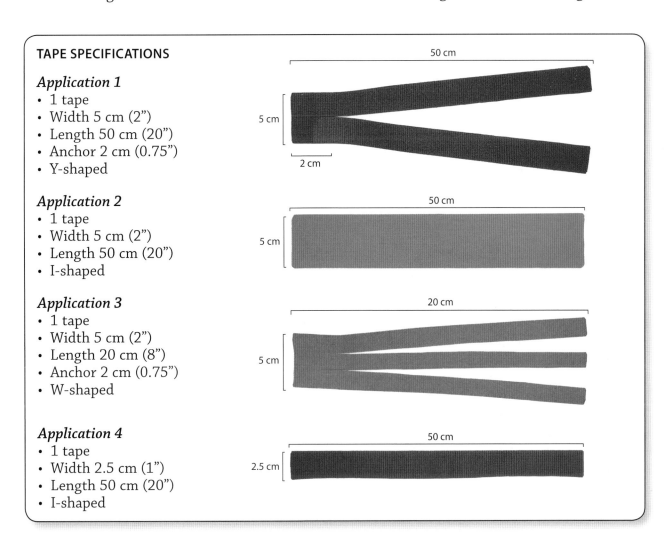

Adductor Muscles - Tape Application

CLINICAL APPLICATIONS

- Coxarthrosis
- Coxitis
- Congenital dislocation of the hip
- Knee joint disorders
- Hip joint disorders
- Pelvic disorders

Combined applications

- Lumbar part of the iliocostalis lumborum ➠ page 192
- Piriformis ➠ page 276
- Quadratus lumborum ➠ page 258
- Rectus abdominis ➠ page 200

Application 1

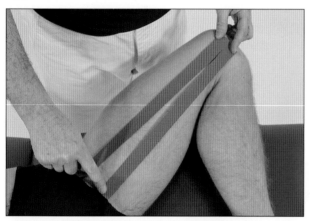
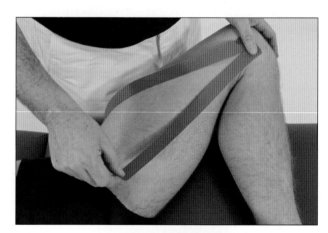
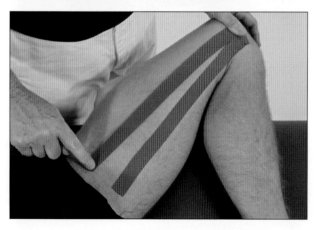
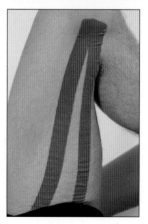

📏 From below the medial condyle of the femur to the groin, plus 2 cm

🧍 Supine, the hip flexed and externally rotated, knee flexed at 90°

1. Apply the tape anchor distally to the medial condyle of the femur.

2. With the hip in full external rotation and keeping the knee flexed at 90°, apply the tape centrally, without tension, outlining the belly of the adductor magnus. End the application just before the muscle's origin on the ischial tuberosity.

Adductor Muscles - Tape Application

Application 2

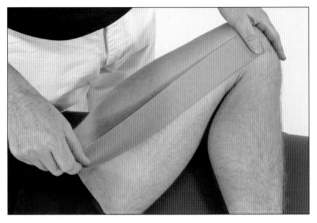 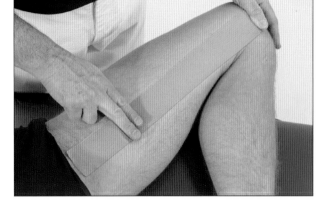

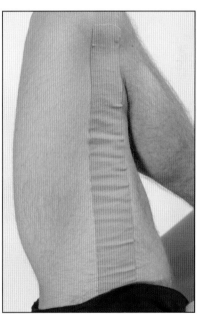

📏 From below the medial condyle of the femur to the groin, plus 2 cm

🧍 Supine, the hip flexed and externally rotated, knee flexed at 90°

1. Apply the tape anchor distally to the medial condyle of the femur.

2. With the hip in full external rotation and keeping the knee flexed at 90°, apply the tape, without tension, along the middle of the belly of the adductor magnus.

Adductor Muscles - Tape Application

Application 3

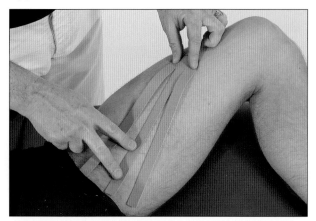

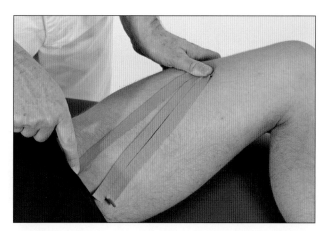

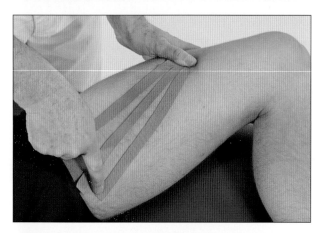

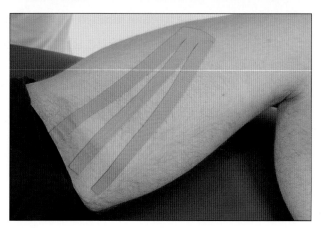

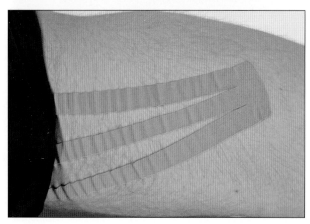

From the linea aspera of the femur, at the level of the middle third of the anteromedial thigh region, to the groin, plus 2 cm

Supine, the hip flexed and externally rotated, knee flexed at 90°

1. Apply the tape anchor on the middle third of the anteromedial thigh region, angled toward the groin.

2. With the hip in full external rotation and keeping the knee flexed at 90°, apply the tape tails spacing them so that they diverge at the groin.

Adductor Muscles - Tape Application

Application 4 - Gracilis

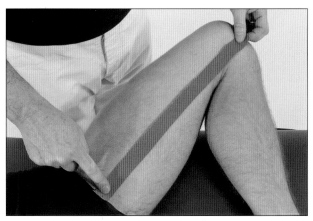 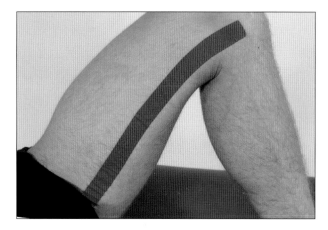

From below the medial condyle of the femur to the side of the pubic symphysis, plus 2 cm

Supine, the hip flexed and externally rotated, knee flexed at 90°

1. Apply the tape anchor distally to the medial condyle of the femur.

2. With the hip in full external rotation and keeping the knee flexed at 90°, apply the tape, without tension, along the course of the gracilis towards the pubic symphysis.

PIRIFORMIS

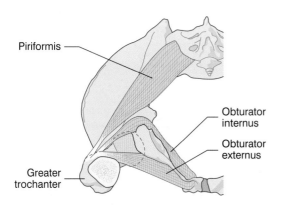

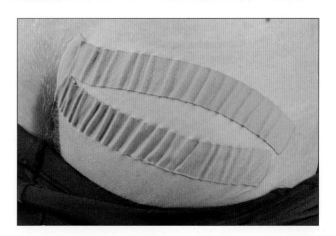

M. piriformis (Latin)

Origin: pelvic surface of the sacrum, margin of the greater sciatic foramen

Insertion: upper margin of the greater trochanter of the femur

Innervation: sacral plexus (L5-S2)

Action: external rotation and extension of the hip joint. The piriformis, together with the external and internal obturator muscles, the superior and inferior gemelli, and the quadratus femoris, holds the head of the femur in the acetabulum.
   A weak piriformis muscle can sometimes result in sciatic nerve problems, pain or paresthesia in the lower limb, frequent micturition, or bladder block.

CLINICAL APPLICATIONS

- Coccydynia
- Postural correction
- Coxarthrosis
- Lumbar discopathy
- Symptomatic lumbar disc herniation
- Hip joint disorders
- Rehabilitation after hip replacement
- Sciatica
- Piriformis syndrome

Combined Applications

- Lumbar part of the iliocostalis lumborum ⇒ page 192
- Rectus abdominis ⇒ page 200
- Rhomboid major ⇒ page 148
- Rhomboid minor ⇒ page 146

TAPE SPECIFICATIONS

- 1 tape
- Width 5 cm (2")
- Length 25 cm (10")
- Anchor 2 cm (0.75")
- Y-shaped

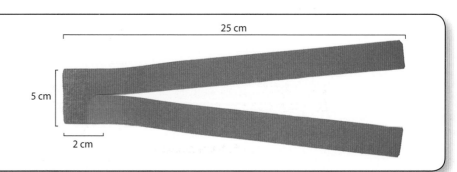

Piriformis - Tape Application

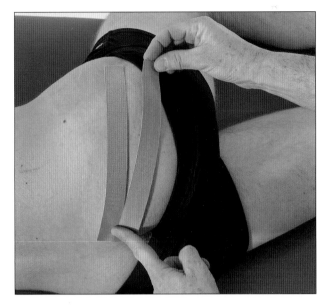 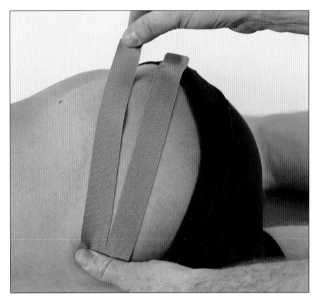

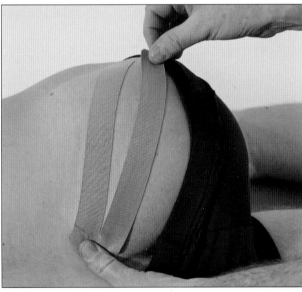 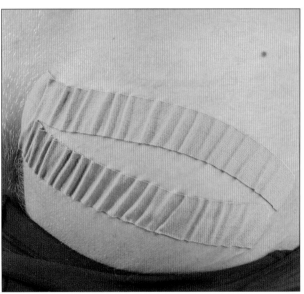

🎗️ From the first sacral foramina to the greater trochanter of the femur, plus 2 cm

🧍 Lateral decubitus, lying on the side opposite to the one to be treated, with the underlying leg extended, the overlying leg flexed, adducted, and internally rotated, and the knee resting on the table

1. Apply the tape anchor on the sacrum, angled toward the greater trochanter of the femur.

2. Apply the upper tail of the Y, without tension, in the direction of the greater trochanter of the femur, following the upper margin of the piriformis, while pulling the skin in the opposite direction.

3. Guide the lower strip of the Y, without applying tension, toward the lower part of the buttock before converging with the first strip towards the greater trochanter of the femur. Again, pull the skin in the opposite direction during application.

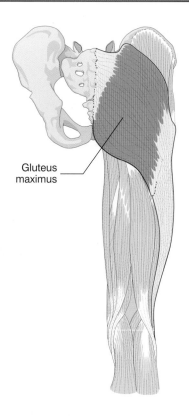

Gluteus
maximus

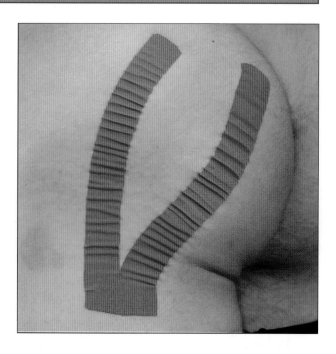

MUSCLE TEST

Patient: prone, with knee flexed at 90° or more; the greater the flexion of the knee, the less the hip will be extended due to tension from the rectus femoris.

Stabilization: the pelvis is stabilized to the trunk, posteriorly by the back muscles, laterally by the lateral abdominal muscles, and anteriorly by the contralateral hip flexors

Test: extension of the hip with the knee flexed

Pressure: against the lower part of the posterior thigh in the direction of the hip flexion.

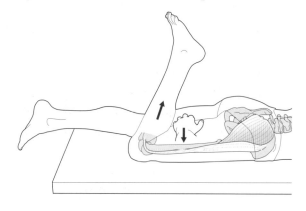

M. gluteus maximus (Latin)

Origin: posterior gluteal line of the ilium and iliac crest, aponeurosis of the erector spinae, posterior surface of the sacrum and lateral surface of the coccyx, sacrotuberous ligament

Insertion: iliotibial tract and gluteal tuberosity

Innervation: inferior gluteal nerve (L5-S2)

Action: extension, external rotation, adduction and abduction of the hip joint. About one-third of the gluteus maximus is responsible for abducting the thigh, whereas the remaining two-thirds adducts it. In other words, this muscle extends (around 15°), adducts (around 20°), externally rotates (around 45°), and abducts the hip joint. In the sitting position, it is responsible for the contraction of the buttocks necessary for correct posture as well as for lateral flexion of the trunk.

Gluteus Maximus - Tape Application

CLINICAL APPLICATIONS

- Trochanteric bursitis
- Coxarthrosis
- Coxitis
- Lumbar discopathy
- Low back pain (myofascial pain syndrome)
- Symptomatic lumbar disc herniation
- Sacroiliitis
- Sciatica
- Scoliosis

Combined applications

- Iliopsoas ➥ page 261
- Lumbar part of the iliocostalis lumborum ➥ page 192
- Quadratus lumborum ➥ page 258
- Rectus abdominis ➥ page 200
- Rhomboid major ➥ page 148
- Rhomboid minor ➥ page 146

TAPE SPECIFICATIONS

- 1 tape
- Width 5 cm (2")
- Length 30 cm (12")
- Anchor 2 cm (0.75")
- Y-shaped

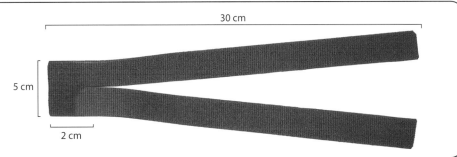

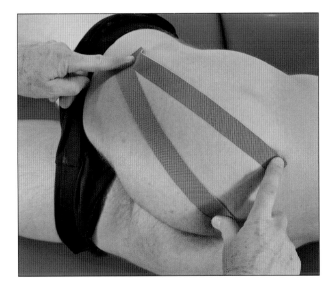
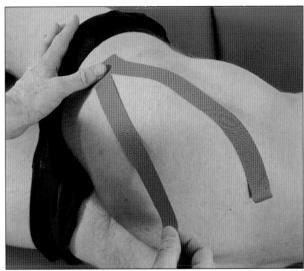

From the gluteal tuberosity of the femur to the posterior part of the iliac crest, plus 2 cm

Lateral decubitus on the side opposite to the one to be treated, with the knee and hip flexed and the knee supported by a cushion to keep the hip neutrally adducted

1. Apply the tape anchor at the level of the gluteal tuberosity of the femur, angled towards the iliac crest.

2. Apply the lateral tape tail, without tension, following the upper margin of the muscle and directing the tape tail toward the iliac crest and the sacrum.

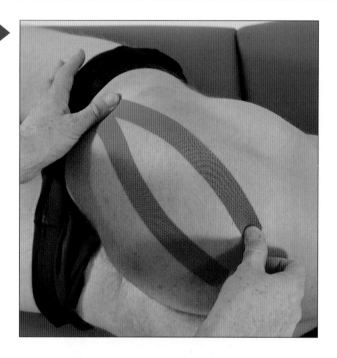 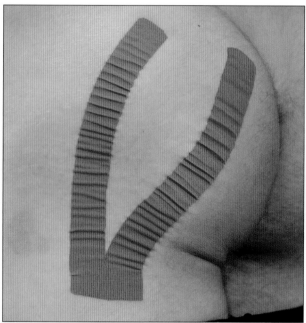

3. Apply the medial tape tail, without tension, following the lower margin of the gluteus maximus and directing the tape tail toward the top of the gluteal cleft.

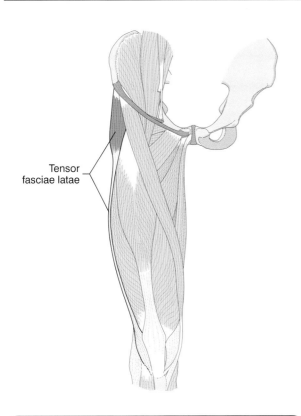

Tensor fasciae latae

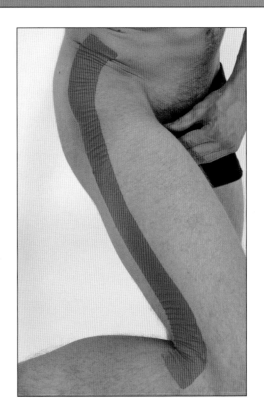

M. tensor fasciae latae (Latin)

Origin: outer lip of the iliac crest, external surface of the anterior superior iliac spine

Insertion: iliotibial tract

Innervation: superior gluteal nerve (L4-L5)

Action: flexion, abduction, and internal rotation of the hip. The tensor fasciae latae, together with the gluteus maximus, stabilizes the hip joint. In addition, this muscle plays an important role in flexion and external rotation of the knee via the iliotibial tract. In the event of impaired function of the tensor fasciae latae, constipation, spastic colon, and colitis are likely to occur.

MUSCLE TEST

Patient: lateral decubitus, with the trunk resting on the table and the legs off the table

Stabilization: the patient generally needs to hold onto the table during the application of pressure.

Test: extension of the hip; the knee is flexed passively by the examiner, or the knee is extended to allow action of the hamstring muscles (semitendinosus, semimembranosus, and biceps femoris).

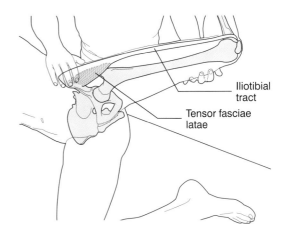

Iliotibial tract

Tensor fasciae latae

Pressure: This test presents a rather complex problem for the application of pressure. If the gluteus maximus is to be isolated as far as possible from the hamstring muscles, then the knee should be held flexed by the examiner. If it is not, the hamstring muscles will inevitably intervene to hold the flexion of the knee against gravity. It becomes difficult to carry out an accurate test when seeking to keep the knee in passive flexion while also exerting pressure on the thigh.

When this test is performed in the presence of marked tension of the hip flexors, it can prove impossible to flex the knee since this would increase the tension of the rectus femoris above the hip joint.

CLINICAL APPLICATIONS

- Hip bursitis
- Coxarthrosis
- Coxitis
- Lumbar discopathy
- Hip joint disorders
- Congenital dislocation of the hip
- Low back pain
- Symptomatic lumbar disc herniation
- Sacroiliitis
- Sciatica
- Scoliosis

Combined Applications

- Gluteus maximus ➥ page 278
- Iliopsoas ➥ page 261
- Lumbar part of the iliocostalis lumborum ➥ page 192
- Quadratus lumborum ➥ page 258
- Rectus abdominis ➥ page 200

TAPE SPECIFICATIONS

- 1 tape
- Width 5 cm (2")
- Length 60 cm (22")
- I-shaped

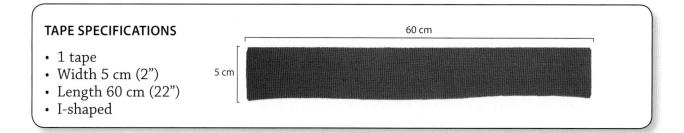

60 cm

5 cm

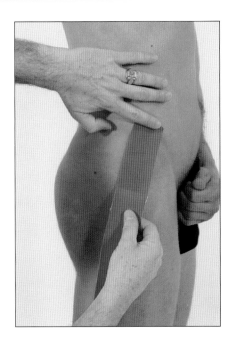 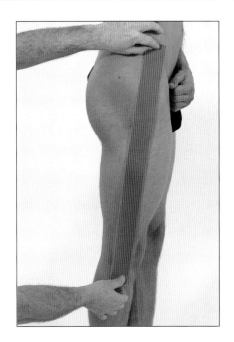

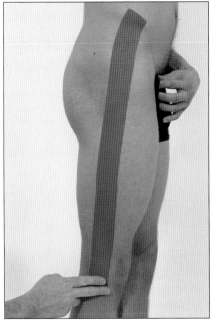 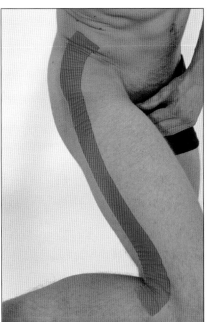

🎞 From 5 cm above the iliac crest to the iliotibial tract, plus 2 cm

🧍 Standing upright, with the leg that is not to be treated bearing the weight, the leg to be treated crossed over the other leg, and the trunk bent in the opposite direction

1. Apply the tape anchor at least 5 cm above the iliac crest.

2. Remove the backing paper from the tape and apply it, without tension, following the course of the tensor fasciae latae and the iliotibial tract, ending below the lateral condyle of the tibia.

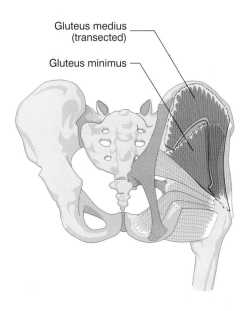

Gluteus medius (transected)

Gluteus minimus

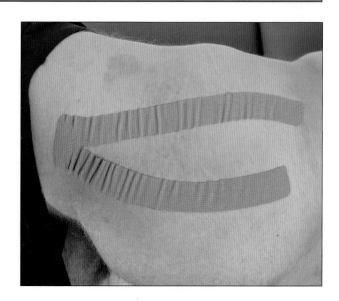

M. gluteus medius (Latin)

(Latin)

Origin
- *Gluteus medius*: external surface of the ilium between the iliac crest and the posterior gluteal line
- *Gluteus minimus*: external surface of the ilium between the greater iliac foramen and the anterior and inferior gluteal lines

Insertion
- *Gluteus medius*: lateral surface of the greater trochanter of the femur
- *Gluteus minimus*: anterolateral surface of the greater trochanter of the femur

Innervation: superior gluteal nerve (L4-L5-S1)

Action: the gluteus medius contributes to the maintenance of correct posture during walking. When it is not functioning correctly, a limping gait results. The gluteus medius abducts the femur at the hip (around 45°). It also helps in flexion (through its anterior fibers) and extension (through its posterior fibers).

The gluteus minimus abducts the femur at the hip joint and medially rotates the thigh. It also assists the gluteus medius in its functions.

MUSCLE TEST - Gluteus medius

Patient: lying on one side with the underlying leg flexed at the hip and knee and the pelvis rotated forward slightly so as to place the posterior part of the gluteus medius in an antigravity position

Stabilization: the patient stabilizes the trunk muscles and the examiner stabilizes the pelvis.

Test: abduction of the hip with slight extension and slight external rotation. The knee is kept extended. It is very important to distinguish the posterior part of the gluteus medius. The hip abductor muscles, evaluated as a group, will generally make themselves felt through the degree of force developed, whereas a test specifically designed to evaluate the gluteus medius can reveal unmistakable weakness.

When external rotation of the hip joint is limited, the pelvis must be prevented from rotating backward, so as not to produce an apparent external rotation. In backward rotation of the pelvis, the tensor fasciae latae and the gluteus minimus participate actively in the abduction. In this condition, even though pressure is applied correctly, in the right direction and

Gluteus Medius and Gluteus Minimus - Tape Application

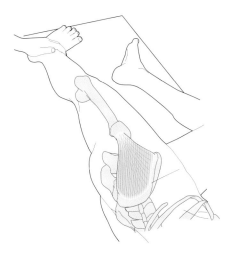

CLINICAL APPLICATIONS

- Hip bursitis
- Coxarthrosis
- Coxitis
- Lumbar discopathy
- Hip joint dysfunction
- Congenital dislocation of the hip
- Low back pain
- Sacroiliitis
- Sciatica
- Scoliosis

Combined Applications

- Iliopsoas ➥ page 261
- Lumbar part of the iliocostalis lumborum ➥ page 192
- Quadratus lumborum ➥ page 258
- Rectus abdominis ➥ page 200
- Rhomboid major ➥ page 148
- Rhomboid minor ➥ page 146
- Tensor fasciae latae ➥ page 281

against gluteus medius, the specificity of the test is reduced significantly. Weakness of the gluteus medius can immediately manifest itself in an individual's inability to properly maintain the test position, with the muscle tending to cramp and the patient attempting to rotate the pelvis backward to allow the tensor fasciae latae and gluteus minimus muscles to take over from the gluteus medius.

Pressure: against the leg, close to the ankle, in the direction of the adduction and slight flexion. Pressure must not be applied against the rotation component. The purpose of applying this pressure to the leg is to have a longer lever to produce the powerful pressure needed to exert the force needed for this muscle test. The risk of damaging the side of the knee joint is relatively low, as this part is reinforced by the strong iliotibial tract.

MUSCLE TEST - Gluteus minimus

Patient: lying on one side

Stabilization: the examiner stabilizes the pelvis

Test: abduction of the hip in a neutral position, between flexion and extension

Pressure: against the leg in the direction of the adduction and very slight extension.

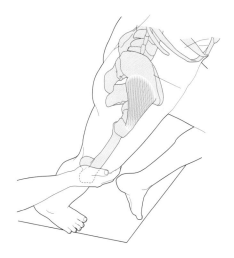

Gluteus Medius and Gluteus Minimus - Tape Application

TAPE SPECIFICATIONS

- 1 tape
- Width 5 cm (2")
- Length 17 cm (6.8")
- Anchor 2 cm (0.75")
- Y-shaped

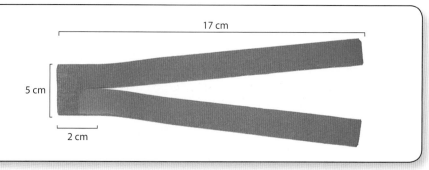

Gluteus medius

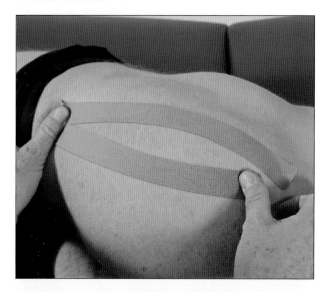

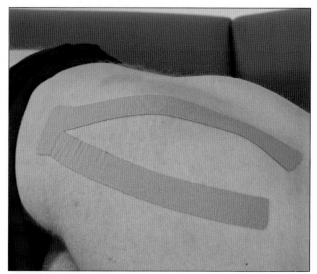

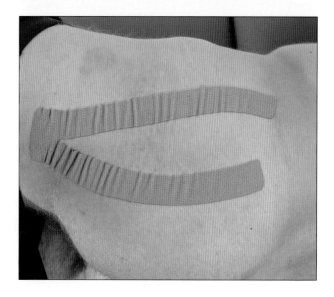

From below the greater trochanter of the femur to the iliac crest, plus 2 cm

Lateral decubitus, on the side opposite to the one to be treated, with the underlying leg adducted and the ipsilateral arm raised

1. Apply the tape anchor below the greater trochanter of the femur.

2. Apply the posterior strip of the Y, without tension, parallel to the curve of the buttock towards the posterosuperior part of the iliac crest.

3. Apply the anterior tape tail, without tension, in an anterior direction towards the ilium before taking it up towards the lateral part of the iliac crest.

Gluteus Medius and Gluteus Minimus - Tape Application

Gluteus minimus

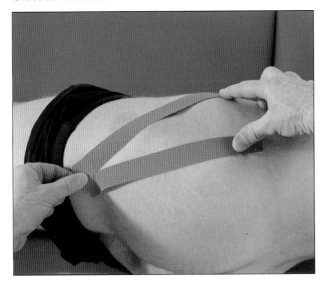

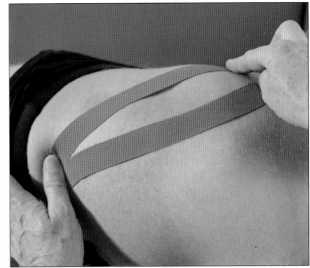

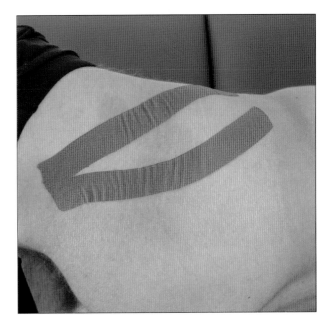

📏 From a point below and posterior to the greater trochanter of the femur to the anterosuperior part of the iliac crest, plus 2 cm

🧍 Lateral decubitus on the side opposite to the one to be treated, with the underlying leg adducted and the ipsilateral arm raised

1. Apply the tape anchor at a point below and posterior to the greater trochanter of the femur, angled toward the anterosuperior part of the iliac crest.

2. Apply the anterior strip of the Y, without tension, towards the anterior superior iliac spine, ending just posterior to it.

3. Apply the posterior tape tail, without tension, making it first diverge from the first strip up to midway along its length and then converge with it towards the upper portion of the iliac crest.

HAMSTRING MUSCLES

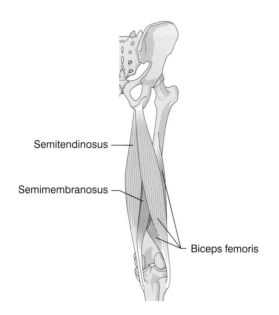

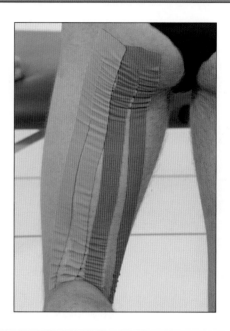

M. biceps femoris, m. semimembranosus, m. semitendinosus (Latin)

Origin
- *Biceps femoris*: ischial tuberosity, sacrotuberous ligament (long head), lateral lip of the linea aspera, and lateral supracondylar line (short head)
- *Semimembranosus*: ischial tuberosity
- *Semitendinosus*: ischial tuberosity

Insertion
- *Biceps femoris*: lateral surface of the head of the fibula, lateral condyle of the tibia
- *Semimembranosus*: medial condyle of the tibia

- *Semitendinosus*: upper part of the medial surface of the tibia

Innervation: sciatic nerve (L5, S1, S2)

Action: the biceps femoris, together with the semimembranosus and semitendinosus (posterior muscles of the thigh), extends and internally rotates the thigh and the hip joint and at the same time assists in flexion of the knee (approximately 150°). The biceps femoris externally rotates the leg at the knee joint while the semimembranosus and semitendinosus rotate it internally in a similar fashion. Together, these three muscles stabilize the lumbar region, extend the thigh from the flexed position, and participate in internal and external rotation.

CLINICAL APPLICATIONS

- Muscle fatigue
- Biceps femoris injury
- Osteoarthritis of the knee
- Knee disorders and dysfunction
- Rehabilitation after knee surgery
- Rehabilitation after knee replacement
- Tendinopathies
- Peripheral ligament injuries of the knee joint
- Knee trauma and dislocation

Combined Applications

- Gastrocnemius ➡ page 305
- Piriformis ➡ page 276
- Quadriceps femoris ➡ page 294
- Sartorius ➡ page 265
- Tensor fasciae latae ➡ page 281

Hamstring Muscles - Tape Application

TAPE SPECIFICATIONS

- 2 tapes
- Width 5 cm (2")
- Length 45 cm (18")
- Anchor 2 cm (0.75")
- Y-shaped

45 cm

5 cm

2 cm

Biceps femoris

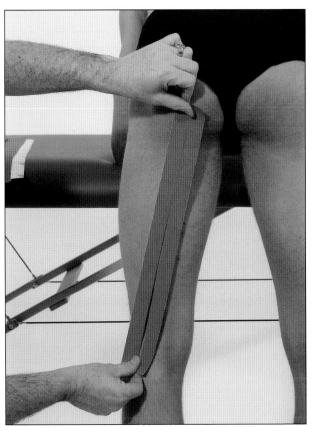 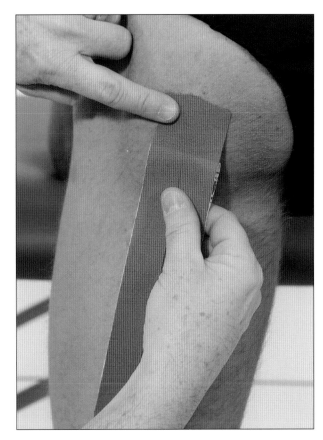

📏 From 5 cm above the ischial tuberosity to 2 cm below the popliteal fossa

🧍 Standing, trunk forward flexed at 90°, knee extended, and forefoot resting on a raised support in order to obtain dorsiflexion of the ankle

1. Apply the tape anchor above and slightly externally to the ischial tuberosity.

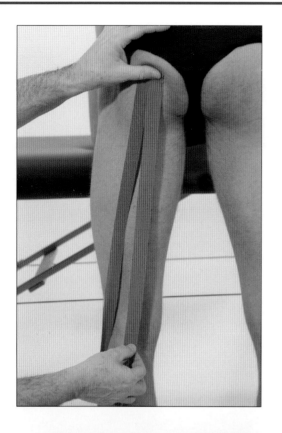

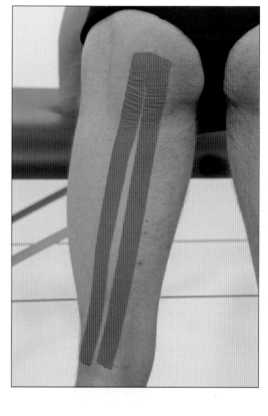

2. Remove the backing paper and, for ease of application, let the tapes hang down, externally to the biceps femoris. Take the internal end of the Y and apply it, without tension, following the internal margin of the muscle downward towards the head of the fibula, while pulling the skin upward.

3. Repeat the procedure with the external strip, this time following the outermost margin of the muscle.

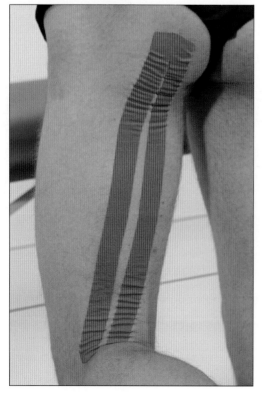

Hamstring Muscles - Tape Application

Semimembranosus and semitendinosus muscles (single tape)

📏 From 5 cm above the ischial tuberosity to 2 cm below the popliteal fossa

🧍 Standing, trunk forward flexed at 90°, knee extended, forefoot resting on a raised support in order to obtain dorsiflexion of the ankle

1. Position the tape anchor above and internally to the ischial tuberosity.

2. Remove the backing paper from the tape tails and, for ease of application, lay them farther down, internally to the semitendinosus and semimembranosus muscles. Take the external strip of the Y and apply it, without imparting tension, following the external margin of the two muscles downward towards the posteromedial surface of the tibia. Pull the skin upward during application.

3. Repeat the procedure with the internal strip, this time following the internal margin of the two muscles.

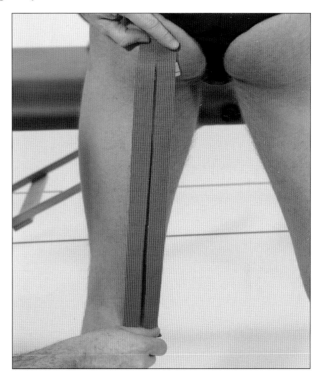

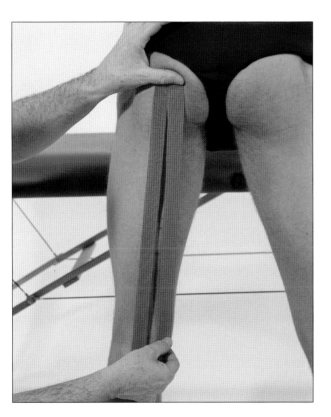

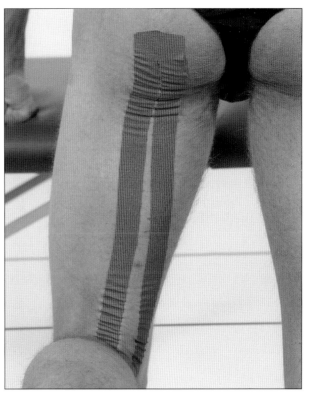

Combined Application 1

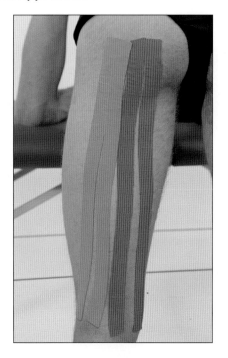 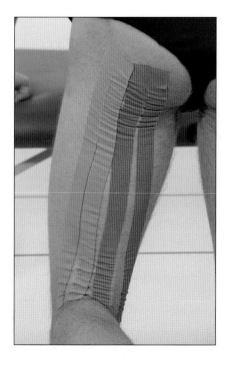

From 5 cm above the ischial tuberosity to 2 cm below the popliteal fossa, two tapes, 5 cm wide, each cut in a Y shape

Standing, trunk forward flexed at 90°, knee extended, forefoot resting on a raised support in order to obtain dorsiflexion of the ankle

1. Carry out the application for the semitendinosus and semimembranosus muscles as described on the previous page, taking care not to cross the midline of the thigh.

2. For application to the biceps femoris, apply the tape anchor above and externally to the ischial tuberosity, so that it lies alongside the first tape. Apply the medial tape tail without tension while pulling the skin upward, so that the tape tail outlines the internal margin of the biceps femoris but does not overlap the first tape. Apply the lateral tape tail, without tension, so that it outlines the external margin of the biceps femoris, again pulling the skin upward. The two ends should converge toward the head of the fibula.

Hamstring Muscles - Tape Application

Combined Application 2

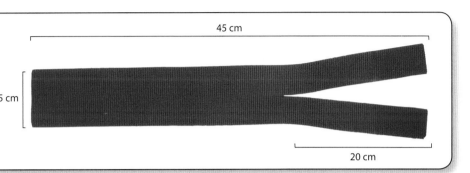

TAPE SPECIFICATIONS

- 1 tape
- Width 5 cm (2")
- Length 45 cm (18")
- Y-shaped,
  with 20 cm strips

45 cm

5 cm

20 cm

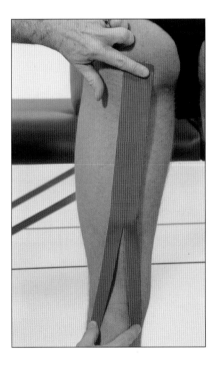
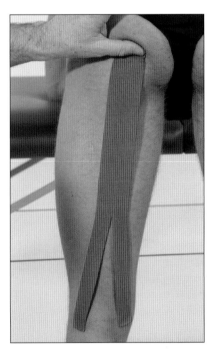
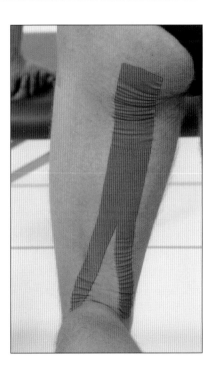

From 5 cm above the ischial tuberosity to 2 cm below the popliteal fossa; the two tails of the Y are to be measured from the musculotendinous junction of the biceps femoris to 2 cm beyond the popliteal fossa (around 20 cm)

Standing, trunk forward flexed at 90°, knee extended, with forefoot resting on a raised support in order to obtain dorsiflexion of the ankle

1. Apply the tape anchor over the ischial tuberosity.

2. Remove the backing paper as far as the bifurcation of the Y and fold it back. Apply the tape, without tension, vertically along the midline of the thigh.

3. Remove the rest of the paper and apply the two tape tails, without tension, towards the lateral and medial angles of the popliteal fossa.

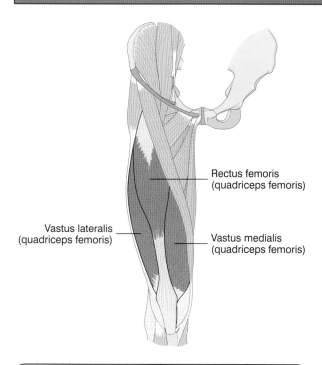

Rectus femoris
(quadriceps femoris)

Vastus lateralis
(quadriceps femoris)

Vastus medialis
(quadriceps femoris)

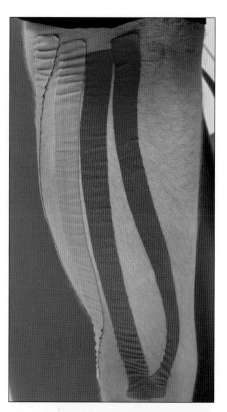

M. quadriceps femoris (m. vastus medialis, m. vastus lateralis, m. vastus intermedius, m. rectus femoris) (Latin)

Origin

- *Vastus medialis*: distal half of the intertrochanteric line, medial lip of the linea aspera, proximal part of the medial supracondylar line
- *Vastus lateralis*: upper half of the intertrochanteric line, lateral part of the gluteal tuberosity, proximal half of the lateral lip of the linea aspera
- *Vastus intermedius*: upper two-thirds of the anterior surface of the body of the femur
- *Rectus femoris*: anterior inferior iliac spine, acetabular notch

Insertion: base of the patella and tibial tuberosity

Innervation: femoral nerve (L2, L3, L4)

Action: the quadriceps femoris, a powerful leg extensor at the knee joint, consists of four muscles, only one of which, the rectus femoris, reaches two joints (i.e., the hip as well as the knee). As a consequence, this muscle is used to move two joints, so the rectus femoris is also a thigh flexor at the hip joint.

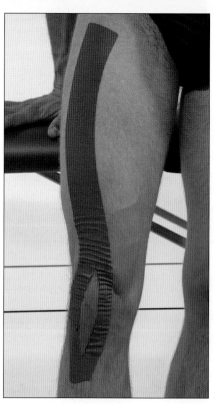

Quadriceps Femoris - Tape Application

MUSCLE TEST

Patient: seated

Stabilization: the examiner holds the thigh firmly on the surface of the table or, since the weight of the trunk is usually sufficient to stabilize the patient during the test, places one hand under the distal end of the thigh to protect it from pressure from the table.

Test: extension of the knee joint without rotation of the thigh

Pressure: against the leg, above the ankle, in the direction of the flexion.

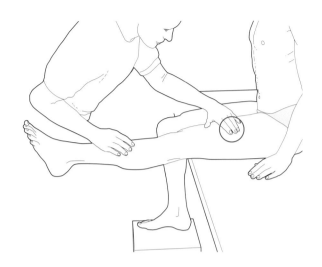

CLINICAL APPLICATIONS

- Muscle fatigue
- Quadriceps femoris injury
- Osteoarthritis of the knee
- Knee disorders and dysfunction
- Rehabilitation after knee surgery
- Rehabilitation after knee replacement
- Patellofemoral pain syndrome
- Tendinopathies
- Peripheral ligament injuries of the knee joint

Combined Applications

- Hamstring muscles ➥ page 288
- Sartorius ➥ page 265
- Tensor fasciae latae ➥ page 281

TAPE SPECIFICATIONS

Vastus medialis and vastus lateralis
- 2 tapes
- Width 5 cm (2")
- Length 45 cm (18")
- Anchor 2 cm (0.75")
- Y-shaped

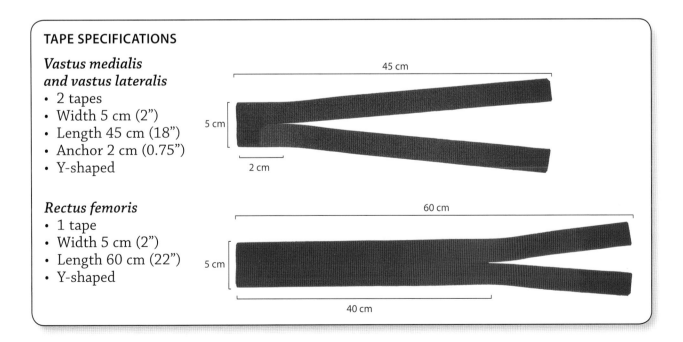

45 cm

5 cm

2 cm

Rectus femoris
- 1 tape
- Width 5 cm (2")
- Length 60 cm (22")
- Y-shaped

60 cm

5 cm

40 cm

Quadriceps Femoris - Tape Application

Vastus medialis (single tape)

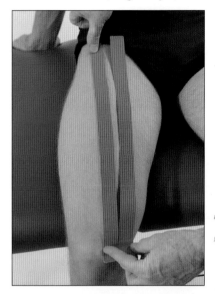 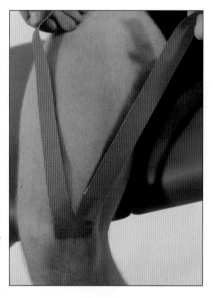 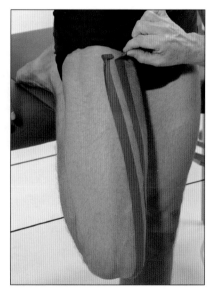

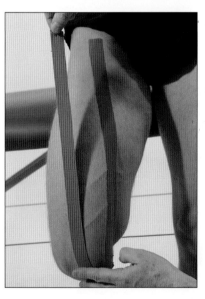 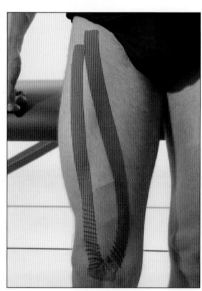

From the medial condyle of the femur to 2 cm above the groin

Standing on the leg that is not to be treated, with the leg to be treated rested posteriorly on the table with the knee fully flexed and the hip extended

1. Apply the tape anchor below the medial condyle of the femur.

2. Apply the medial strip of the Y, without tension, skirting the medial margin of the vastus medialis, following a more lateral direction on reaching the origin of the muscle.

3. Apply the lateral tape tail, without tension, away from the first to outline the lateral margin of the vastus medialis. The two strips should converge again at the level of the origin of the muscle.

Quadriceps Femoris - Tape Application

Vastus lateralis (single tape)

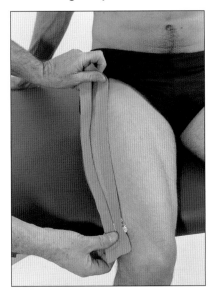

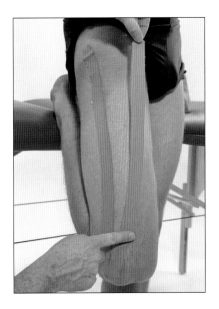

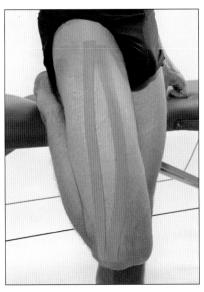

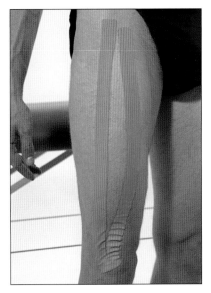

From below the lateral condyle of the femur to 2 cm above the groin

Standing on the leg that is not to be treated, with the leg to be treated resting posteriorly on the table with the knee fully flexed and the hip extended

1. Apply the tape anchor below the lateral condyle of the femur.

2. Apply the medial strip of the Y, without tension, along the medial margin of the vastus lateralis.

3. Apply the lateral tape tail, without tension, along the medial margin of the vastus lateralis. The two strips should converge again at the level of the muscle's origin.

Quadriceps Femoris - Tape Application

Combined Application

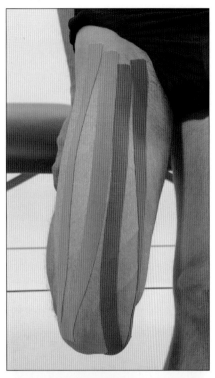

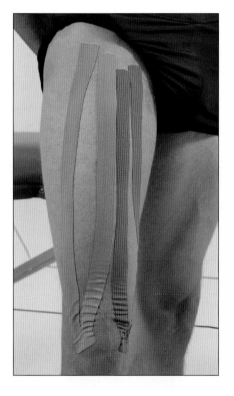

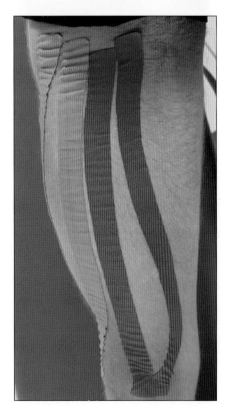

📏 From below the lateral and medial condyles of the femur to 2 cm above the groin

🧍 Standing on the leg that is not to be treated, with the leg to be treated resting posteriorly on the table with the knee fully flexed and the hip extended

1. Apply the anchors of the two tapes below the lateral and medial condyles of the femur. The tape anchor to be applied to the vastus lateralis should be positioned slightly higher than the anchor for the vastus medialis.

2. Apply the tape tails of the two Ys so that they outline the edges of the muscle bellies without allowing either application to cross the centerline of the quadriceps femoris.

Rectus femoris

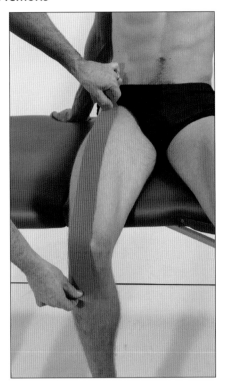

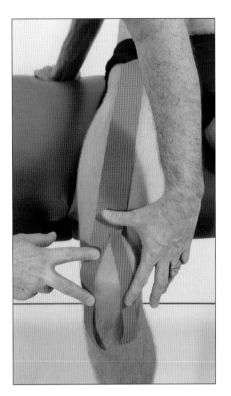

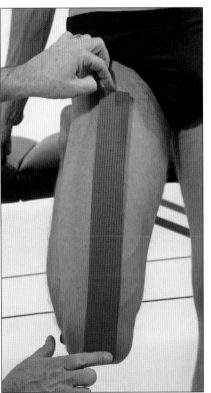

📏 From the anterior margin of the tibia to 2 cm above the groin; the two strips of the Y are to be measured from the anterior margin of the tibia to 6 cm above the patella.

⚕ Standing on the leg that is not to be treated, with the leg to be treated resting posteriorly on the table with the knee fully flexed and the hip extended

1. Tear the backing paper just above the bifurcation of the Y and position the bifurcation 6 cm above the patella. Remove the backing paper from the upper part of the tape.

2. Take hold of the upper portion of the tape and apply it, without tension, along the rectus femoris muscle as far as the anterior superior iliac spine.

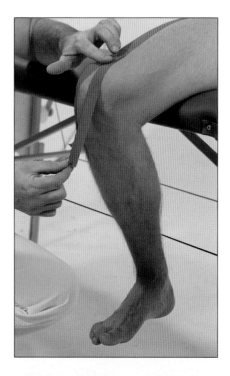

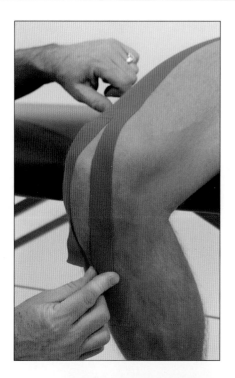

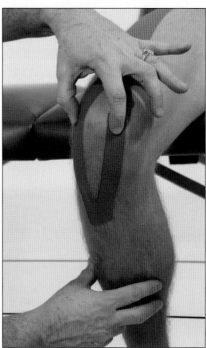

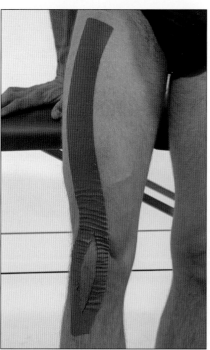

3. Remove the backing paper from the two lower strips and, for ease of application, rest the strips on the center of the patella. Ask the patient to sit on the table and to flex the knee to 110°. Apply the two tape tails following the lateral and medial margins of the patella and then inward towards the anterior margin of the tibia. Cover the margins of the patella with a third of the width of each tape.

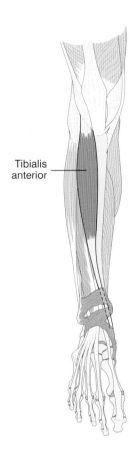

Tibialis anterior

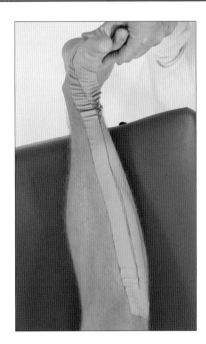

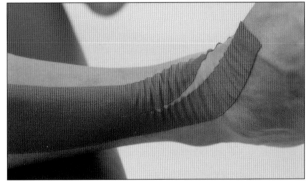

M. tibialis anterior (Latin)

Origin: lateral condyle and proximal half of the lateral surface of the tibia, interosseous membrane of the leg, crural fascia

Insertion: on the medial and plantar surface of the medial cuneiform bone, on the base of the first metatarsal bone

Innervation: deep fibular (peroneal) nerve (L4, L5, S1)

Action: the tibialis anterior dorsally flexes the foot at the ankle joint and aids inversion of the foot.

CLINICAL APPLICATIONS

- Knee joint disorders
- Talipes equinus
- Neurological and motor rehabilitation of the leg or foot
- Anterior tibial compartment syndrome

Combined Applications

- Achilles tendon ➥ page 61
- Adductor muscles ➥ page 270
- Gastrocnemius ➥ page 305
- Plantaris ➥ page 331
- Soleus ➥ page 308
- Tibialis posterior ➥ page 311

Tibialis Anterior - Tape Application

TAPE SPECIFICATIONS

Application 1
- 1 tape
- Width 5 cm (2")
- Length 40 cm (16")
- Anchor 2 cm (0.75")
- Y-shaped

5 cm

40 cm

2 cm

Application 2
- 1 tape
- Width 5 cm (2")
- Length 40 cm (16")
- Y-shaped,
  with 15 cm strips

5 cm

40 cm

15 cm

Application 1

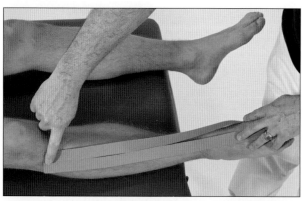

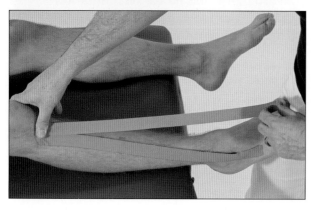

📏 From below the lateral condyle of the femur to the base of the big toe

🧍 Supine, with the feet extended off the table and the foot plantar flexed

1. Apply the tape anchor below the lateral condyle of the femur.

2. Remove the backing paper from the tape and, for ease of application, rest the two strips on the base of the big toe and by the side of the foot. Apply the internal tape tail, without tension, in a medial direction, following the anterior margin of the tibia as far as the ankle (instep), and then in a more markedly medial direction to end below the medial margin of the foot at the level of the cuboid bone.

3. Apply the lateral tape tail, without tension, approximately 1 cm away from first tape as far as the ankle, following the first metatarsal bone thereafter. ▶

NEUROMUSCULAR TAPING from Theory to Practice

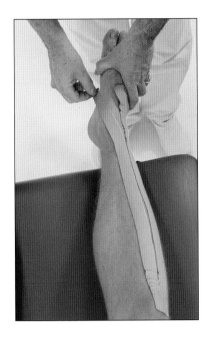

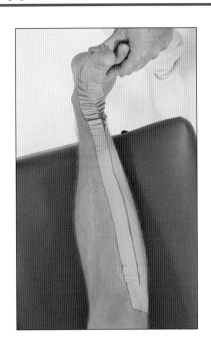

Tibialis Anterior - Tape Application

Application 2

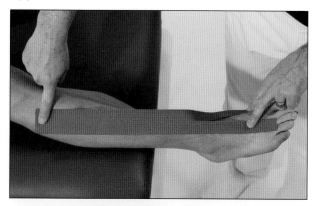

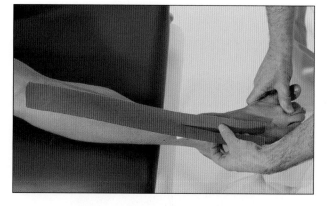

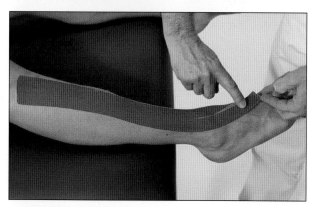

From the head of the fibula to the base of the toes, measure the two tails of the Y from the base of the toes to the ankle (instep)

Supine, with the feet extended off the table and the ankle in plantar flexion and inversion

1. Place the tape anchor over the head of the fibula.

2. Remove the backing paper as far as the bifurcation of the Y and fold it back. Apply the first tape tail, without tension, in a medial direction, following the anterior margin of the tibia as far as the ankle.

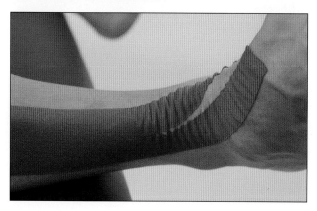

3. Apply the medial tape tail, without tension, wrapping it round the medial margin of the foot, without imparting tension to the tape.

4. Apply the lateral tape tail, without tension, following the first metatarsal bone.

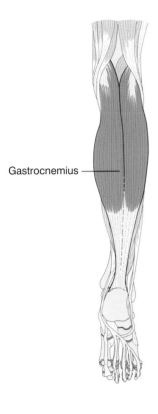

Gastrocnemius

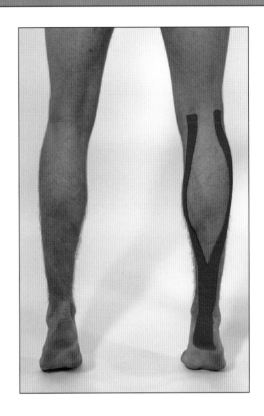

M. gastrocnemius (Latin)

Origin
- *Lateral head*: posterior surface of the lateral condyle of the femur
- *Medial head*: medial epicondyle and posterior surface of the medial condyle of the femur

Insertion: middle of the posterior surface of the calcaneus by way of the calcaneal tendon (Achilles tendon)

Innervation: tibial nerve (S1, S2)

Action: the gastrocnemius plantar flexes the foot at the ankle joint and is involved in inversion of the foot. It is also a strong knee flexor.

CLINICAL APPLICATIONS

- Bursitis
- Pain in the plantar surface of the heel
- Muscle fatigue
- Achilles tendon injuries
- Gastrocnemius injuries
- Ankle disorders
- Rehabilitation after Achilles tendon surgery
- Rehabilitation after knee replacement
- Neurological and motor rehabilitation of the foot or knee
- Posterior tibial compartment syndrome

Combined Applications

- Extensor digitorum longus ➡ page 329
- Tibialis anterior ➡ page 301

Gastrocnemius - Tape Application

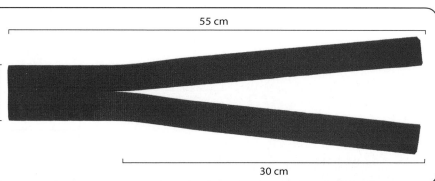

55 cm

5 cm

30 cm

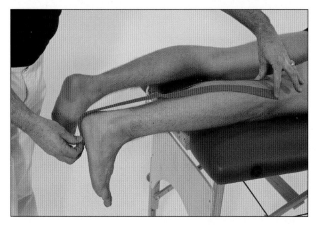

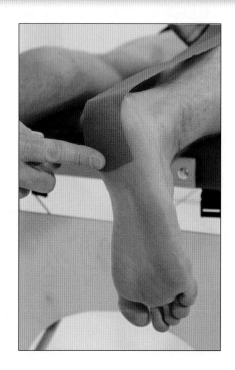

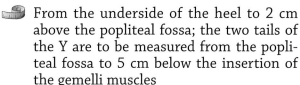 From the underside of the heel to 2 cm above the popliteal fossa; the two tails of the Y are to be measured from the popliteal fossa to 5 cm below the insertion of the gemelli muscles

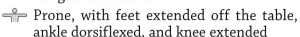 Prone, with feet extended off the table, ankle dorsiflexed, and knee extended

1. Apply the 5 cm tape anchor on the underside of the heel.

2. Have the patient place toes and forefoot just below the anterior surface of your (the therapist's) quadriceps femoris. This allows passive dorsiflexion of the patient's ankle to be achieved by pushing the patient's toes forward.

3. Remove the backing paper as far as the bifurcation of the Y and, with no tension, apply the tape centrally to the Achilles tendon as far as the junction with the lateral and medial heads of the gastrocnemius.

4. Rub the center of the tape to make it adhere properly and then check that it is well wrapped around the tendon laterally.

5. Take hold of the inner strip and apply it, without tension, following the internal margin of the medial head of the gastrocnemius, stopping just before the popliteal fossa.

6. Repeat the procedure for the lateral head of the gastrocnemius, carefully following the outermost margin of the muscle.

Gastrocnemius - Tape Application

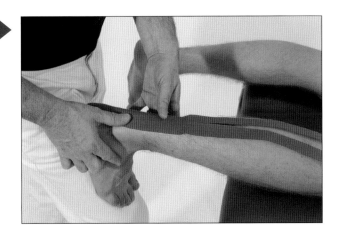 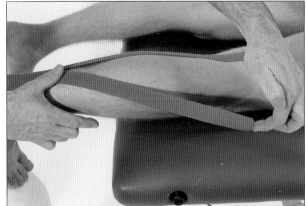

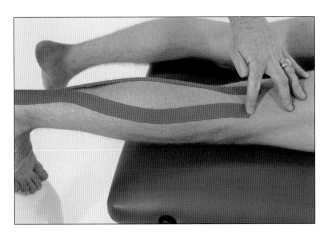 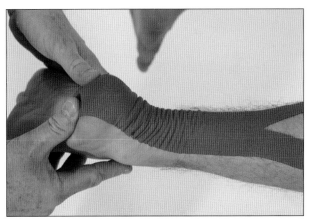

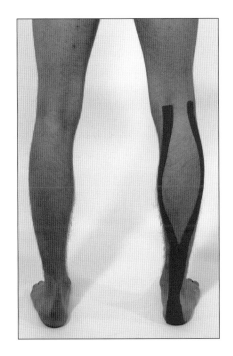 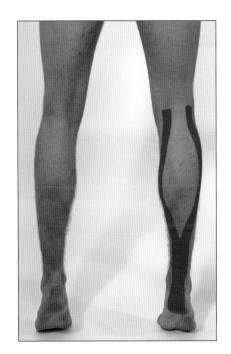

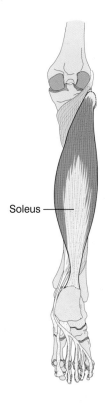

Soleus

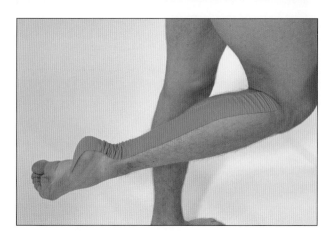

MUSCLE TEST

Patient: prone, with the knee flexed to at least 90°

Stabilization: the examiner supports the leg, holding it near the ankle.

Test: plantar flexion of the ankle without inversion or eversion of the foot

Pressure: against the forefoot, pulling it in a caudal direction (i.e., in the direction of ankle dorsiflexion). In cases of severe muscle weakness, the patient may not be able to withstand the pressure exerted on the heel. With slight weakness, a greater lever action will be needed. This is obtained by simultaneously applying pressure against the sole of the foot.

M. soleus (Latin)

Origin
- Posterior surface of the head of the fibula
- Proximal fourth of the posterior surface of the body of the fibula
- Soleal line and middle third of the medial surface of the fibula

Insertion: posterior surface of the calcaneus via the calcaneal tendon (or Achilles tendon)

Innervation: tibial nerve (S1, S2)

Action: the soleus, gastrocnemius, and plantar muscles are involved in plantar flexion of the foot when considerable muscular force is required. The soleus is also important in inversion of the foot.

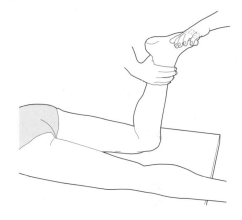

Soleus - Tape Application

CLINICAL APPLICATIONS

- Bursitis
- Pain in the plantar surface of the heel
- Muscle fatigue
- Achilles tendon injuries
- Gastrocnemius injuries
- Ankle disorders
- Rehabilitation after Achilles tendon surgery
- Rehabilitation after knee replacement
- Neurological and motor rehabilitation of the foot or knee
- Posterior tibial compartment syndrome

Combined Applications

- Extensor digitorum longus ➠ page 329
- Tibialis anterior ➠ page 301

TAPE SPECIFICATIONS

- 1 tape
- Width 5 cm (2")
- Length 50 cm (20")
- I-shaped

50 cm

5 cm

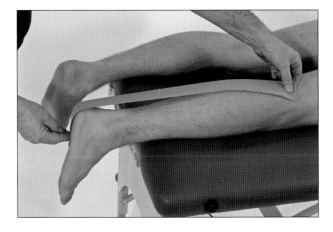

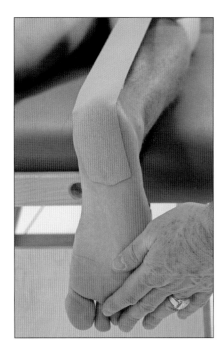

From the underside of the heel to the popliteal fossa

Prone, with feet extended off the table, ankle dorsiflexed, and knee extended

1. Apply the tape anchor to the underside of the heel.

Soleus - Tape Application

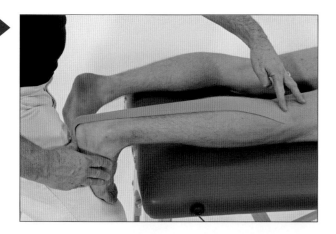

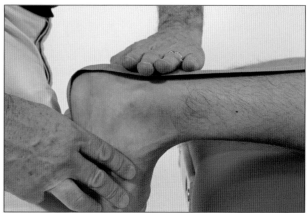

2. Have the patient place toes and forefoot just below the anterior surface of your (the therapist's) quadriceps femoris. This allows passive dorsiflexion of the patient's ankle to be achieved by pushing the patient's toes forward.

3. With the patient in this position, remove the backing paper from the tape, except for the last 5 cm. Taking hold of its distal end, apply the tape, with no tension, along the soleus, ending on the posterior aspect of the head of the fibula.

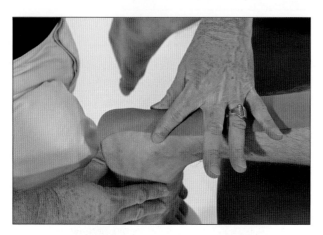

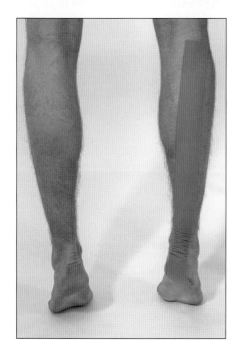

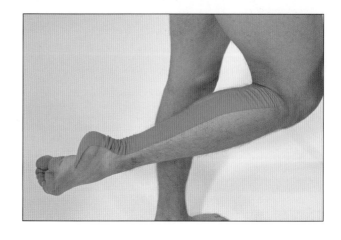

TIBIALIS POSTERIOR

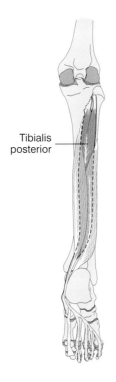

Tibialis posterior

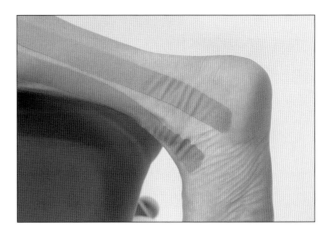

M. tibialis posterior (Latin)

Origin: posterior aspect of the tibia, medial face of the fibula; interosseous membrane of the leg

Insertion: navicular (or scaphoid) bone, calcaneus, the three cuneiform bones, cuboid bone, bases of the second, third, and fourth metatarsal bones

Innervation: tibial nerve (L4, L5, S1)

Action: the tibialis posterior supinates the foot and contributes to flexion of the ankle.

MUSCLE TEST

Patient: lateral decubitus, with the underlying leg externally rotated

Stabilization: the examiner stabilizes the leg above the ankle

Test: inversion of the foot with plantar flexion of the ankle

Pressure: against the medial side and plantar surface of the foot, in the direction of ankle dorsiflexion and eversion of the foot.

CLINICAL APPLICATIONS

- Tendon injuries
- Knee joint disorders
- Talipes equinus
- Neurological and motor rehabilitation of the leg or foot
- Posterior tibial compartment syndrome

Combined applications

- Achilles tendon ➥ page 61
- Adductor muscles ➥ page 270
- Extensor hallucis longus ➥ page 327
- Plantaris ➥ page 331
- Tibialis anterior ➥ page 301

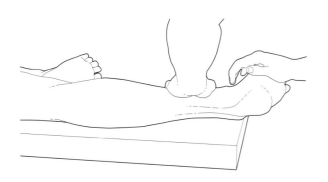

Tibialis Posterior - Tape Application

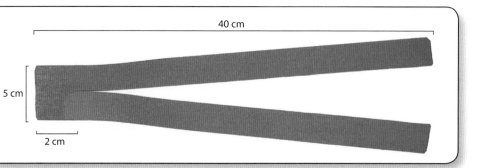

TAPE SPECIFICATIONS

- 1 tape
- Width 5 cm (2")
- Length 40 cm (16")
- Anchor 2 cm (0.75")
- Y-shaped

40 cm

5 cm

2 cm

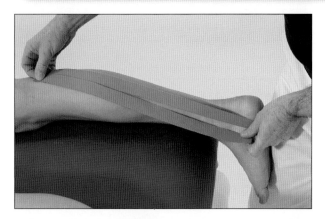
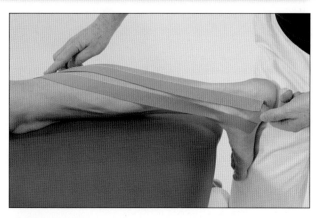
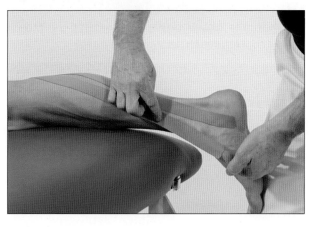
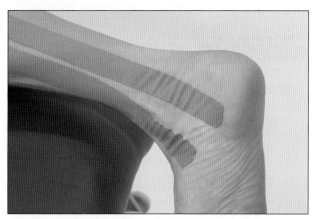

From below the popliteal fossa to the medial margin of the foot

Prone, with foot off the table and ankle in plantar flexion and eversion

1. Position the tape anchor below and slightly medially to the popliteal fossa, angled toward the medial margin of the foot.

2. Apply the internal strip following the course of the tibialis posterior, then direct it medially to pass just in front of the medial malleolus. End on the medial aspect of the first metatarsal bone.

3. Apply the external strip following a course parallel to that of the first but passing dorsally to the medial malleolus. End on the medial process of the calcaneal tuberosity.

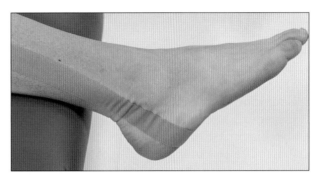

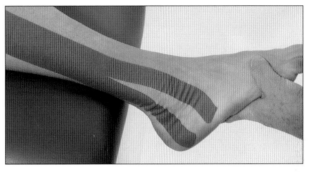

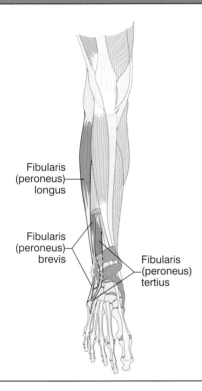

Fibularis (peroneus) longus

Fibularis (peroneus) brevis

Fibularis (peroneus) tertius

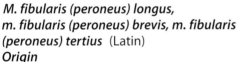

*M. fibularis (peroneus) longus,
m. fibularis (peroneus) brevis, m. fibularis
(peroneus) tertius* (Latin)

Origin

- *Peroneus longus*: lateral condyle of the tibia and head, proximal two-thirds of the fibula
- *Peroneus brevis*: distal two-thirds of the lateral surface of the fibula
- *Peroneus tertius*: lower third of the anterior surface of the fibula and interosseous membrane of the leg

Insertion

- *Peroneus longus*: lateral surface of the base of the first metatarsal bone and of the medial and intermediate cuneiform bones
- *Peroneus brevis*: lateral surface of the base of the fifth metatarsal
- *Peroneus tertius*: dorsal surface of the base of the fifth metatarsal

Innervation: peroneal nerve (L4, L5, S1)

Action: the peroneus longus and peroneus tertius muscles contribute to eversion of the foot and the peroneus brevis contributes to eversion of the ankle. The peroneus longus is also involved in plantar flexion of the ankle and the peroneus tertius is involved in its dorsiflexion.

MUSCLE TEST

Patient: supine, with the leg rotated internally; alternatively, lying on the side opposite the muscle to be treated

Stabilization: the examiner stabilizes the leg above the ankle

Test: eversion of the foot with plantar flexion of the ankle

Pressure: against the lateral margin and sole of the foot in the direction of the inversion of the foot and dorsiflexion of the ankle.

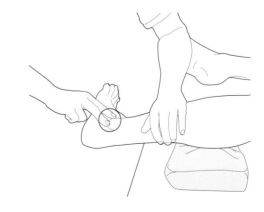

Fibularis (Peroneus) Longus, Brevis and Tertius - Tape Application

CLINICAL APPLICATIONS

- Hallux valgus
- Ankle sprains
- Fractures of the foot
- Neuropathy of the common fibular (peroneal) nerve
- Osteoarthritis of the ankle
- Rehabilitation following trauma to the foot or ankle
- Neurological and motor rehabilitation
- of the leg or foot
- Tendon injuries

Combined Applications

- Achilles tendon ➡ page 61
- Flexor digitorum longus and hallucis longus ➡ page 321
- Gastrocnemius ➡ page 305
- Plantaris ➡ page 331
- Soleus ➡ page 308
- Tibialis posterior ➡ page 311

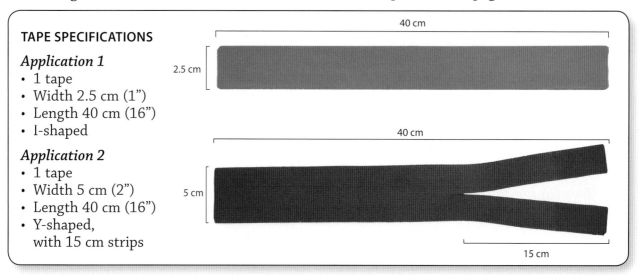

TAPE SPECIFICATIONS

Application 1
- 1 tape
- Width 2.5 cm (1")
- Length 40 cm (16")
- I-shaped

Application 2
- 1 tape
- Width 5 cm (2")
- Length 40 cm (16")
- Y-shaped, with 15 cm strips

40 cm

2.5 cm

40 cm

5 cm

15 cm

Application 1

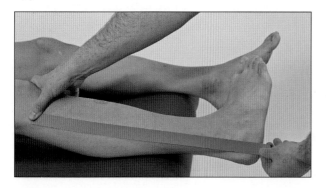 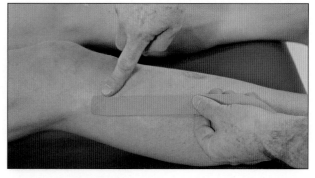

 From 2 cm above the head of the fibula to 2 cm beyond the heel

Supine, with feet extended off the table and the foot to be treated in dorsiflexion and inversion

1. Apply the tape anchor 2 cm above the head of the fibula.

2. Apply the tape, without tension, downward and vertically along the lateral surface of the leg. Bring it behind the lateral malleolus and end under the heel. ▶

Fibularis (Peroneus) Longus, Brevis and Tertius - Tape Application

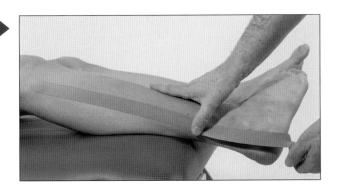 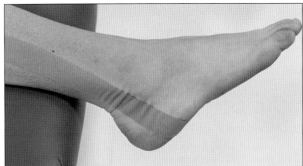

Application 2

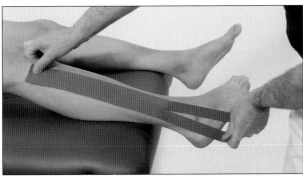 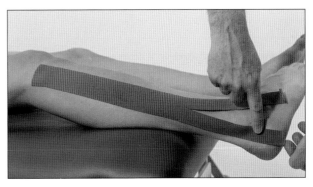

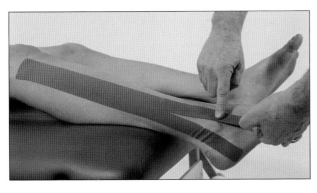 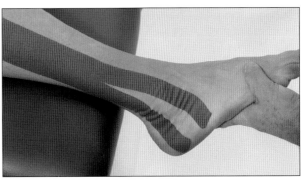

From 2 cm above the lateral condyle of the tibia to 2 cm beyond the lateral margin of the foot; the tails of the Y are to be measured from 5 cm above the lateral malleolus to 2 cm beyond the lateral margin of the foot

Supine, with feet extended off the table and the foot to be treated in dorsal flexion and inversion

1. Apply the tape anchor 2 cm above the lateral condyle of the tibia.
2. Remove the backing paper as far as the bifurcation of the Y and fold it back. Apply the tape, with no tension, vertically along the length of and anterior to the fibula.
3. Remove the backing paper from the tails of the Y. With the foot in dorsiflexion, apply the posterior tape tail dorsally to the lateral malleolus, with no tension and ending under the heel. With the foot in plantar flexion, apply the anterior strip, without tension, outlining the front of the lateral malleolus and ending on the base of the fifth metatarsal bone.

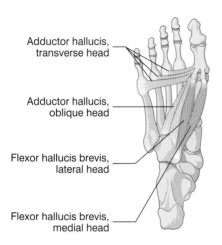

Adductor hallucis, transverse head

Adductor hallucis, oblique head

Flexor hallucis brevis, lateral head

Flexor hallucis brevis, medial head

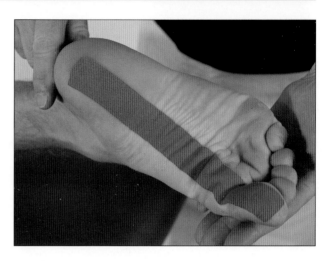

M. flexor hallucis brevis (Latin)

Origin: medial part of the cuboid bone; lateral cuneiform bone

Insertion: medial and lateral part of the base of the proximal phalanx of the big toe

Innervation: medial plantar nerve (S2, S3)

Action: the flexor hallucis brevis flexes the big toe, maintains balance, and supports the longitudinal arch of the foot.

CLINICAL APPLICATIONS

- Hallux valgus
- Fallen longitudinal arch of the foot
- Ankle sprains
- Calcaneal tuberosity pain
- Neuropathy of the fibular (peroneal) nerve
- Rehabilitation after trauma to the foot or ankle
- Neurological and motor rehabilitation of the leg or foot
- Tendinopathies

Combined Applications

- Achilles tendon ➡ page 61
- Gastrocnemius ➡ page 305
- Soleus ➡ page 308
- Tibialis anterior ➡ page 301
- Tibialis posterior ➡ page 311

MUSCLE TEST

Patient: supine or seated

Stabilization: the examiner stabilizes the foot proximally to the metatarsophalangeal joint of the big toe and keeps the foot and ankle in a neutral position. Plantar flexion of the foot can constitute a limitation to this test due to the tension exerted by the antagonist extensor digitorum longus muscles

Test: flexion of the metatarsophalangeal joint of the big toe

Pressure: against the plantar surface of the proximal phalanx in the direction of the extension.

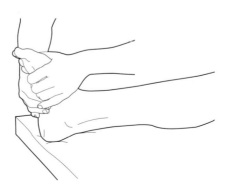

Flexor Hallucis Brevis - Tape Application

TAPE SPECIFICATIONS

- 1 tape
- Width 2.5 cm (1")
- Length 20-25 cm (8-10")
- I-shaped

2.5 cm

20-25 cm

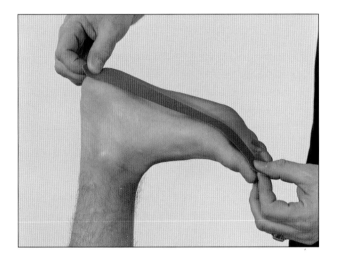
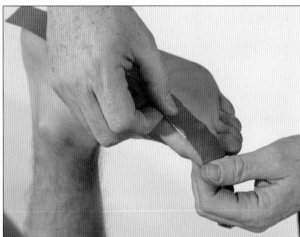
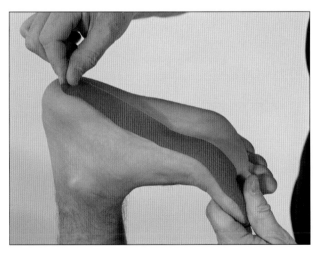
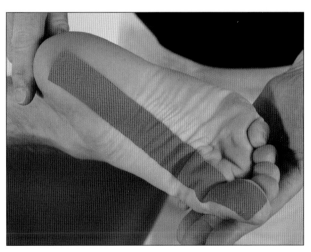

From the tip of the big toe to 2 cm beyond the heel

Prone, with knee flexed through 90°, ankle dorsiflexed, and big toe extended

1. Apply the tape to the tip of the big toe.

2. Remove the backing paper from the tape, except for the last 2.5 cm. Use one of your (the therapist's) hands to help extend the big toe, holding it by the distal phalanx, while using the other hand to direct the tape toward the cuboid bone, ending beyond this bone.

FLEXOR DIGITORUM BREVIS

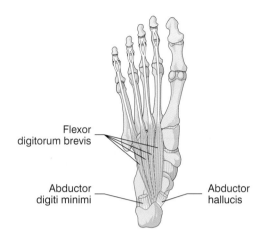

Flexor digitorum brevis

Abductor digiti minimi

Abductor hallucis

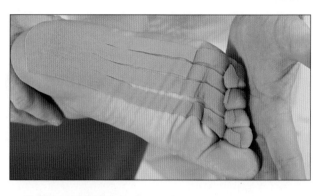

M. flexor digitorum brevis (Latin)

Origin: calcaneal tuberosity, plantar aponeurosis

Insertion: middle phalanges of the second, third, fourth, and fifth toes

Innervation: plantar nerve (S1, S2)

Action: flexion of the last four toes.

CLINICAL APPLICATIONS

- Ankle sprains
- Hammer toes
- Claw toes

- Calcaneal tuberosity pain
- Inflammation of the common fibular (peroneal) nerve
- Rehabilitation after trauma to the foot or ankle
- Neurological and motor rehabilitation of the leg or foot
- Tendinitis

Combined Applications

- Achilles tendon ➠ page 61
- Extensor digitorum brevis and hallucis brevis ➠ page 325
- Extensor digitorum longus ➠ page 329
- Gastrocnemius ➠ page 305
- Soleus ➠ page 308
- Tibialis anterior ➠ page 301
- Tibialis posterior ➠ page 311

TAPE SPECIFICATIONS

Flexor digitorum brevis
- 1 tape
- Width 5 cm (2")
- Length 27 cm (11")
- Anchor 5 cm (2")
- Fan-shaped with four strips

Flexor digitorum brevis and hallucis brevis
- 1 tape
- Width 5 cm (2")
- Length 25 cm (10")
- Anchor 5 cm (2")
- Fan-shaped with five strips

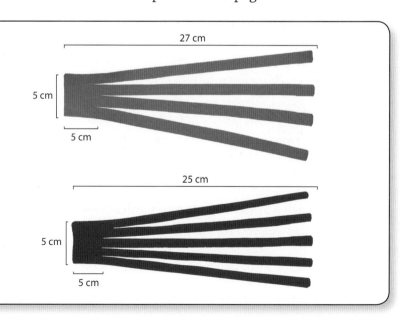

Flexor Digitorum Brevis - Tape Application

Application 1 - Flexor digitorum brevis

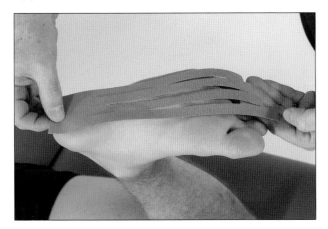
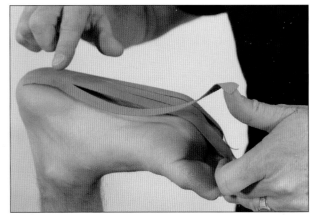

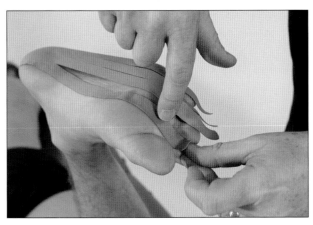
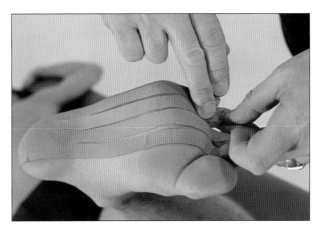

From the heel to 2 cm beyond the tip of the second toe; each strip is then cut to the length of the respective toe

Prone, with knee flexed at 90°, ankle dorsiflexed, and toes extended

1. Apply the tape anchor under the heel. Remove the backing paper from the tape and, for ease of application, lay the ends of the strips on the tips of the outer toes.

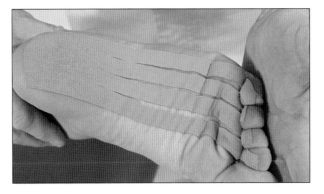

2. Attach the end of the first tape tail (the tail for the second toe) to your thumb for the moment and, with the middle finger, extend the patient's toe, pushing the distal phalanx downward. Then apply the tape with your free hand, with no tension, along the second metatarsal bone and the phalanges of the second toe, ending on the toe pad.

3. Repeat the procedure described in point 2 for the third, fourth, and fifth toes.

Flexor Digitorum Brevis - Tape Application

Application 2 - Flexor digitorum brevis and flexor hallucis brevis

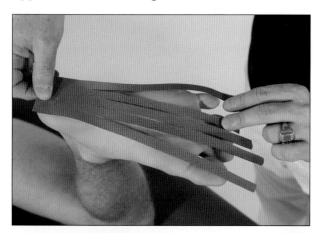 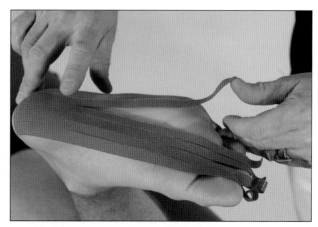

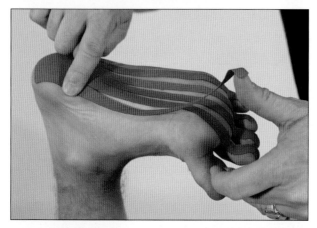 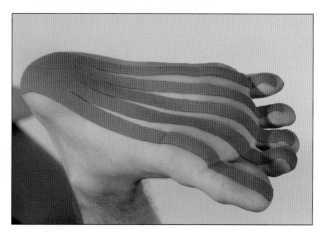

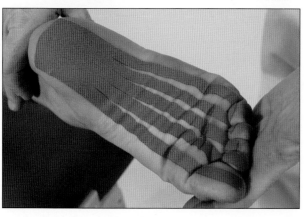

From the heel to 2 cm beyond the tip of the big toe. Each strip is then cut to the length of the respective toe.

Prone, with knee flexed at 90°, ankle dorsiflexed, and toes extended

1. Apply the tape anchor on the underside of the heel. Remove the backing paper from the tape and, for ease of application, lay the strips on the tips of the medial toes.

2. Attach the end of the first tape tail (the tail for the fifth toe) to your thumb for the moment and with your middle finger help extend the toe, pushing the distal phalanx downward. Then apply the tape with your free hand, with no tension, along the fifth metatarsal bone and the phalanges of the fifth toe, ending on the toe pad.

3. Repeat the procedure described in point 2 for the fourth, third, second, and first toes.

NEUROMUSCULAR TAPING from Theory to Practice

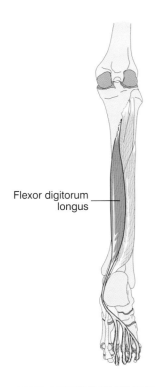
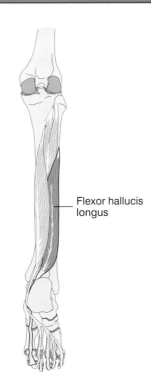

Flexor digitorum longus

Flexor hallucis longus

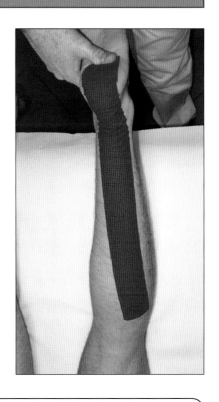

M. flexor digitorum longus (Latin)

Origin: medial part of the posterior surface of the tibia

Insertion: bases of the distal phalanges of the second, third, fourth, and fifth toes

Innervation: tibial nerve (L5, S1)

Action: this muscle flexes the last four toes and assists plantar flexion of the foot.

M. flexor hallucis longus (Latin)

Origin: distal two-thirds of the posterior surface of the fibula, posterior surface of the interosseous membrane

Insertion: base of the distal phalanx of the big toe

Innervation: tibial nerve (S1-S3)

Action: plantar flexion of the big toe

MUSCLE TEST

Patient: supine or seated

Stabilization: the examiner stabilizes the foot proximally to the metatarsophalangeal joint of the big toe and keeps the foot and ankle in a neutral position. Plantar flexion can constitute a limitation to this test due to the tension exerted by the antagonist extensor digitorum longus muscles.

Test: flexion of the metatarsophalangeal joints of the toes

Pressure: against the plantar surface of the proximal phalanx in the direction of the extension

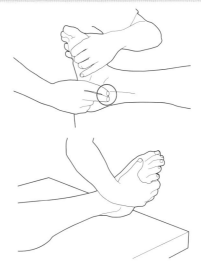

Flexor Digitorum Longus and Hallucis Longus - Tape Application

CLINICAL APPLICATIONS

- Ankle sprains
- Hammer toes
- Claw toes
- Calcaneal tuberosity pain
- Neuropathy of the common fibular (peroneal) nerve
- Rehabilitation after trauma to the foot or ankle

- Neurological and motor rehabilitation of the leg or foot
- Tendon injuries

Combined Applications

- Extensor digitorum longus ➥ page 329
- Extensor hallucis longus ➥ page 327
- Tibialis anterior ➥ page 301

TAPE SPECIFICATIONS

- 1 tape
- Width 5 cm (2")
- Length 50 cm (20")
- I-shaped

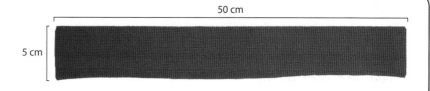

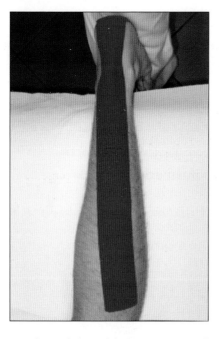
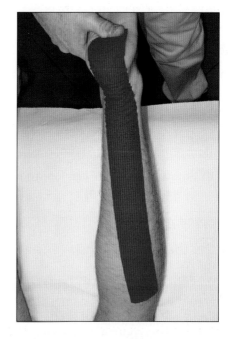

From the calcaneal tuberosity to the proximal third of the posterior aspect of the fibula

Prone, with foot extended off the edge of the table, foot in dorsiflexion and inversion, and big toe extended

1. Apply the tape anchor proximally to the middle third of the fibula.

2. Apply the tape, without tension, taking it down vertically as far as the distal third of the fibula, then directing it medially toward the medial margin of the Achilles tendon.

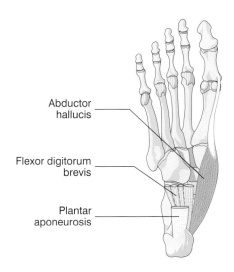

Abductor
hallucis

Flexor digitorum
brevis

Plantar
aponeurosis

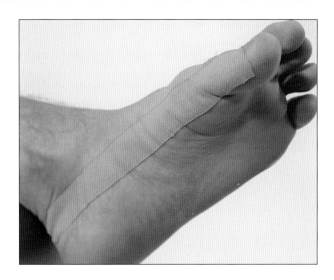

M. abductor hallucis (Latin)

Origin: calcaneal tuberosity, plantar aponeurosis, flexor retinaculum

Insertion: medial surface of the base of the proximal phalanx of the big toe

Innervation: medial plantar nerve (L4, L5, S1)

Action: abducts and helps to flex the metatarsophalangeal joint of the big toe. It is also involved in adduction of the forefoot.

CLINICAL APPLICATIONS

- Hallux valgus
- Sprains of the metatarsophalangeal joint of the big toe
- Hammer toes
- Claw toes
- Rehabilitation after trauma to the foot or ankle
- Neurological and motor rehabilitation of the leg or foot
- Tendinitis

Combined applications
- Achilles tendon ➥ page 61
- Extensor hallucis longus ➥ page 327
- Flexor digitorum brevis ➥ page 318
- Flexor hallucis brevis ➥ page 316
- Gastrocnemius ➥ page 305
- Soleus ➥ page 308

MUSCLE TEST

Patient: supine or seated

Stabilization: the examiner grips the heel firmly

Test: if possible, abduction of the big toe from the axial line of the foot. This is usually a difficult movement, as the patient opposes the pressure exerted by the examiner, pulling the forefoot in the direction of the adduction.

Pressure: against the medial side of the first metatarsal bone and the proximal phalange of the big toe; the muscle may be palpated, and it is often possible to observe it along the medial margin of the foot.

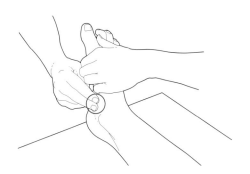

Abductor Hallucis - Tape Application

TAPE SPECIFICATIONS

- 1 tape
- Width 2.5 cm (1")
- Length 25 cm (10")
- I-shaped

25 cm

2.5 cm

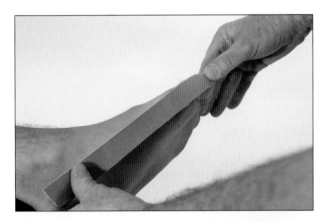

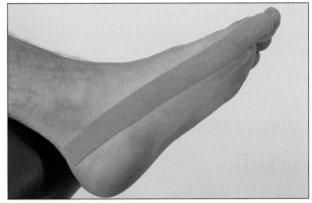

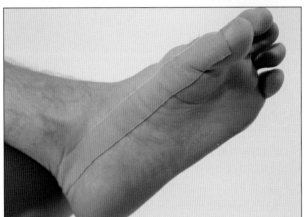

From the base of the distal phalanx of the big toe to 2 cm beyond the calcaneal tuberosity

Supine

1. Apply the tape anchor to the base of the distal phalanx of the big toe.

2. Remove the backing paper from the tape, except for the last 2.5 cm. With one hand, help to extend and adduct the big toe by holding it by the distal phalange, while using the other hand to apply the tape, without tension, taking it beyond the medial process of the calcaneal tuberosity.

NOTE: To increase the stability of the application, cut the tape 3 cm longer and cut a hole in one end into which to insert the big toe.

EXTENSOR DIGITORUM BREVIS AND HALLUCIS BREVIS

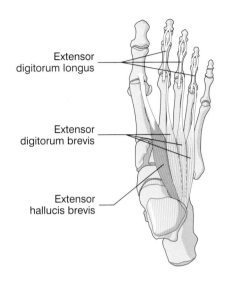

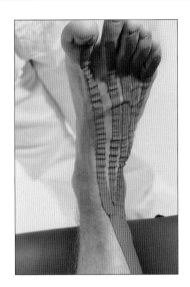

M. extensor digitorum brevis (Latin)

Origin: upper surface of the calcaneus

Insertion: base of the proximal phalanx of the big toe, lateral sides of the tendons of the extensor

Innervation: deep fibular (peroneal) nerve (L4, L5, S1)

Action: extends the phalanges.

CLINICAL APPLICATIONS

- Hallux valgus
- Hammer toes
- Claw toes
- Ankle sprains
- Metatarsalgia
- Osteoarthritis of the ankle
- Neurological and motor rehabilitation of the leg or foot
- Tendon injuries

Combined Applications

- Achilles tendon ➥ page 61
- Gastrocnemius ➥ page 305
- Plantaris ➥ page 331
- Soleus ➥ page 308
- Tibialis posterior ➥ page 311

TAPE SPECIFICATIONS

- 1 tape
- Width 5 cm (2")
- Length 30 cm (12")
- Anchor 5 cm (2")
- Fan-shaped with five strips

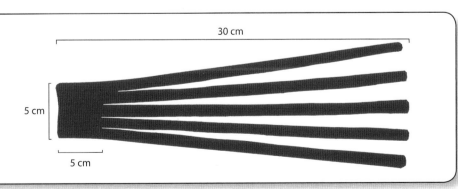

Extensor Digitorum Brevis and Hallucis Brevis - Tape Application

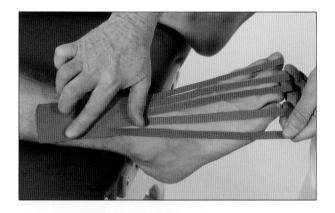 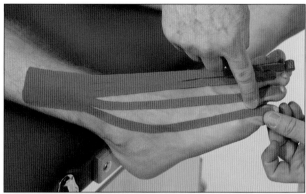

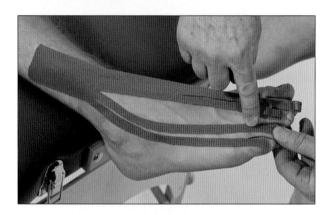 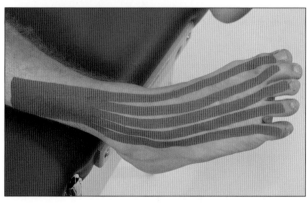

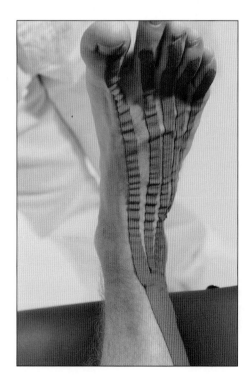

From 10 cm above the lateral malleolus to the tip of the big toe: each strip is cut to the length of the respective toe.

Supine, with foot extended off the table, the ankle in plantar flexion, the foot in inversion, and the toes flexed

1. Apply the tape anchor on the side of the leg 10 cm above the heel and angled toward the back of the toes.

2. Remove the backing paper and, for ease of application, lay the tapes on the backs of the toes. With one hand, help flex each toe, holding it by its distal phalanx, while using the other hand to apply the tape, without tension, along the surface of the respective metatarsal bone and phalanges. Each strip ends at the base of the toenail.

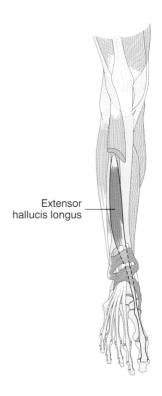

Extensor
hallucis longus

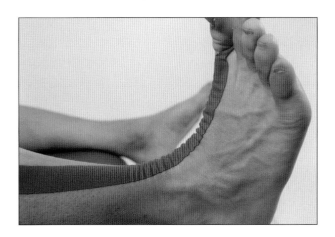

M. extensor hallucis longus (Latin)

Origin: middle two-quarters of the anterior surface of the fibula, interosseous membrane of the leg

Insertion: base of the distal phalanx of the big toe

Innervation: deep fibular (peroneal) nerve (L4, L5, S1)

Action: extends the big toe and assists in dorsiflexion of the first toe and ankle.

CLINICAL APPLICATIONS

- Hallux valgus
- Hallux bursitis
- Ankle sprains
- Hammer toes
- Claw toes
- Osteoarthritis of the ankle
- Neurological and motor rehabilitation of the leg or foot
- Tendon injuries

Combined Applications

- Achilles tendon ➥ page 61
- Fibularis (peroneus) longus, brevis and tertius ➥ page 313
- Gastrocnemius ➥ page 305
- Plantaris ➥ page 331
- Soleus ➥ page 308
- Tibialis posterior ➥ page 311

MUSCLE TEST

Patient: supine or seated

Stabilization: the examiner stabilizes the foot in slight plantar flexion

Test: extension of the metatarsophalangeal and interphalangeal joints of the big toe

Pressure: against the dorsal surfaces of the distal and proximal phalanges of the big toe in the direction of the flexion.

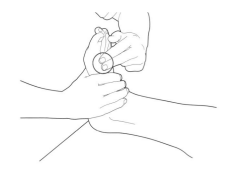

Extensor Hallucis Longus - Tape Application

TAPE SPECIFICATIONS

40 cm

2.5 cm

- 1 tape
- Width 2.5 cm (1")
- Length 40 cm (16")
- I-shaped, with a hole for the big toe

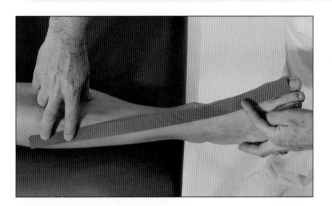
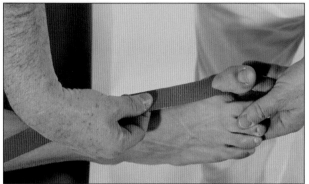

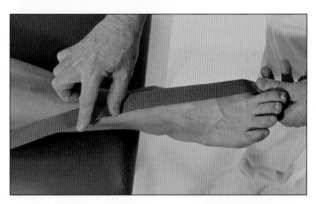
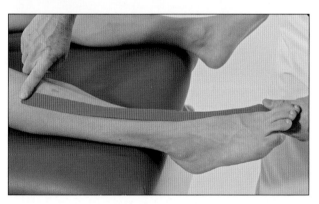

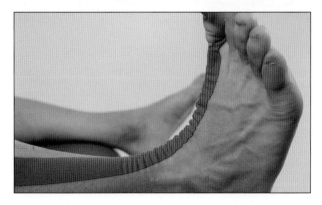

From 3 cm beyond the base of the big toe to 5 cm below the head of the fibula

Supine, with the foot extended off the table and the ankle plantar flexed

1. Insert the big toe through the hole in the tape.

2. Ask the patient to bend the big toe toward the sole of the foot. Remove the backing paper from the tape, except for the last 2.5 cm, and apply it without tension in an upward direction, following the course of the muscle and deviating laterally toward the head of the fibula. End beyond the middle two-quarters of the anterior surface of the fibula.

EXTENSOR DIGITORUM LONGUS

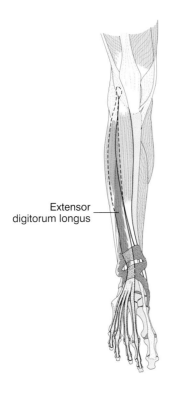

Extensor digitorum longus

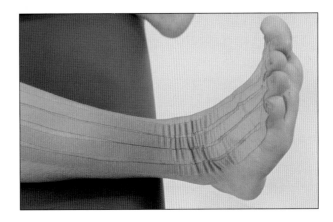

M. **extensor digitorum longus** (Latin)

Origin: lateral condyle of the tibia, upper part of the anterior surface of the fibula, upper part of the interosseous membrane of the leg

Insertion: bases of the medial and distal phalanges of the last four toes

Innervation: deep fibular (peroneal) nerve (L4, L5, S1)

Action: extends the toes on the metatarsophalangeal and interphalangeal joints and assists in dorsiflexion of the ankle and eversion of the foot.

MUSCLE TEST

Patient: supine or seated

Stabilization: the examiner stabilizes the foot in slight plantar flexion

Test: extension of the metatarsophalangeal and interphalangeal joints

Pressure: against the dorsal surface of the distal and proximal phalanges in the direction of the flexion.

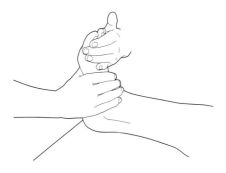

CLINICAL APPLICATIONS

- Hallux valgus
- Ankle sprains
- Hammer toes
- Claw toes
- Metatarsalgia
- Osteoarthritis of the ankle
- Neurological and motor rehabilitation of the leg or foot
- Tendon injuries

Combined Applications

- Achilles tendon ➡ page 61
- Gastrocnemius ➡ page 305
- Plantaris ➡ page 331
- Soleus ➡ page 308
- Tibialis posterior ➡ page 311

Extensor Digitorum Longus - Tape Application

TAPE SPECIFICATIONS

- 1 tape
- Width 5 cm (2")
- Length 55 cm (21")
- Anchor 2 cm (0.75")
- Fan-shaped with four strips

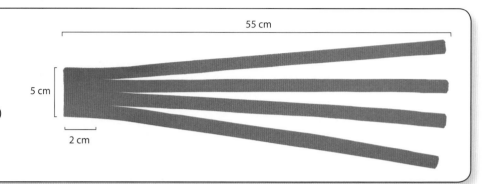

55 cm

5 cm

2 cm

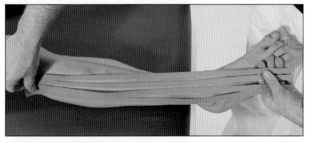
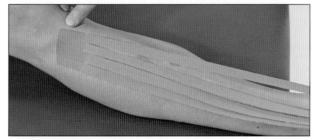
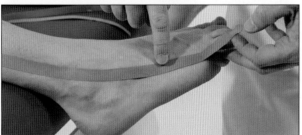
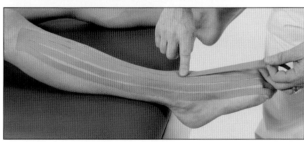
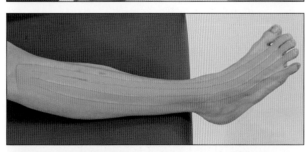

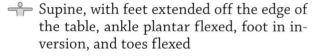 From the lateral condyle of the tibia to the tips of the toes

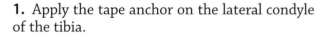 Supine, with feet extended off the edge of the table, ankle plantar flexed, foot in inversion, and toes flexed

1. Apply the tape anchor on the lateral condyle of the tibia.

2. Apply the tape tails, without tension, distributing them over the anterolateral surface of the leg and then over the corresponding metatarsal bone and phalanges (i.e., of the second, third, fourth, and fifth toes). End each tape tail at the base of the respective toenail. During this procedure, help to flex each toe in turn by pressing on its distal phalanx.

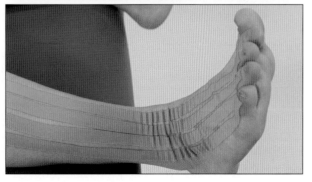

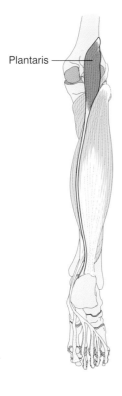

Plantaris

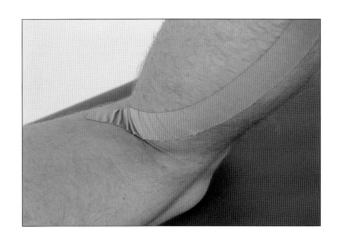

CLINICAL APPLICATIONS

- Baker's cysts
- Tendon injuries
- Knee joint disorders
- Talipes equinus
- Neurological and motor rehabilitation of the leg or foot
- Anterior tibial compartment syndrome
- Calcaneal spurs
- Achilles tendon injuries

Combined applications

- Adductor muscles ➥ page 270
- Extensor digitorum longus ➥ page 329
- Extensor hallucis longus ➥ page 327
- Tibialis anterior ➥ page 301

M. plantaris (Latin)

Origin: lateral supracondylar line of the femur, posterior surface of the capsule of the knee joint

Insertion: medial process of the calcaneal tuberosity

Innervation: tibial nerve (L4, L5, S1)

Action: plantar flexion of the ankle or talocrural joint. This muscle also weakly flexes the knee.

TAPE SPECIFICATIONS

- 1 tape
- Width 2.5 cm (1")
- Length 50 cm (20")
- I-shaped

50 cm

2.5 cm

Plantaris - Tape Application

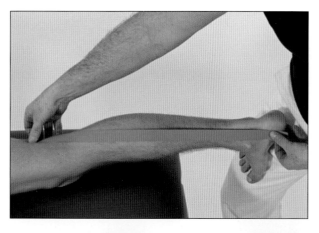
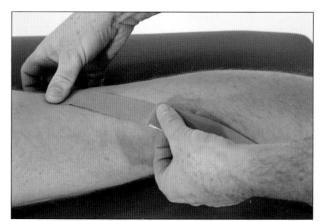
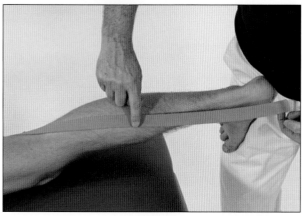
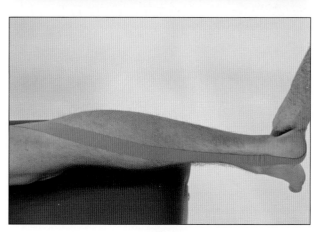
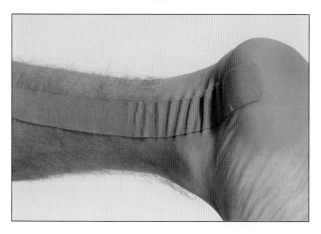
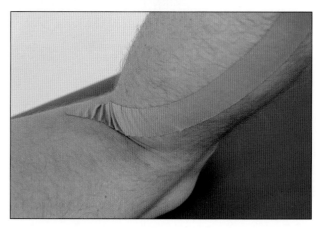

From 5 cm above the lateral condyle of the femur to the heel

Prone, with the foot extended off the table in dorsiflexion and eversion

1. Apply the tape anchor 5 cm above the lateral condyle of the femur, on the back of the thigh.

2. Apply the tape, without tension, downward along the calf before deviating slightly in the direction of the medial malleolus.

9

Some Primary Conditions

- Cervical spine pain syndromes
- Forward shoulder
- Shoulder impingement syndromes
- Adhesive capsulitis
- Epicondylitis
- Carpal tunnel syndrome

- Lumbar spine pain syndromes
- Sciatica
- Gonarthrosis
- Calcaneal spur
- Plantar fasciitis

CERVICAL SPINE PAIN SYNDROMES

Damage to the brachial plexus gives rise to paresthesia (numbness) or pain in the upper extremities, expressed through symptoms such as those of cervical disc syndrome or cervical vertebra syndrome.

It can cause stiffness in the neck and shoulders, as in peripheral nerve inflammation, without necessarily being linked to the cervical vertebrae. Excessive use of the upper limbs can lead to chronic inflammation of the brachial plexus.

In general, brachial plexus syndrome and pain or numbness affecting the cervical spine, shoulders and arms are grouped together under the umbrella term for the shoulder, arm and neck area: cervical syndrome.

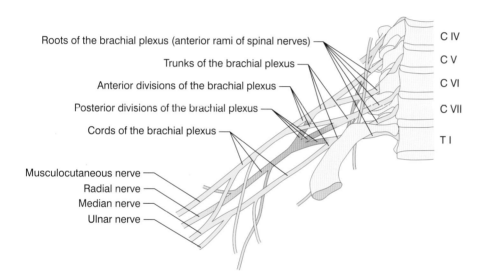

Roots of the brachial plexus (anterior rami of spinal nerves)
Trunks of the brachial plexus
Anterior divisions of the brachial plexus
Posterior divisions of the brachial plexus
Cords of the brachial plexus
Musculocutaneous nerve
Radial nerve
Median nerve
Ulnar nerve

C IV
C V
C VI
C VII
T I

BRACHIAL PLEXUS

The brachial plexus is formed by the anterior branches of the lower four cervical and first thoracic nerves (C5, C6, C7, C8 and T1) and in part by C4 and T2. The brachial plexus has three primary trunks – superior, middle and inferior – which split into three secondary trunks or cords – posterior, lateral and medial.

TAPE SPECIFICATIONS

- 1 tape
- Width 2.5 cm (1")
- Length 90 cm (36")
- Y-shaped, with 15 cm strips

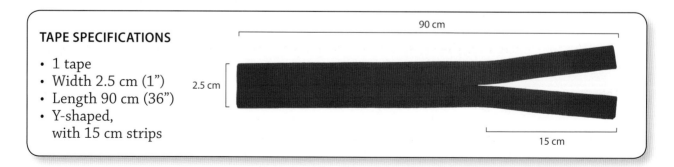

90 cm

2.5 cm

15 cm

Cervical Spine Pain Syndromes - Tape Application

Depending on the location of the patient's peripheral symptoms, either a posterior or anterior application is performed along the course of the nerves making up the brachial plexus.

Posterior application

If the patient has a posterior disorder, taping is applied along the posterior course of the nerves that supply the extensor muscles of the arm. Apply the tape with no tension starting from the most distal area supplied by the nerves to the most central projection of their origin with the arm in as closed a position as possible.

Anterior application

If the patient has an anterior disorder, an unloading application is made along the course of the nerves that innervate the flexor muscles of the arm. Apply the tape from the most distal point supplied by the nerves to the most central projection of their origin, with the arm in as open a position as possible.

Posterior application

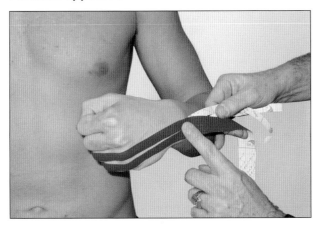 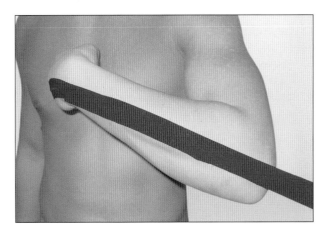

From the metacarpophalangeal joints of the ring and little fingers to the spinous process of the first thoracic vertebra

The arm is adducted in front of the chest, the elbow is bent around the chest and the wrist and fingers are flexed.

1. Apply the tape anchor on the dorsum of the metacarpophalangeal joints of the flexed ring and little fingers. The patient's arm is forward flexed.

2. After removing 10 cm of backing paper and with the patient's wrist flexed, apply the tape to the back of the hand and wrist.

3. With the patient's elbow and wrist flexed as far as possible, apply the tape on the posterior surface of the forearm and arm, taking it over the lateral tip of the olecranon.

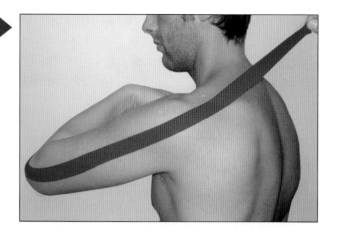
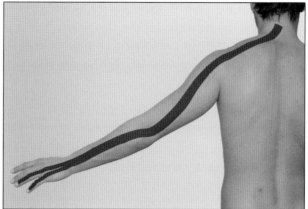

4. Keeping the elbow flexed, the patient now brings the arm horizontally across their chest by adducting the shoulder. Apply the tape to the back of the shoulder, taking it over the upper part of the scapula as far as the spinous process of the first thoracic vertebra.

5. The patient flexes their wrist and the elbow as far as possible; apply the tape, taking it over the lateral tip of the olecranon.

6. With the patient's elbow still flexed, apply the tape, without tension, as far as the posterior part of the shoulder.

7. The patient gradually crosses the arm in a parallel line across the chest.

8. The patient flexes the elbow, keeping the arm in a parallel line around their chest. Apply the tape to the upper part of the scapula as far as the spinous process of the first thoracic vertebra.

Anterior application

From the carpometacarpal joints of the ring and little fingers

Arm is abducted to 90° and extended with elbow and wrist also extended.

1. Apply the tape distally attaching the strips anteriorly to the carpometacarpal joints of the extended ring and little fingers.

2. The patient extends the elbow and abducts the shoulder, bringing the arm backward and outwards. Apply the tape, without tension, on the anterior forearm and arm, passing the axilla laterally up to the medial third of the clavicle.

TAPE SPECIFICATIONS

Correction in external rotation
- 1 tape
- Width 5 cm (2")
- Length 20 cm (8")
- Anchor 2 cm (0.75")
- Y-shaped

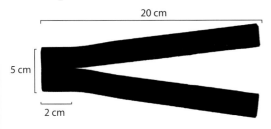

Correction with the deltoid in a state of compression
- 1 tape
- Width 5 cm (2")
- Length 25 cm (10")
- Anchor 5 cm (2")
- Y-shaped

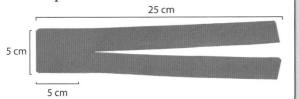

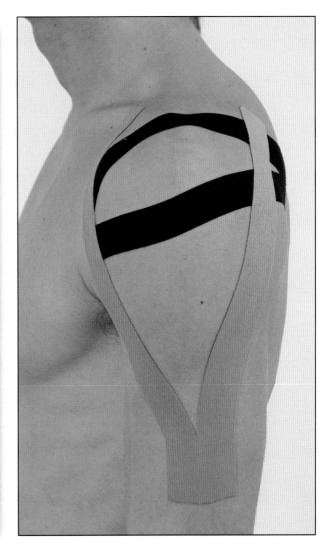

NOTE: This application, which exerts a certain amount of compression, cannot be left in place continuously for long periods of time. It is to be used only during sporting activity.

Forward Shoulder - Tape Application

Correction in external rotation

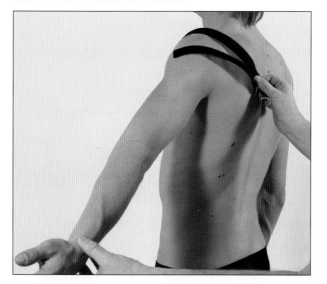

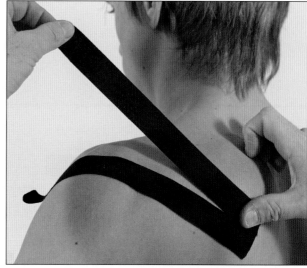

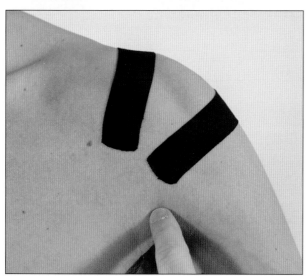

From below the spine of the scapula to 2 cm beyond the acromion

Arm abducted to 45° and externally rotated

1. Position the tape in the center of the scapula and, exerting 25-50% tension, apply it in a forward direction so that the upper strip passes over the acromion and the lower strip goes horizontally below the acromion, surrounding the mass of the deltoid.

Forward Shoulder - Tape Application

Correction with the deltoid in a state of compression

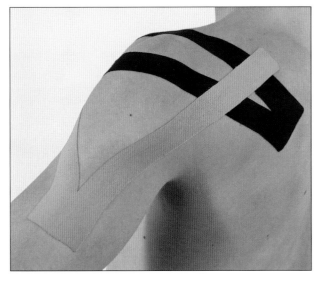
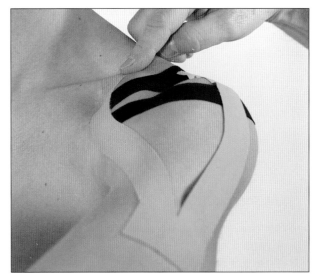

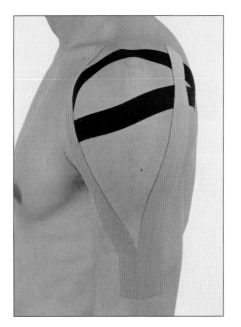

From the insertion of the deltoid to the acromion

The patient has their arm against their side.

1. Apply the tape anchor below the insertion of the deltoid.

2. Ask the patient to forward flex the arm slightly to 25° and actively hold the position; apply the anterior strip, without tension, to outline the anterior margin of the muscle.

3. Ask the patient to extend their arm slightly to 25° and actively hold the position; apply the posterior strip, without tension, outlining the posterior margin of the deltoid.

NOTE: Different levels of stabilization may be achieved. Muscles slightly shortened and tape without tension; posterior strip applied with the arm extended 25° and anterior strip applied with the arm flexed through 25°. For greater stabilization, flex and extend the arm by more than 25° to 45°, 60°, 70° or 90°. A greater angle of flexion and extension creates greater shortening of the muscles. (This stabilization is to be maintained only for a short time, i.e. for the duration of sporting activities or during rehabilitation exercises.)

**Combined application
for the deltoid and the supraspinatus**

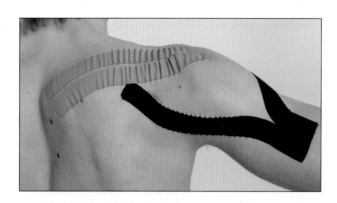

TAPE SPECIFICATIONS

With the deltoid in decompression
- 1 tape
- Width 5 cm (2")
- Length 25 cm (10")
- Anchor 5 cm (2")
- Y-shaped

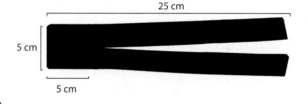

With the supraspinatus in decompression
- 1 tape
- Width 5 cm (2")
- Length 25 cm (10")
- Anchor 2 cm (0.75")
- Y-shaped

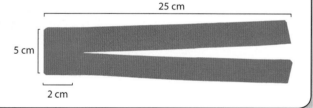

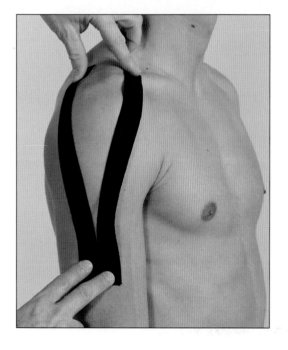

Application for the deltoid

🏷 From 5 cm below the deltoid tuberosity, or "deltoid V", of the humerus to 2 cm beyond the acromioclavicular joint

🧍 The patient has their arm down against their side.

1. Apply the tape anchor below and slightly in front of the deltoid V.

2. The patient abducts the arm to 90° and extends it. With no tension, apply the anterior strip, to outline the anterior margin of the deltoid, ending on the distal third of the clavicle.

3. The patient forward flexes the arm to 90°. With no tension, apply the posterior strip outlining the posterior margin of the deltoid.

Application for the supraspinatus

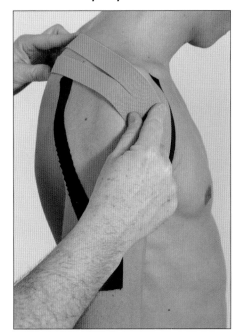
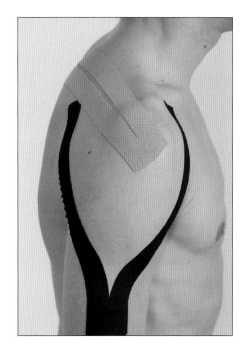

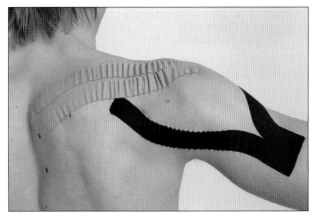

🩹 From the greater tubercle of the humerus to the upper angle of the scapula, plus 2 cm

🧍 The patient's arm is naturally adducted by their side and rotated internally, with the elbow flexed and the forearm resting on the abdomen.

1. Position the tape anchor over the greater tubercle of the humerus.

2. With no tension, apply the upper strip just above the supraspinous fossa of the scapula, outlining the upper angle of the scapula.

3. With no tension, apply the lower strip parallel to the first, just below the spine of the scapula.

**Combined application
for the deltoid and the descending part
of the trapezius**

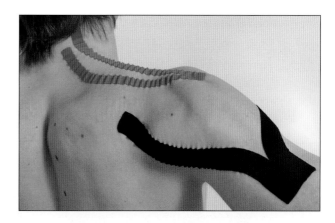

TAPE SPECIFICATIONS

With the deltoid in decompression
- 1 tape
- Width 5 cm (2")
- Length 25 cm (10")
- Anchor 5 cm (2")
- Y-shaped

With the trapezius in decompression
- 2 tapes
- Width 2.5 cm (1")
- Length 25 cm (10")
- Anchor 2 cm (0.75")
- Y-shaped
- Bilateral application

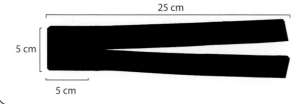

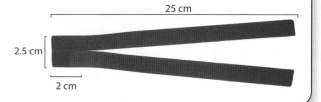

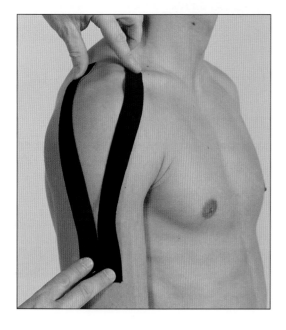

Application for the deltoid

🔖 From 5 cm below the deltoid V of the humerus to 2 cm beyond the acromioclavicular joint

👤 The patient has their arm down along their side

1. Apply the tape anchor below and slightly in front of the deltoid V.

2. The patient abducts the arm to 90° and extends it. With no tension, apply the anterior strip to outline the anterior margin of the deltoid ending on the distal third of the clavicle.

3. The patient forward flexes the arm to 90°. With no tension, apply the posterior strip outlining the posterior margin of the deltoid.

Shoulder Impingement Syndromes - Tape Application

Application for the descending part of the trapezius

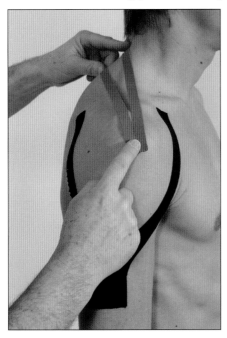

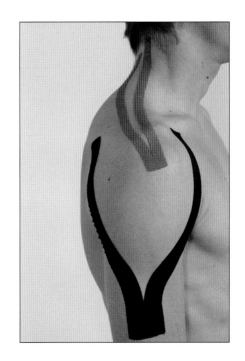

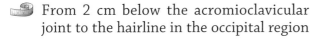 From 2 cm below the acromioclavicular joint to the hairline in the occipital region

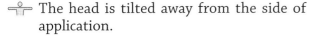 The head is tilted away from the side of application.

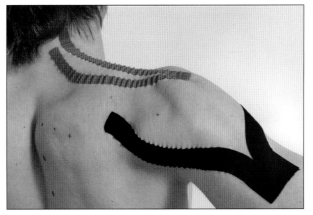

1. Position the tape anchor 2 cm below the acromioclavicular joint.

2. With no tension, apply the upper strip following the upper margin of the descending part of the trapezius and ending at the hairline in the occipital region.

3. The head, still tilted in the opposite direction, is then flexed forward and rotated slightly toward the side of the application. Apply the lower strip to outline the posterior margin of the descending part of the trapezius.

4. Apply on the descending part of the muscle on the opposite side also because this muscle is connected with the spinal column; applications should therefore always be bilateral and symmetrical.

Shoulder Impingement Syndromes - Tape Application

Combined application
for the biceps brachii and descending part
of the trapezius

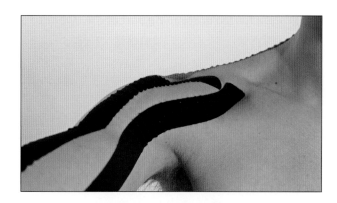

TAPE SPECIFICATIONS

With the biceps brachii in decompression
- 1 tape
- Width 5 cm (2")
- Length 35 cm (14")
- Anchor 2 cm (0.75")
- Y-shaped

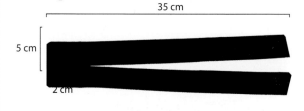

With the trapezius in decompression
- 2 tapes
- Width 2.5 cm (1")
- Length 25 cm (10")
- Y-shaped
- Anchor 2 cm (0.75")
- Bilateral application

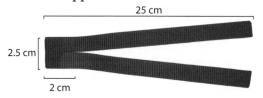

Application for the biceps

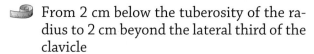 From 2 cm below the tuberosity of the radius to 2 cm beyond the lateral third of the clavicle

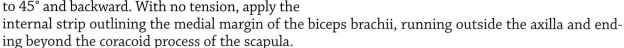 The patient's arm is against their side, forearm in supination.

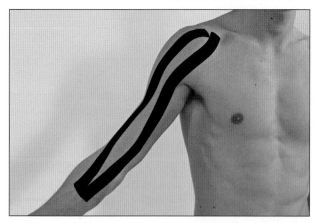

1. Apply the tape anchor just below the tuberosity of the radius.

2. The patient extends their elbow and abducts the arm and shoulder, drawing the arm outward to 45° and backward. With no tension, apply the internal strip outlining the medial margin of the biceps brachii, running outside the axilla and ending beyond the coracoid process of the scapula.

3. The patient reduces the abduction of the arm and shoulder slightly to 25°; with no tension, apply the lateral strip outlining the lateral margin of the biceps brachii and end beyond the supraglenoid tubercle of the scapula.

Shoulder Impingement Syndromes - Tape Application

Application for the descending part of the trapezius

🗍 From 2 cm below the acromioclavicular joint to the hairline in the occipital region

👤 The head is tilted away from the side of application.

1. Position the tape anchor 2 cm below the acromioclavicular joint.

2. With no tension, apply the upper strip following the upper margin of the fibers of the descending part of the trapezius and ending at the hairline in the occipital region.

3. The head, still tilted, is then forward flexed and rotated slightly toward the side of the application. Apply the lower strip outlining the posterior margin of the descending part of the superior muscle.

4. Carry out an application also on the descending part of the same muscle on the opposite side. As this muscle is connected to the spinal column, applications should always be bilateral and symmetrical.

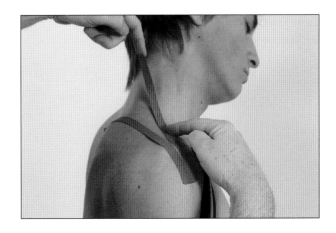

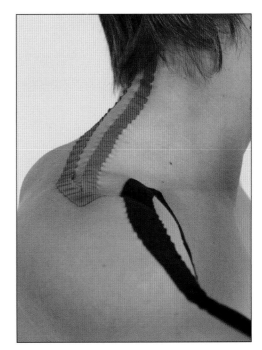

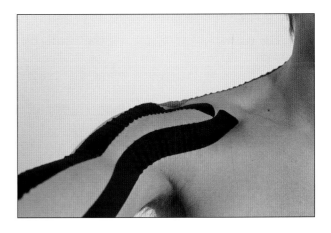

Shoulder Impingement Syndromes - Tape Application

Combined application for the biceps brachii and supraspinatus

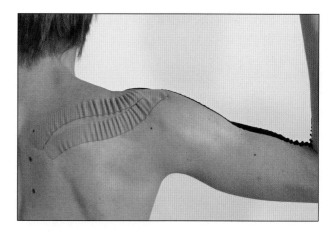

TAPE SPECIFICATIONS

With the biceps brachii in decompression
- 1 tape
- Width 5 cm (2")
- Length 35 cm (14")
- Anchor 2 cm (0.75")
- Y-shaped

35 cm

5 cm

2 cm

With the supraspinatus in decompression
- 1 tape
- Width 2.5 cm (1")
- Length 25 cm (10")
- Anchor 2 cm (0.75")
- Y-shaped

25 cm

2.5 cm

2 cm

Application for the biceps brachii

From 2 cm below the tuberosity of the radius to 2 cm beyond the lateral third of the clavicle

The patient's arm is against their side, forearm in supination.

1. Apply the tape anchor just below the tuberosity of the radius.

2. The patient extends their elbow and abducts the shoulder, drawing the arm outward and backward. With no tension, apply the internal strip outlining the medial margin of the biceps brachii, passing outside the axilla and ending beyond the coracoid process of the scapula.

3. The patient reduces the abduction of the shoulder slightly; with no tension, apply the lateral strip outlining the lateral margin of the biceps brachii and ending beyond the supraglenoid tubercle of the scapula.

NEUROMUSCULAR TAPING from Theory to Practice

Shoulder Impingement Syndromes - Tape Application

Application for the supraspinatus

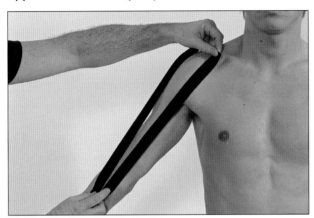 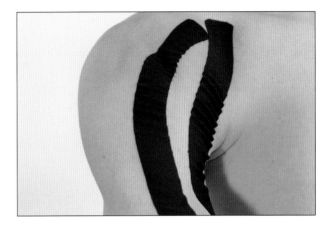

📏 From the greater tubercle of the humerus to the upper angle of the scapula, plus 2 cm

👤 The patient's arm is naturally adducted by their side and internally rotated with the elbow flexed and the forearm resting on the abdomen.

1. Position the tape anchor over the greater tubercle of the humerus.

2. With no tension, apply the upper strip just above the supraspinous fossa of the scapula, outlining the upper angle of the scapula.

3. With no tension, apply the lower strip parallel to the first, just below the spine of the scapula.

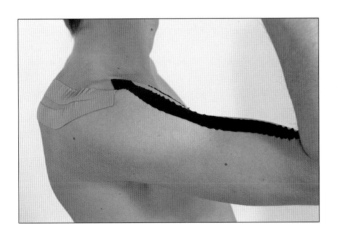 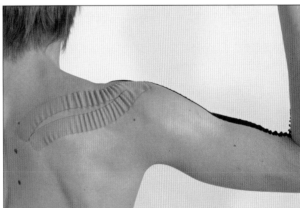

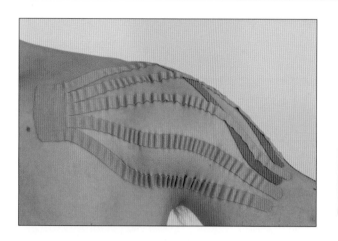

NOTE: The aim of this application is to create space in the joint. It may also be indicated in cases of shoulder pain, inflammation of the rotator cuff, bursitis, or after surgery.

TAPE SPECIFICATIONS

- 2 tapes
- Width 5 cm (2")
- Length 25-30 cm (10-12")
- Anchor 2 cm (0.75")
- Fan-shaped with five strips

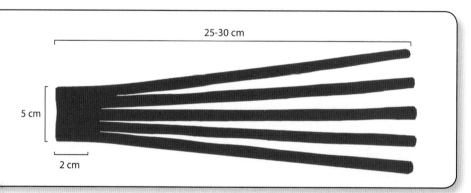

25-30 cm

5 cm

2 cm

Application of the anterior fan

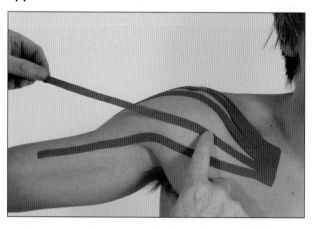

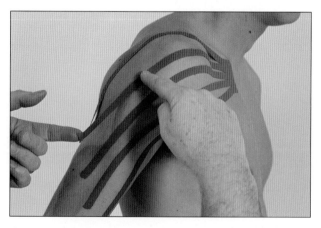

 25-30 cm: a standard-sized fan to cover the region to be treated

Arm abducted to 90°, externally rotated and slightly extended

1. Apply the tape anchor just below the clavicle so that the middle of the central strip is positioned over the anterior aspect of the head of the humerus.

2. With no tension, apply the lower strip directing it toward the angle of the axillary fossa and then along the medial margin of the biceps brachii.

3. Apply the second and third strips parallel to the first, 1 cm apart.

4. The patient lowers their arm to 45° of abduction. Apply the fourth and fifth strips following a course parallel to the others, and again with the strips 1 cm apart; the last strip runs just in front of the acromion.

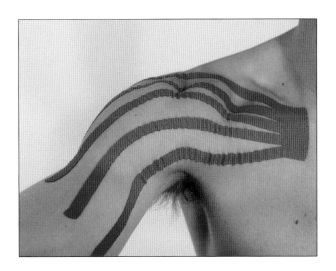

Application of the posterior fan

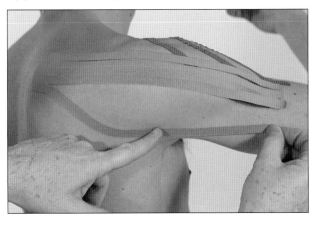
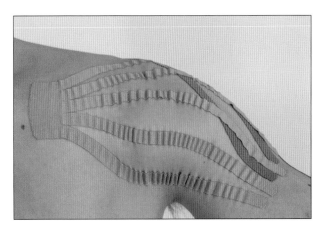

🔖 25-30 cm; a standard-sized fan to cover the region to be treated

⊤ Arm forward flexed to 90° and slightly adducted

1. Apply the tape anchor just below the spine of the scapula so that the middle of the central strip is positioned over the posterior aspect of the head of the humerus.

2. With no tension, apply the lower strip directing it toward the axillary fossa and then along the lateral margin of the triceps brachii.

3. Apply the second and third strips parallel to the first, 1 cm apart from each other. The patient lowers the arm to 45° of flexion; apply the fourth and fifth strips, parallel to the others, 1 cm apart.

EPICONDYLITIS

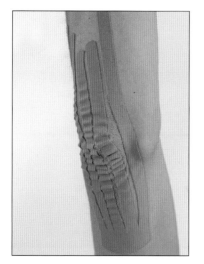
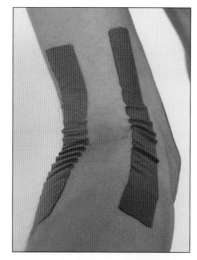
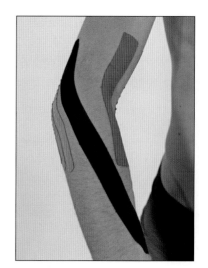

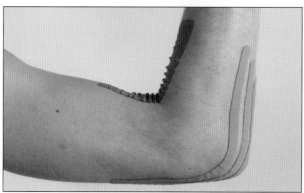

TAPE SPECIFICATIONS

Posterior drainage of the elbow joint
- 1 tape
- Width 5 cm (2")
- Length 25 cm (10")
- Anchor 2 cm (0.75")
- Fan-shaped with five strips

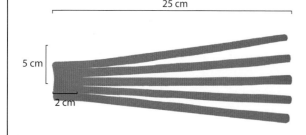

25 cm

5 cm

2 cm

Anterior drive for the joint axis
- 2 tapes
- Width 2.5 cm (1")
- Length 20 cm (8")
- I-shaped

20 cm

2.5 cm

Correction using the decompressive technique on the lateral epicondyle of the humerus
- 1 tape
- Width 2.5 cm (1")
- Length 30 cm (12")
- I-shaped

30 cm

2.5 cm

Epicondylitis - Tape Application

Posterior drainage of the elbow joint

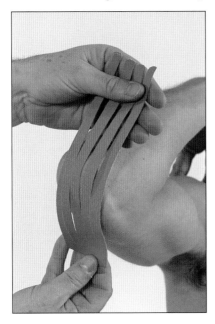 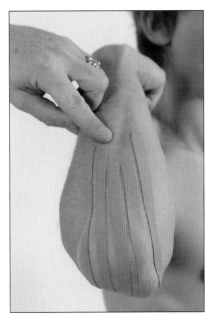 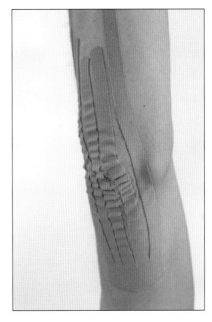

25 cm; a standard-sized fan to cover the posterior side of the elbow

The patient's arm is forward flexed, elbow fully flexed and forearm in supination.

1. Apply the tape anchor on the posterior surface of the arm so that the mid-point of the tape length coincides with the olecranon.

2. Distribute the strips of tape along the axis of the arm and forearm so that the outer ones outline the trochlea of the humerus. In this way, the ends of the tape will form a 'U' shape on the posterior surface of the forearm, as the central ones will end closer to the elbow than the others.

Epicondylitis - Tape Application

Anterior guide for the joint axis

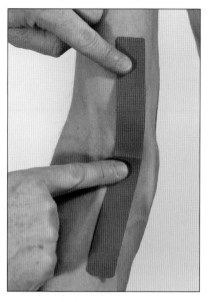 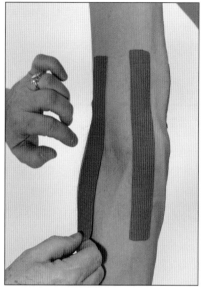 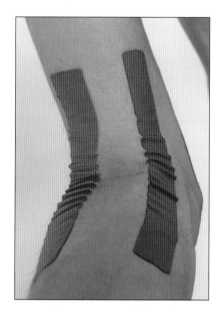

🔖 20 cm: 2 strips, each 2.5 cm wide

🔧 Elbow is extended: forearm in supination with hand extended

1. Apply the ends of the two tapes medially and laterally on the anterior surface of the arm, so that the middle of each tape is positioned over the anterior region of the elbow.

2. With no tension, apply the tapes in a downward vertical direction.

Correction using the decompressive technique on the lateral epicondyle of the humerus

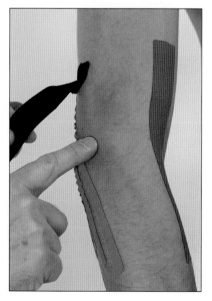 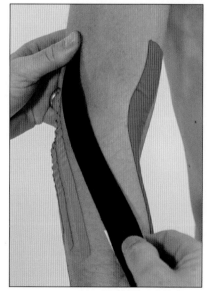 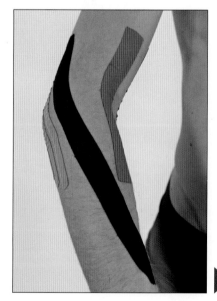

NEUROMUSCULAR TAPING from Theory to Practice

Epicondylitis - Tape Application

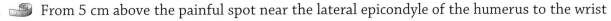

▶ 🖊️ From 5 cm above the painful spot near the lateral epicondyle of the humerus to the wrist

👤 The patient's arm is flexed forward, the elbow slightly flexed, forearm in pronation and wrist flexed.

1. Apply the tape anchor 5 cm above the painful spot near the lateral epicondyle of the humerus.

2. After removing 10 cm of backing paper and folding it back, stretch the skin and with no tension, apply the tape over the painful spot.

3. Remove the remaining backing paper and apply the tape, without tension, on the posterior margin of the brachioradialis, ending close to the radial side of the wrist.

Complete application

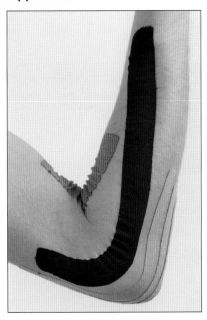

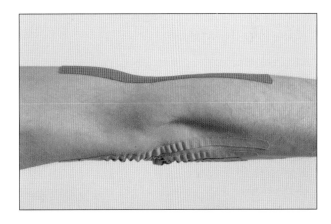

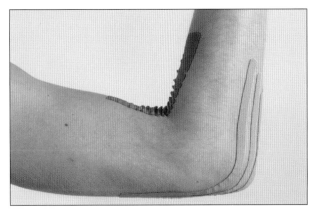

CARPAL TUNNEL SYNDROME

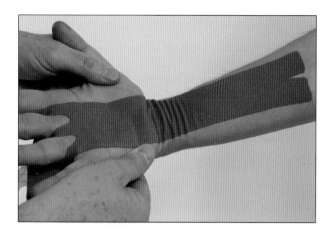 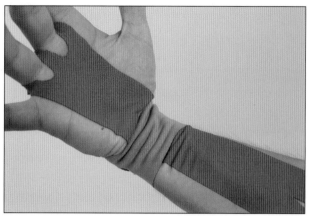

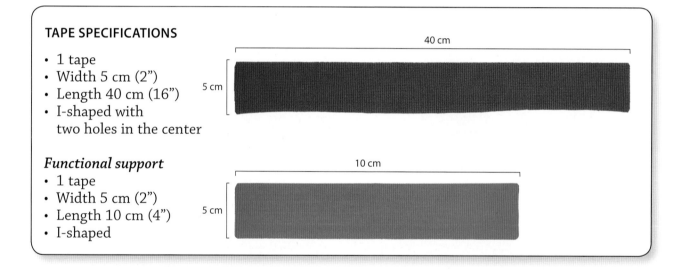

TAPE SPECIFICATIONS

- 1 tape
- Width 5 cm (2")
- Length 40 cm (16")
- I-shaped with two holes in the center

Functional support

- 1 tape
- Width 5 cm (2")
- Length 10 cm (4")
- I-shaped

40 cm

5 cm

10 cm

5 cm

NOTE: This application may also be indicated in cases of wrist instability and in rehabilitation after trauma to the wrist. The transverse tape (the blue tape in the photograph) is used in carpal tunnel syndrome in the functional phase, for example during manual work and sporting activities. The glove technique yields good results in acute conditions.

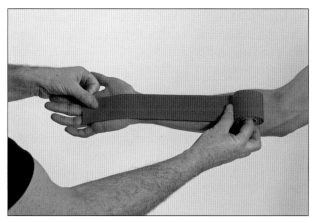
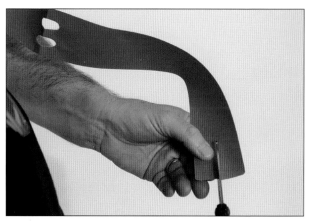
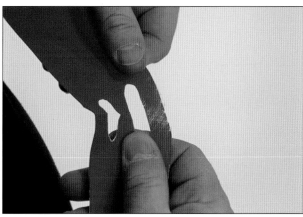
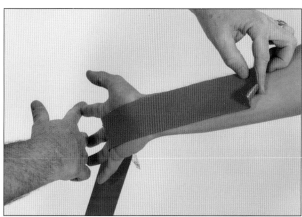
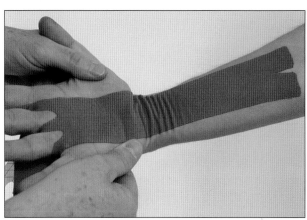
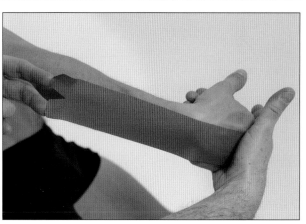

From the palmar side of the bases of the fingers to the distal third of the forearm: this length is then doubled and holes are cut in the center fold.

The forearm is in supination, the wrist in neutral position between flexion and extension.

1. Cut two holes mid-way along the tape, into which the patient's third and fourth fingers are inserted. Cut another hole, 1.5 cm long, centrally at each end of the tape.

2. The patient holds out their arm with the palm facing upward.

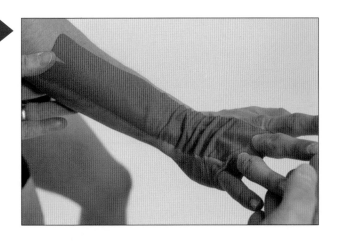

3. Insert the third and fourth fingers through the two holes and, with the wrist extended, apply the first half of the tape, with no tension, along the anterior surface of the forearm.

4. The patient then turns the palm downward and hyperflexes the wrist; apply the second half of the tape, with no tension, along the posterior surface of the forearm.

Functional support

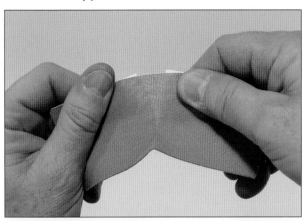

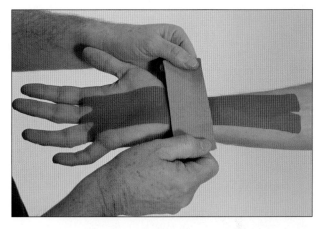

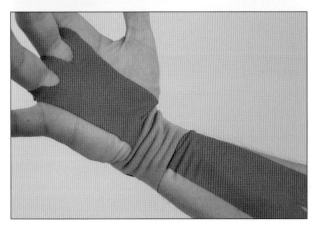

5. Apply a further strip of tape anteriorly to cover three quarters of the circumference of the wrist, stretching it by 25% between the ulnar and radial margins. Make sure that the wrist is well aligned in the correct position. This tape serves to provide protection and support. In view of its transverse course and tension, this tape can be left in place only for a limited amount of time.

LUMBAR SPINE PAIN SYNDROMES

TAPE SPECIFICATIONS

- 2 tapes
- Width 5 cm (2")
- Length 25-30 cm (10-12")
- I-shaped

25-30 cm

5 cm

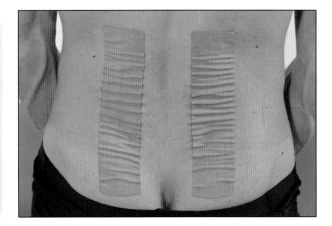

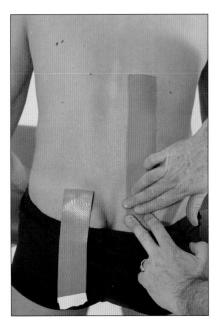 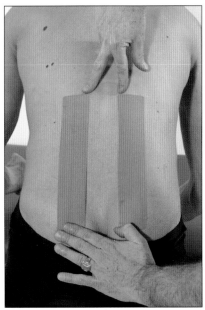 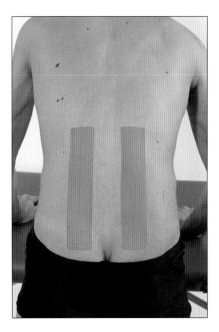

From the iliolumbar ligament, 2 cm laterally from the gluteal cleft, to the transverse process of the tenth thoracic vertebra

The patient stands or, preferably, sits with trunk forward flexed to 45°, head also flexed forward.

1. Apply the two tape anchors 2 cm to the right and 2 cm to the left of the gluteal cleft.

2. Apply each tape, without tension, in a vertical direction, parallel to the spinal column. If the patient is unable to achieve adequate forward flexion of the trunk, the operator should pull the patient's skin downward.

Application in postoperative rehabilitation

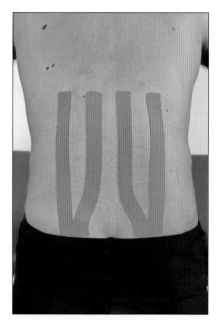
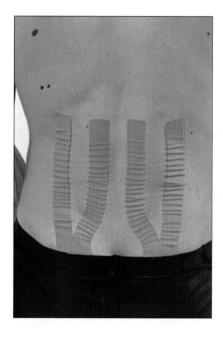

3. Following surgery, apply two Y-shaped tapes to the muscles to relieve tension; make sure that the tape is not placed over the scar.

SCIATIC NERVE

The sciatic nerve arises from the anterior branches of L4 and L5 and of S1, S2 and S3. The branches of L4 and L5 form the superior gluteal nerve, while the branches of S1 and S2 form the posterior femoral cutaneous nerve.

The sciatic nerve splits into the tibial (L4, L5, S1, S2, S3) and common fibular (peroneal) (L4, L5, S1, S2) nerves. Branches from the former innervate the biceps femoris (long head), semitendinosus, semimembranosus, and adductor magnus (posterior portion) muscles, while the latter supplies the biceps femoris (short head).

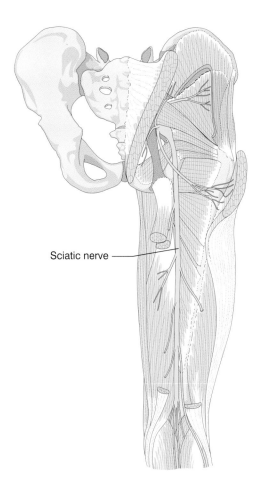

Sciatic nerve

If the intervertebral disc between L4 and L5 exerts pressure on the L5 nerve root, this can result in pain in the posterior, anterior and lateral thigh, in the lateral malleolus, the hindfoot and the big toe.

In some situations, sensation at the level of the lateral malleolus is altered and the extensor capacity of the extensor hallucis longus and extensor hallucis brevis muscles is reduced. Furthermore, if the intervertebral disc between L5 and S1 exerts pressure on the S1 nerve root, this can result in pain in the back of the thigh, calf and lateral malleolus or extreme pain in the calcaneal or Achilles tendon, the heel, the lateral margin of the foot and the fourth and fifth toes. In the presence of altered sensation on the posterior surface of the lateral malleolus and weakness of the Achilles tendon, a decrease in muscle strength may be noticed.

TAPE SPECIFICATIONS

- 1 tape
- Width 2.5 cm (1")
- Length 90 cm (36")
- I-shaped

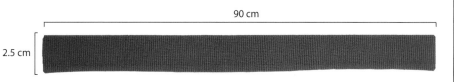

90 cm

2.5 cm

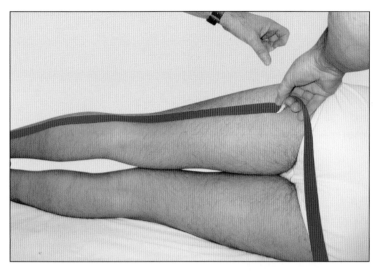

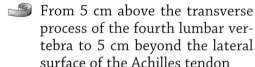 From 5 cm above the transverse process of the fourth lumbar vertebra to 5 cm beyond the lateral surface of the Achilles tendon

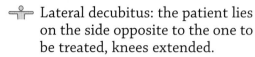 Lateral decubitus: the patient lies on the side opposite to the one to be treated, knees extended.

1. The patient lies on the side opposite to that of the sciatic nerve to be treated, with legs relaxed and ankles dorsiflexed. Apply the tape, without tension, starting from a point 5 cm below the lateral surface of the Achilles tendon.

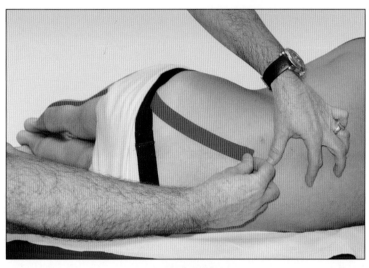

2. With the patient's knee extended, continue the application along the course of the nerve, making sure the tape adheres to the posterolateral surface of the knee joint.

3. Keeping the knee extended, the patient performs a hip flexion and adduction; in other words, remaining on their side, the patient has to move closer to the edge of the couch and bring the underlying straightened and adducted leg off the couch. The operator fixes the tape along the central axis of the sciatic nerve, in the middle of the hamstring muscles.

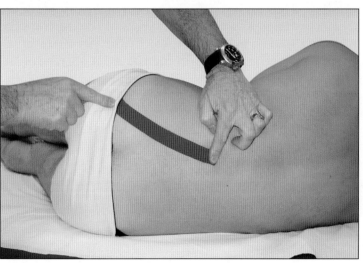

4. At this point the patient may stand upright, extend their knee and adduct the hip, crossing the knee over the other leg. The patient then flexes the trunk forward, toward the leg that is not to be treated. With no tension, apply the tape in the direction of the lumbar vertebrae anchoring it beyond the fourth lumbar vertebra.

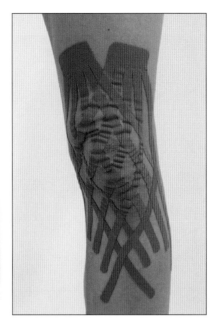

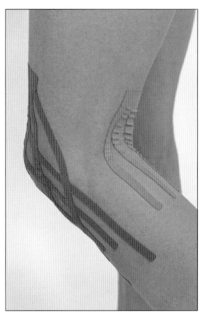

NOTE: This application can also be used after knee replacement or cruciate ligament surgery; in both cases only after the stitches have been removed (the wound must be well closed).

TAPE SPECIFICATIONS

Double anterior fan
- 2 tapes
- Width 5 cm (2")
- Length 30 cm (12")
- Anchor 2 cm (0.75")
- Fan-shaped with five strips

30 cm

5 cm

2 cm

Posterior fan
- 1 tape
- Width 5 cm (2")
- Length 20 cm (8")
- Anchor 2 cm (0.75")
- Fan-shaped with five strips

20 cm

5 cm

2 cm

Double anterior fan

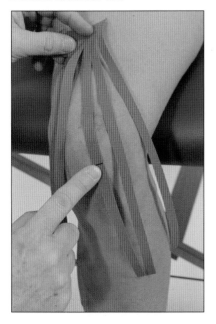 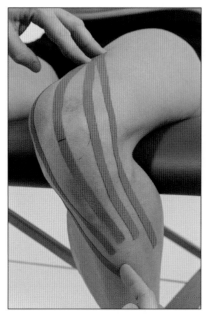 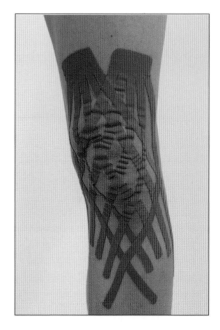

If any edema is present, the anchor is to be positioned 5 cm higher. This means that the tape tails will have to be longer.

The patient is seated with the knee flexed to 110°.

1. Apply the anchor of the first fan 1 cm laterally to the centerline of the quadriceps muscle, so that the middle of the central strip is positioned over the center of the patella.

2. With no tension, apply the lateral strip so that it wraps around the anterolateral surface of the knee before descending vertically. Apply the next strip by wrapping it around the lateral margin of the patella.

3. With no tension, apply the medial strip so that it wraps around the anteromedial surface of the knee before descending vertically. Apply the next strip by wrapping it around the medial margin of the patella.

4. Finally, apply the central strip, running over the center of the patella.

5. Repeat the sequence for the medial fan, positioning the tape 1 cm medially to the center line of the quadriceps femoris and reversing the references.

Posterior fan

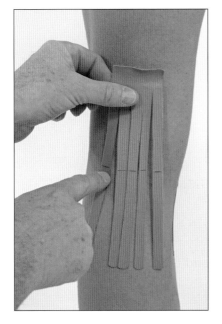 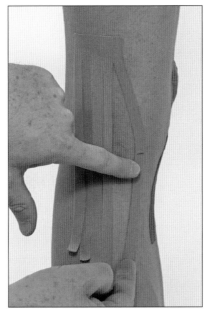 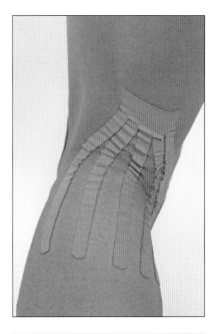

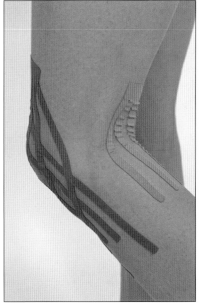

🎞 20 cm

The patient is standing, knee extended.

1. Apply the tape anchor on the anterior surface of the thigh so that the middle of the tape's length corresponds to the posterior region of the knee.

2. With no tension, apply the strips about 1 cm apart. Wrap the external ones around the margins of the popliteal fossa.

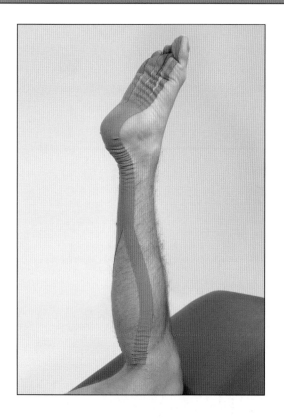

TAPE SPECIFICATIONS

- 1 tape
- Width 5 cm (2")
- Length 65 cm (26")
- Combined Y and fan shape

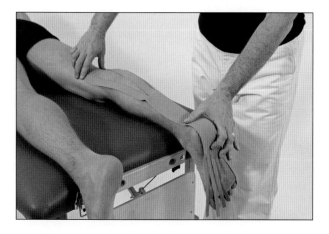

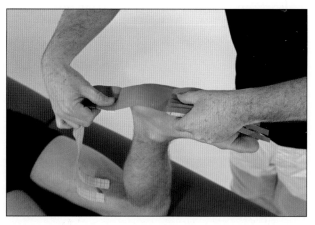

From 2 cm above the popliteal fossa to the tips of the toes; the two strips of the Y are measured from 2 cm above the popliteal fossa to 5 cm below the insertions of the lateral and medial heads of the gastrocnemius. The strips of tape are to be measured from the tips of the toes to the base of the heel. Each strip is then cut according to the length of the respective toe.

The patient is prone with feet extended off the couch, knee extended, ankle dorsiflexed.

Calcaneal Spur - Tape Application

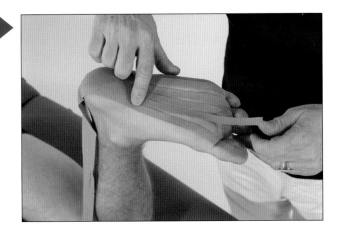
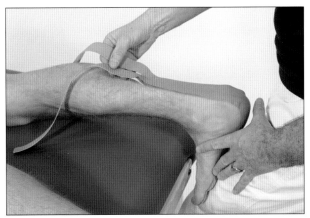
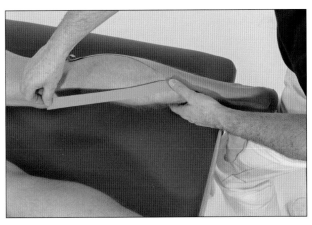
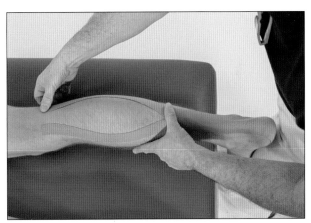

1. The patient flexes their knee to 90°, keeping the ankle dorsiflexed. Apply the 5-cm fan anchor on the underside of the heel.

2. With one hand, help to extend the toe, pushing it downward. Meanwhile, with the other hand, apply each strip of tape, without tension, along the respective metatarsal bone and toe phalanges.

3. The patient extends their knee and places the forefoot against the therapist's thigh. In this way, by pushing forward with the knee, the therapist can assist with the dorsiflexion of the ankle. Apply the tape, without tension, as far as the bifurcation, covering the calcaneal or Achilles tendon. Use the two strips of the Y to outline the medial and lateral margins of the gastrocnemius, ending at the margins of the popliteal fossa.

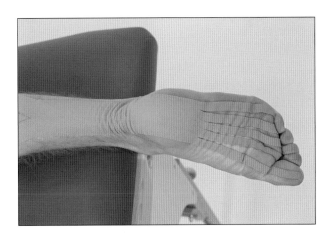

NOTE: This application is a standard protocol for neurological rehabilitation of the leg and foot; it may also be indicated in cases of calcaneal inflammation.

PLANTAR FASCIITIS

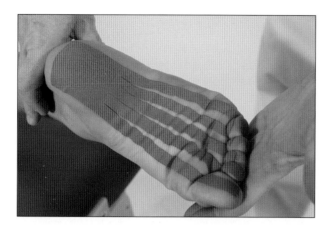

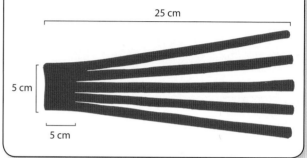

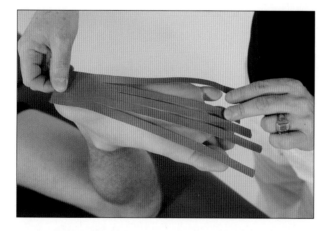

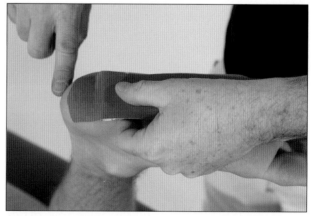

From the heel to 2 cm beyond the tip of the big toe; each strip is then cut to the length of the respective toe.

Prone: the knee is flexed to 90°, ankle dorsiflexed, toes extended.

1. Apply the tape anchor under the heel. Remove the backing paper and, for ease of application, lay the ends of the strips on the tips of the medial toes.

2. Attach the end of the first strip (the one for the fifth toe) to your thumb. Meanwhile, use your middle finger to assist the extension of the toe by pushing the distal phalanx downward. With the free hand apply the strip of tape, without tension, over the fifth metatarsal bone and the phalanges of the fifth toe. The strip ends on the toe pad.

3. Repeat the procedure described in point 2 for the fourth, third, second and first toes.

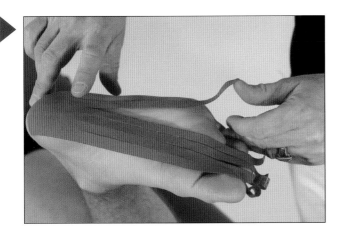
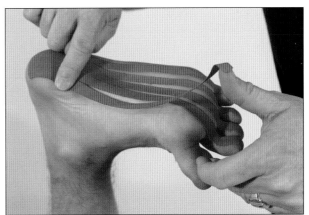
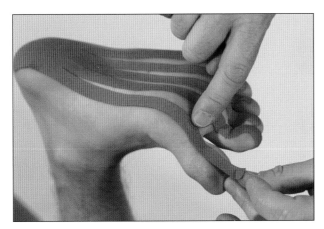
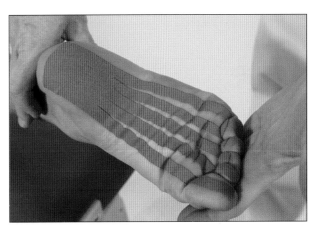

Frequently Asked Questions

Exactly how long should the tape be?

Make sure that the length of the tape is appropriate for the area and the muscle to be treated. The length calculation should be based on the course of the muscle, beginning several centimeters (usually 2 cm) before its start (either its insertion or its origin) and ending a few centimeters after its end. A tape that is too short can reduce the exteroceptive stimulus and therefore yield poorer results. Conversely, a tape that is too long may unintentionally involve other areas of skin or muscle.

Exactly what size and shape should the tape be?

The shape of the tape depends on the shape of the muscle and the area to be treated. Bear in mind that too much tape present on the skin overlying the course of the muscle will provide more compressive stimulus rather than decompressive. To ensure a correct decompressive stimulus only 30-50% of the surface area over the muscle fibre should be covered with tape. Covering 100% of the surface area over muscle fibre produces a compressive effect.

How should the tape be made to adhere to the skin?

Pay attention to the following points:
- To ensure good adherence to the skin, you should smooth and rub the tape along its course using the palm of your hand (only in the direction of its length).
- Make sure the tape adheres well to the skin before the patient changes position.
- The patient's skin should be perfectly clean and free of oil, creams or ointments. It should therefore first be washed with soap and water or cleaned with other suitable products and then dried.
- The skin must also be free of hairs, and should be shaved if necessary.

Should the patient be screened before tape application?

A complete patient screening process before the application of the NeuroMuscular Taping will enhance overall results and give the therapist an overview on expected results. Patients with infections or cancer should not be taped. Skin alterations, skin inflammation or skin irritations may also be a factor for excluding patients from tape treatment. Being a biomeccanical, non pharmacological treatment, NeuroMuscular Taping has very few treatment exclusions. Medical advice is advised before taping.

How can skin irritation be prevented?

The patient should be questioned about skin allergies prior to the application. If the patient has a known skin allergy, the extent of the allergy must be evaluated. If there is any concern about irritation, a patch test of tape may be applied on the underside of the forearm. The tape product may be tested to ensure its quality does not cause an allergic reaction. Sunbathing with the tape on may cause irritation. Skin creams, lotions and perfumes may be a source of irritation.

What should be done in the event of irritation following application of the tape?

If the tape irritates the skin, it is important to consider the following points:
- If a skin allergy is known to be extensive, the application may not be recommended. If the

skin irritation is minimal, the tape should only be left in place for a few days, a single day, several hours or only during physical therapy.
- If only certain areas of skin are prone to irritation, those areas should be avoided or the tape should be left in place for a limited number of hours or during physical therapy only.
- Wait one hour after shaving before applying the tape, or use an electric razor to avoid irritating the skin.
- If the tape irritates the patient's skin even when it has been applied correctly and with due precaution, change the color or brand of tape used, as coloring dyes in the tape or the quality of the adhesive glue may be causing the irritation.
- Avoid skin irritation by removing the tape while gently pulling the skin in the opposite direction. The tape may also be removed by gently placing a finger over the tape as it is removed. The tape may be removed while showering or bathing to minimize irritation.
- Seek medical advice if the irritation persists.

Was the tape applied with the patient's body in the correct position?

Don't forget that to obtain *decompressive stimulus* on the muscle, the tape is to be applied to the skin along the course of the muscle being treated with the muscle elongated. On the other hand, to obtain *compressive stimulus* on the muscle, the tape is to be applied to the skin along the course of the muscle in question with the muscle shortened.

Was the tape applied with tension?

To obtain *decompressive stimulus* on the muscle, the tape is to be applied to the skin without stretching it in any way whatsoever. Remember that the tape often comes pre-stretched by 10% on its paper backing.

Only in special circumstances in order to obtain *compressive stimulus* on the muscle should the tape be applied over the course of the muscle, with no more than 25% tension.

Is this the correct muscle course?

This volume includes descriptions of muscle tests in order to ensure correct identification of muscle courses and therefore correct positioning of tapes.

What if the tape comes off during movement?

If the tape comes off the skin during movement this may mean that:
- It was applied with too much tension.
- The skin was not cleaned well prior to the application.
- The skin is too dry or too damp.
- There was excessive sweating due to physical activity.

Should the patient notice improvement immediately after application?

If the tape was applied correctly, the patient should immediately obtain a greater ROM and a reduction of the pain. If this does not happen, the diagnosis and therapeutic aim and so the tape application used need to be reassessed immediately. If after initial improvement the patient's condition worsens, the tape must be removed and the patient reassessed.

The basic principle behind the application of Neuromuscular Taping is to normalize ROM and reduce pain.

What if the patient perceives an increase in pain after the application?

An increase in pain levels following an application means that the tape has not been applied properly. This may be due to one of three reasons:
- The tape must be applied using the decompressive technique in order to increase the interstitial spaces and thereby reduce compression on the skin receptors; if it is applied using compressive technique, the pain will increase.
- The application has not allowed for the patient's normal physiological joint range of motion and is therefore producing excessive stimulation.

– The tape has not been applied to the area of origin of the pain. The patient should undergo renewed diagnostic assessment in order to arrive at a new and correct application.

How long should the tape be left in place on the patient?

The tape can be left in place for three or four days consecutively, after which the patient should be reassessed and a fresh tape applied. In an acute phase, the tape is left in place only 1 to 3 days. Whereas during rehabilitation it may be left in place for longer from 3 to 7 days. The application of NMT in therapeutic settings follows these stages: going from acute and post-acute phases through the functional phase.

From what age can NeuroMuscular Taping be used?

The youngest patient to undergo taping was one day old and presented obstetric torticollis. There is no upper age limit for the use of this technique.

Can the patient wash?

The patient can wash, taking care not to rub the tape. The skin and tape may be patted dry with a towel and a hair dryer may be used to dry the tape.

Is the application similar to the one described in the text?

Make sure that the application is true to what is described in the text. A makeshift application or incorrect assessment of the patient will not ensure the desired result.

What if the patient feels a tingling sensation in the site of the application?

A tingling sensation felt locally during application of the tape is quite normal. However, an increase in blood flow should be distinguished from skin irritation. If the skin is irritated then the tape should be removed and the skin washed clean.

Do the different colors indicate different tape characteristics?

The different colors do not denote different tape characteristics. The choice of colored tape may be indicated during neurological rehabilitation to assist a patient in recognizing movement. Remember that the therapeutic stimulus is due to the method of application, not to the color of the tape used.

Should the tape be applied starting from the point of origin or the point of insertion?

Follow the instructions given in the text. In any case, as the tape is applied onto the skin overlying the muscle course and not directly on the muscle fascia, it makes no difference whether it begins at the origin or the insertion. Being larger, the base anchor of the tape will always create a slight compression, however pay close attention to not compress the joint or other neighboring muscles.

What if the tape appears to have been applied correctly, but no skin folds appear?

A stretched elastic tape always imparts a concentric return stimulus. If no skin folds are formed, this means that a compressive stimulus is created, which reduces muscle elasticity, increases pain and limits mobility.

Recommended Readings

Anatomical illustrations used are original art work from the Editorial Department of Edi.Ermes.

AA.VV. Anatomia Umana Trattato, 4ª ed. Milan: Edi.Ermes, 2006-2007.

Basaglia N. Progettare la riabilitazione. Il lavoro in team interprofessionale. Milan: Edi.Ermes, 2002.

Blow D. Frattura omerale: trattamento in fase di immobilizzazione. Il Fisioterapista 2011; 1: 13-6.

Blow D. Taping NeuroMuscolare & sport. Sport&Medicina 2010; 6: 25-33.

Castano P, Donato RF (eds). Anatomia dell'uomo. Milan: Edi.Ermes, 2006.

Chisotti L. Spalla: valutazione di capacità "propriocettive" con il Taping NeuroMuscolare. Il Fisioterapista 2011; 1: 23-27.

Conti F (ed). Fisiologia Medica, 2ª ed. 2 vols. Milan: Edi.Ermes, 2011.

di Prampero PE, Veicsteinas A (eds). Fisiologia dell'uomo. Milan: Edi.Ermes, 2002.

Ferrario A, Monti GB, Jelmoni GP. Traumatologia dello sport - Clinica e terapia. Milan: Edi.Ermes, 2005.

Gerhardt JJ, Cocchiarella L, Randall L. The Practical Guide to Range of Motion Assessment. 1st Edition. Chicago (IL): American Medical Association Press, 2002.

Giammatteo S, Giammatteo T. Integrative Manual Therapy for Muscle Energy: For Biomechanics Application of Muscle Energy and & Beyond Technique. 1st Edition. Berkeley (CA): North Atlantic Books, 2003.

Hislop HJ, Montgomery J. Daniels and Worthingham's Muscle Testing: Techniques of Manual Examination. 8th Edition. Philadelphia (PA): WB Saunders Co., 2007.

Knott M, Voss I, Myers JW, Voss DE. Proprioceptive Neuromuscular Facilitation: Patterns and Techniques. 3rd Revised edition. Philadelphia (PA): Lippincott Williams & Wilkins, 1985.

Neumann DA. Kinesiology of the Musculoskeletal System. 1st Edition. St. Louis (MO): Mosby, 2002.

Niel-Asher S. The Concise Book of Trigger Points. Chichester (EN): Lotus Publishing, 2005

Pascucci T. Protesi di gomito: il Taping NeuroMuscolare nel trattamento riabilitativo. Il Fisioterapista 2011; 1: 19-22.

Pirola V. Cinesiologia. Il movimento umano applicato alla rieducazione e alle attività sportive. Milan: Edi.Ermes, 1998

Pirola V. Memo Cinesiologia. Milan: Edi.Ermes, 2004.

Sahrmann S. Diagnosis and Treatment of Movement Impairment Syndromes. 1st Edition. St. Louis (MO): Mosby, 2001.

Schmidt R, Wrisberg C. Motor Learning and Performance. 4th Edition. Champaign (IL): Human Kinetics, 2008.

Stella L (ed.). Bendaggio funzionale: moderne applicazioni. 4 vols. Milan: Edi.Ermes, 2002

Tomson D, Schuchhardt C. Drenaggio linfatico. Teoria, tecniche di base e applicate & fisioterapia decongestionante. Milan: Edi.Ermes, 2010.

Wolf U. Bildatlas der Manuellen Therapie. 2 vols. Marburg: KVM, 2007.